Essentials of Perioperative Nursing

Second Edition

Cynthia Spry, RN, MA, MSN, CNOR
Regional Clinical Advisor
Advanced Sterilization Products
Irvine, California

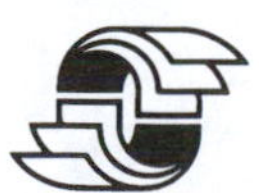

AN ASPEN PUBLICATION®
Aspen Publishers, Inc.
Gaithersburg, Maryland
1997

Library of Congress Cataloging-in-Publication Data

Spry, Cynthia.
Essentials of perioperative nursing/
Cynthia Spry.—2nd ed.
p. cm.
Includes bibliographical references and index.
ISBN 0-8342-0581-5
1. Operating room nursing—Programmed instruction.
I. Title. [DNLM: 1. Perioperative
Nursing—programmed instruction.
WY 18.2 S771e 1997]
RD32.3.S65 1997
610.73′677—dc20
DNLM/DLC
for Library of Congress
96-18621
CIP

Orders: (800) 638-8437
Customer Service: (800) 234-1660

About Aspen Publishers • For more than 35 years, Aspen has been a leading professional publisher in a variety of disciplines. Aspen's vast information resources are available in both print and electronic formats. We are committed to providing the highest quality information available in the most appropriate format for our customers. Visit Aspen's Internet site for more information resources, directories, articles, and a searchable version of Aspen's full catalog, including the most recent publications: **http://www.aspenpub.com**

Aspen Publishers, Inc. • The hallmark of quality in publishing
Member of the worldwide Wolters Kluwer group

The authors have made every effort to ensure the accuracy of the information herein. However, appropriate information sources should be consulted, especially for new or unfamiliar procedures. It is the responsibility of every practitioner to evaluate the appropriateness of a particular opinion in the context of actual clinical situations and with due consideration to new developments. Authors, editors, and the publisher cannot be held responsible for any typographical or other errors found in this book.

Editorial Resources: Jane Colilla
Library of Congress Catalog Card Number: 96-18621
ISBN: 0-8342-0581-5

Printed in the United States of America

1 2 3 4 5

Table of Contents

Introduction

PURPOSE—OVERVIEW

Operating room experience during nursing school is generally minimal and in many cases is absent. The nursing curriculum frequently does not include a course in perioperative nursing. One or two operating room experiences may be all that the student acquires before becoming a registered nurse (RN) and subsequently being hired for the operating room. Coupled with this unfortunate reality is the fact that many operating rooms do not have an educator on staff. As a result, the nurse, new to the operating room, may be assigned to work with a senior nurse or preceptor who demonstrates excellence in practice but who may not have been schooled as an educator.

Essentials of Perioperative Nursing is designed to be a resource for the orientee and a resource for the person responsible for educating the orientee. It is an introductory perioperative nursing text that presents information and concepts that are essential to perioperative nursing practice. It is definitely not intended to be an inclusive perioperative text. Rather, it covers essential elements that are encountered at an entry level and that require early mastery. The text is intended to be used by the entry-level perioperative nurse during the orientation period. It will also be useful to the advanced practitioner wishing to review or validate previous learning or to assess learning needs in preparation for certification.

Chapters are organized under broad headings that suggest desired patient outcomes. An example of a broad heading is prevention of infection. Absense of infection is a desired patient outcome. Chapters grouped under prevention of infection include the subjects of sterilization, asepsis, scrubbing, gowning, gloving, and so forth. The content of these chapters provides the essential knowledge that one needs to perform nursing interventions that will promote the desired outcome of absence of infection.

Each chapter contains learning objectives, an outline, lesson content, programmed instructional exercises, a test, additional references, and where appropriate, a competency checklist. Learners may progress independently through the text and refer to the competency checklists to identify those competencies that must be accomplished to complete their learning of the specific topic as presented. As information beyond the scope of this text is presented, additional required competencies will need to be identified and checklists developed. Learning activities are located throughout each chapter. The questions in the learning activities are designed to test retention, comprehension, and the ability to synthesize and apply the information. Questions should be completed by referring to the preceding instructional material. Answers to the learning activities are located at the back of the book.

The content of each chapter includes information that is most significant and essential to that topic. It is basic information meant to be supplemented as the nurse progresses from entry level to competency. It is also content that lends itself to a programmed instruction format. Essential behavioral skills, such as scrubbing, are best learned through a live-demonstration, return-demonstration format rather than through a programmed instruction format. Although the concepts related to essential behavioral skills are included in this text, the skills themselves are best identified in the skills checklists, which are designed to be used with a clinical instructor. It is suggested that the orientee complete the programmed-instruction unit related to a particular skill prior to the skill practicum.

The educator may find it most appropriate to use the learning objectives and chapter outline to prepare a lesson, and the chapter content and references to supplement other instructional materials. The test following each chapter may be used to evaluate learning. The chapter post tests may also be used as a learning assessment tool for the nurse who has some operating room knowledge or as a starting point for ongoing inservice presentations.

OBJECTIVES

At the completion of this text the learner will be able to

- describe the essential elements of perioperative nursing practice
- identify desired patient outcomes of perioperative care
- recognize common nursing diagnoses for the surgical patient
- identify the role of the perioperative nurse in the achievement of desired patient outcomes
- demonstrate understanding of basic principles of perioperative nursing by attaining a passing score on all tests contained in the text
- identify behavioral skills necessary to demonstrate competency in essential perioperative practice

ASSUMPTIONS ABOUT THE LEARNER

It is assumed that the learner

- is a registered nurse
- has varied clinical experience
- is self-motivated
- has limited knowledge of perioperative nursing practice
- views knowledge of perioperative nursing practice as desirable and useful
- desires immediate feedback to identify additional learning needs
- understands and utilizes the nursing process
- is familiar with nursing diagnoses
- is capable of completing a patient assessment

SECOND EDITION REVISIONS

In addition to updated and expanded content, this second edition of *Essentials of Perioperative Nursing* differs in its conceptual framework. The first edition was task oriented and provided a step-by-step progression of those tasks inherent to perioperative nursing. Knowledge of desired patient outcomes and nursing process was assumed; however, the information was not presented within these frameworks. Without the umbrella of desired patient outcomes or the nursing process, the technical procedures became isolated tasks. In this second edition, the content is presented in the framework of desired patient outcomes with particular attention given to the Outcome Standards that have been identified by the Association of Operating Room Nurses (AORN). Desired patient outcomes represent the desired goal of perioperative nursing activities. Achievement of the outcome standards is supported through the use of the nursing process. Mastery of the content is needed to achieve desired patient outcomes.

Today, cost considerations and the demand to reduce operating expenses have brought about major changes in the workplace. Less costly unlicensed personnel are being recruited to perform tasks previously performed by the registered nurse. Although there is little research to demonstrate the wisdom of these changes or the true impact to the quality of patient care and patient outcomes, the drive to hire the least expensive worker persists. The operating room has not gone untouched. The ratio of registered nurses to patients has decreased while the ratio of other unlicensed personnel to patients has increased. More than at any other time in the history of perioperative nursing practice, operating room nurses are being asked to define and describe what they do that should not be done by a less skilled ancillary health care worker at a lower cost. The ability of the nurse to master isolated perioperative tasks is not the answer. The answer lies in the nurse's ability to assess the patient, diagnose, plan, intervene, coordinate, and manage the patient's surgical experience, perform interventions, and evaluate the outcome, all with the goal of achieving specific identified patient outcomes. With this in mind, the second edition is structured around the patient's surgical experience and progresses through the pre-, intra-, and postoperative phases of patient care. Unlike the first edition in which nursing diagnoses were presented in a dedicated chapter, nursing diagnoses and nursing process provide the structure for the learner's progression throughout this text and throughout the three phases of the patient's surgical experience. In summary, nursing as a process, and desired patient outcomes as a perioperative nursing goal, were not evident in the first edition. In this second edition they are the framework.

Several other changes include the learning objectives at the beginning of each chapter, the skills checklists, the content on patient assessment, the scope of perioperative nursing, the phases of the surgical experience, and the roles of the surgical team members.

CHAPTER 1

Introduction to Perioperative Nursing

Learner Objectives

At the end of Introduction to Perioperative Nursing, the learner will

- define the three phases of the surgical experience
- describe the scope of perioperative nursing practice
- identify members of the surgical team
- discuss the roles of surgical team members
- list patient outcome standards for perioperative care

Lesson Outline

I. **PHASES OF THE SURGICAL EXPERIENCE**
   A. Preoperative
   B. Intraoperative
   C. Postoperative

II. **NURSING PROCESS THROUGHOUT THE PERIOPERATIVE PERIOD**
   A. Assessment
   B. Nursing Diagnoses
   C. Planning
   D. Intervention
   E. Evaluation

III. **PATIENT OUTCOMES: STANDARDS OF PERIOPERATIVE CARE**

IV. **ROLES OF THE PERIOPERATIVE NURSE**

V. **PRACTICE SETTINGS**

VI. **MEMBERS AND RESPONSIBILITIES OF THE SURGICAL TEAM**

CHAPTER 1

Introduction to Perioperative Nursing

PHASES OF THE SURGICAL EXPERIENCE

1. The surgical experience can be segregated into three phases: (1) preoperative, (2) intraoperative, and (3) postoperative. The word *perioperative* encompasses and is used to describe all three.

Preoperative

2. The preoperative phase begins at the point in time when the patient, or someone acting on the patient's behalf, makes the decision to have surgery. This phase ends when the patient is transferred to the operating room bed.
3. The preoperative phase is the period that is used to physically and psychologically prepare the patient for surgery. The length of the preoperative period varies. For the patient whose surgery is elective, the period may be lengthy. For those patients whose surgery is emergent, the period is brief or there may be no awareness of this period on the part of the patient.
4. Diagnostic studies and medical regimens are initiated in the preoperative period. Information obtained from preoperative assessment and interview in this period is used to prepare a plan of care for the patient.
5. Nursing activities in the preoperative phase are directed toward patient support, teaching, and preparation for the procedure.

Intraoperative

6. The intraoperative phase begins when the patient is transferred to the operating room bed and ends with transfer to the postanesthesia care unit or other area where immediate postsurgical recovery care is given.
7. During the intraoperative period the patient is monitored, anesthetized, prepped, and draped, and the operation is performed.
8. Nursing activities in the intraoperative period center on patient safety, prevention of infection, and satisfactory physiologic response to anesthesia and surgical intervention.

Postoperative

9. The postoperative phase begins with the patient's transfer to the recovery unit and ends with the resolution of surgical sequelae. The postoperative period may be brief or extensive and most commonly ends outside the facility where the surgery was performed. Although the perioperative nurse cares for the patient in the postoperative period, it is uncommon for the perioperative nurse to provide care beyond the time of transfer to the recovery unit or home. Care in the recovery unit is assumed by postanesthesia care nurses, and care at home, if required, is delivered by home health care nurses. Recently, however, in an effort to better utilize nursing re-

sources, many perioperative nurses are being given training in postanesthesia care, and increasingly, perioperative nurses are responsible for care in both the operating room and postanesthesia care units.

10. Perioperative nursing activities in the immediate postoperative phase center on support of the patient's physiologic systems.

NURSING PROCESS THROUGHOUT THE PERIOPERATIVE PERIOD

11. The words *perioperative* and *perioperative nursing* are accepted and utilized in nursing and medical literature. Perioperative nursing was formerly referred to as "operating-room nursing." Indeed, until recently, patient care took place in the intraoperative period and was administered within the operating room itself. However, as the responsibilities of the nurse who specialized in this arena expanded to include care in the pre- and postoperative phases, as well as the intraoperative phase, the term *perioperative* has become more appropriate.
12. The perioperative nurse is a nurse who specializes in perioperative practice and who provides nursing care to the surgical patient throughout the continuum of care.
13. Perioperative nurses provide patient care within the framework of the nursing process. They use the tools of patient assessment, care planning, intervention, and evaluation of patient outcomes to meet the needs of patients who are undergoing operative or other invasive procedures. Much of perioperative nursing is technical. Equipment, instrumentation, and surgical techniques are major areas of responsibility. The patient, however, is the focus of the perioperative nurse's activities. Technical skills and responsibilities are purposeful within the nursing process during the implementation phase.

Assessment

14. Nursing assessment of the patient may take place in a number of settings and time frames. Assessment may be performed a week or more before surgery or just prior to the procedure. Assessment may occur in the patient's inpatient hospital unit, the surgeon's office, the preadmission testing unit of the surgical facility, or the same day/ambulatory surgery unit. In some instances the assessment process is initiated in a phone conversation with the patient several days prior to surgery and completed on the day of surgery at the surgical facility. Often the initial nursing assessment is performed by a nurse who is not assigned to the operating room. Although the perioperative nurse may perform the initial nursing assessment it is more likely that the perioperative nurse will perform an assessment just prior to patient entry into the operating room. Assessment at this time will include a brief interview, a quick inspection of the patient, and a review of the patient's record, including assessment data obtained previously by other care givers.

Nursing Diagnoses

15. Assessment data provide information that the perioperative nurse uses to formulate nursing diagnoses and desired outcomes. Although there are several nursing diagnoses that are typical of the surgical patient, such as knowledge deficit and high risk for infection, assessment data form the foundation for patient-specific nursing diagnoses and individualized care tailored to meet individual and unique patient needs.

Planning

16. The perioperative nurse uses knowledge of the patient, the proposed procedure, patient needs, related nursing diagnoses, and desired outcomes to plan care for the patient.
17. Care planning usually begins before the patient is seen. The perioperative nurse begins the care planning prior to interviewing the patient by combining knowledge of the planned procedure, needed resources, and common nursing diagnoses related to surgical intervention. Knowledge of the individual patient that is obtained during the assessment stage is combined with this previous planning to prepare for the unique needs of the patient and to provide care that is individually tailored to each patient.

Intervention

18. In the intervention stage of the nursing process the perioperative nurse provides, coordinates, supervises, and documents care within the framework of accepted standards of nursing care, such as the standards of clinical practice and professional performance developed by the Association of Operating Room Nurses (AORN).

Evaluation

19. In the final evaluation stage of the nursing process, the perioperative nurse evaluates the results of given care in relation to how well expected patient outcomes have been met.

PATIENT OUTCOMES: STANDARDS OF PERIOPERATIVE CARE

20. Nursing care of the surgical patient is directed toward achieving specified desired patient outcomes. The Association of Operating Room Nurses has identified patient outcomes that describe the results that a patient can expect to achieve during surgical interventions. These standards reflect the responsibilities of the perioperative nurse. They are as follows:
    - The patient demonstrates knowledge of the physiological and psychological responses to surgical intervention.
      Criterion:
      Dependent upon physical and psychological status, the patient:
      a. confirms, verbally or in writing, consent for the operative procedures,
      b. describes the sequence of events during the perioperative period, and
      c. expresses feelings about the surgical experience.
    - The patient is free from infection.
      Criterion:
      Dependent upon physical and psychological status, the patient will be free from infection following the operative procedure (AORN, 1995, p. 125).
      Criterion might include the absence of elevated temperature, redness, heat, unusual pain, purulent drainage, and swelling. (Because these signs may be evident immediately postoperative, the time frame for meeting the criterion might be 72 hours.)
    - The patient's skin integrity is maintained.
      Criterion:
      Dependent on physical and psychological status, the patient is free from evidence of skin breakdown or altered state.
    - The patient is free from injury related to positioning, extraneous objects, or chemical, physical, and electrical hazards.
      Criterion:
      Dependent upon physical and psychological status, the patient is free from injury during the intraoperative phase and any sequelae during the postoperative phase (AORN, 1995, p. 126).
      Criterion will be dependent on the risk to which the patient is exposed. Examples of criterion are the absence of an unintended foreign body, absence of burn, absence of numbness, and evidence of postoperative range of motion equal to that of the preoperative status.
    - The patient's fluid and electrolyte balance is maintained.
      Criterion:
      Dependent on physical and psychological status, the patient's
      a. mental orientation is consistent with the preoperative level,
      b. elimination processes correlate with activities related to the operative procedure, and
      c. fluid and electrolyte balance is consistent with preoperative status.
    - The patient participated in the rehabilitation process.
      Criterion:
      Dependent upon physical and psychological status, the patient
      a. identifies problem areas related to surgical experience, and
      b. performs activities related to care (AORN, 1995, p. 126).

    Other desired patient outcomes not specifically listed in the AORN Outcome Standards may be identified by the perioperative nurse and included in the plan of care. Outcomes such as managed pain, maintenance of dignity and privacy, and maintenance of normal body temperature are appropriate and should be planned for. New knowledge regarding patient response to surgery and the effect of nursing interventions will lead to new desired patient outcomes that have implications for perioperative nursing practice. The perioperative nurse who plans patient care should be guided by, but not limited by, established patient outcome standards.

ROLES OF THE PERIOPERATIVE NURSE

21. Perioperative nurses function in various roles including those of manager, clinical practitioner, educator, and researcher. In these roles responsibilities include but are not limited to
    - peer education and patient-family teaching
    - patient support and reassurance
    - patient advocacy
    - control of the environment
    - efficient provision of resources
    - maintenance of asepsis
    - monitoring patient physiological and psychological status
    - supervision of ancillary personnel
    - exploration and validation of current and future practice
    - integration and coordination of care
    - collaboration and consultation ("Report," 1994, p. 85)

PRACTICE SETTINGS

22. Technological advances have resulted in dramatic changes in surgical technique within the last 15 years. Many procedures that once involved utilizing a hospital-based operating room, that necessitated a large incision, and that required a hospital stay and an extended recovery can now be performed in same-day or ambulatory settings. New, minimally invasive, surgical techniques in which surgery is performed through a small puncture hole with specialized instruments and equipment facilitate rapid recovery and same-day discharge. Reimbursement guidelines also encourage same-day or ambulatory surgery and early discharge. As a result, surgery has moved into settings outside the acute-care hospital-based operating room. These settings include free-standing surgical centers, satellite surgery facilities, mobile surgical units, surgeon office-based operating rooms, and clinics. Surgery in physicians' offices is growing dramatically and this trend can be expected to continue as managed care grows (Patterson, 1996, p. 1).
23. Perioperative nursing, once practiced exclusively within the hospital, is now practiced in a variety of settings. However, the needs of the patient who is undergoing surgery transcend the setting and in all settings the perioperative nurse brings specialized skills, technical competence, knowledge, and caring that is essential to a successful surgical experience.

MEMBERS AND RESPONSIBILITIES OF THE SURGICAL TEAM

24. Safe and effective care of the patient in surgery requires a team effort. Each member of the surgical team brings unique skills that must be coordinated to achieve the desired patient outcomes.
25. Team members may be categorized according to their responsibilities during the procedure. Sterile team members are those who scrub their hands and arms, don sterile attire, contact sterile instruments and supplies, and work in the sterile field, i.e., the area immediately surrounding the surgical site.
26. Members of the sterile surgical team may include the primary surgeon; assistants to the surgeon, i.e., other surgeons, residents, physician assistants, and registered nurse first assistants (RNFA); and the scrub person, who may also be a registered nurse, a licensed practical nurse, a surgical technologist, or a surgical technician.
27. Members of the nonsterile surgical team carry out their responsibilities outside the sterile field and do not wear sterile attire. Members of the nonsterile surgical team may include the anesthesiologist, the nurse anesthetist, the circulating nurse, and others.
28. The primary surgeon is responsible for the preoperative diagnosis, selection of the procedure to be performed, and the actual performance of surgery.
29. The assistants work under the direction of the primary surgeon and are responsible for providing assistance during surgery, such as exposing the site, suctioning, tissue handling, and suturing. The nature of the surgery, the state, the medical board and the boards of nursing regulations, the surgeon preference, and the hospital policies are factors that determine who may function as an assistant.
30. The scrub person works primarily with instruments and equipment. Responsibilities of the scrub person include
    - selecting instruments, equipment, and other supplies appropriate for the surgery
    - preparing the sterile field and arranging instruments on the back table prior to surgery
    - maintaining integrity and sterility of the sterile field throughout the procedure
    - having knowledge of the procedure and anticipating the surgeon's needs throughout
    - providing instruments, sutures, and supplies to the surgeon in an appropriate and timely fashion
    - implementing procedures that contribute to patient safety, i.e., surgical counts for instruments, sponges, and sharps
31. Factors that determine the most appropriate scrub person include the nature of the surgery, the skills required for the procedure, the staffing skill mix, and hospital policy.
32. The anesthesiologist is responsible for assessing the patient prior to surgery and for administering anesthetic agents to facilitate surgery and provide pain relief. The certified registered nurse anesthetist administers anesthesia under the direct supervision of the anesthesiologist, or in some cases, the surgeon.
33. The perioperative nurse in the circulating role coordinates the care of the patient, is the patient's advocate throughout the intraoperative experience, and has responsibility for managing and implementing activities outside the sterile field. Activities are directed toward achieving desired patient outcomes. The nursing process is used as a framework for these activities. Examples of activities performed by the perioperative nurse in the circulating role include
    - providing emotional support to the patient prior to the induction of anesthesia
    - performing ongoing patient assessment
    - documenting patient care

- obtaining appropriate surgical supplies and equipment
- creating and maintaining a safe environment
- implementing and enforcing policies and procedures that contribute to patient safety, e.g., surgical counts for instruments, sponges, and sharps, as well as performing equipment checks
- preparing and disposing specimens
- communicating relevant information to other team members and to the patient's family

34. Perfusionists, radiology and laboratory technicians, perioperative educators, pathologists, nurse's aides, clerks, and personnel from materials management, environmental services, and central service are some of the other personnel that are necessary to achieve desired patient outcomes. All have a role in ensuring a safe surgical experience. It is the perioperative nurse who coordinates the contributions of each team member.

NOTES

Association of Operating Room Nurses (AORN). (1995). *Standards and recommended practices* (pp. 125–126). Denver, CO: AORN.

Patterson, P. (1996). Office surgery is gaining market share. *OR Manager*, *12*(2), 1, 12.

Report of the project team to redefine/reconceptualize perioperative nursing of the Association of Operating Room Nurses. (1994, January). *AORN Journal*, *59*, 83–85.

Appendix 1–A

Chapter 1 Post Test

Instructions: Fill in the blanks, mark the correct answer(s), or answer the question as appropriate.

1. Explain why the term *perioperative nurse* is more appropriate than the term *operating-room nurse*. (Ref. 11)

 ____

 ____

2. The preoperative period may be as long as 3 weeks or as short as a half hour. (Ref. 2, 3)

 True False

3. The perioperative nurse may begin planning care for the scheduled surgical patient prior to performing a nursing assessment; however, the plan of care can only be individualized after the assessment. (Ref. 17)

 True False

4. List two criteria that may be used to evaluate whether the desired outcome of the patient demonstrates knowledge of the physiological and psychological responses to surgical intervention has been achieved. (Ref. 20)

 ____

 ____

5. List two criteria that may be used to evaluate whether the desired outcome that the patient is free from infection has been achieved. (Ref. 20)

 ____

 ____

6. List four desired patient outcomes other than the two listed in questions 4 and 5. (Ref. 20)

 ____

 ____

 ____

 ____

7. The nurse providing patient care to a patient undergoing a surgical procedure in a physician's office-based procedure room is technically not a perioperative nurse. (Ref. 23)

 True False

8. Although the perioperative nurse must be skilled in technology, responsibilities related to technical equipment are outside the scope of the nursing process. (Ref. 13)

 True False

9. Arrangements of instruments on the sterile back table prior to surgery is the responsibility of (Ref. 26, 30):
   a. the perioperative nurse in the scrub role
   b. the perioperative nurse in the circulating role
   c. the scrub person who is not a nurse
   d. all of the above

10. Responsibilities of the perioperative nurse in the circulating role would appropriately include (Ref. 27, 33):
    a. communicating with the patient's family to provide a report of the patient during surgery
    b. sending specimens to the laboratory
    c. testing a tourniquet
    d. donning sterile attire to assist the surgeon
    e. informing the surgeon that his or her glove has become contaminated and needs to be changed

Chapter 2

Preparing the Patient for Surgery

Learner Objectives

At the end of Preparing the Patient for Surgery, the learner will

- discuss purposes of preoperative assessment
- state desired patient outcomes related to the preoperative phase
- identify the critical factors included in a preoperative patient assessment
- recognize nursing diagnoses common to the surgical patient in the preoperative phase
- describe interventions in the preoperative phase to achieve desired patient outcomes

Lesson Outline

I. DESIRED PATIENT OUTCOME—PREOPERATIVE PERIOD

II. PREOPERATIVE PREPARATION

III. PATIENT ADVOCACY

IV. PREOPERATIVE ASSESSMENT

- A. Overview
- B. Sources of Patient Information
- C. Assessment Parameters
  1. Physiologic
  2. Psychosocial

V. NURSING DIAGNOSES

VI. NURSING INTERVENTIONS FOR PATIENT PREPARATION

- A. Patient-Family Teaching
- B. Communication of Relevant Data

CHAPTER 2

Preparing the Patient for Surgery

DESIRED PATIENT OUTCOME—PREOPERATIVE PERIOD

1. A well-prepared patient will have an understanding of the events that can be anticipated to occur in the preoperative and immediate postoperative periods. The Association of Operative Nurses (AORN) Outcome Standard states, "The patient demonstrates knowledge of the physiological and psychological responses to surgical intervention" (AORN, 1995, p. 125). The patient should have knowledge of the procedure to be performed and should confirm the consent. The patient should also be prepared for discharge and demonstrate some essential understanding of expected participation in his or her own recovery. The patient should feel supported in the preoperative period and be encouraged to express feelings about the surgical experience. Finally, the patient's level of anxiety or fear should be reduced to a minimum.

PREOPERATIVE PREPARATION

2. Preparations for surgery are begun in the preoperative period as the patient is psychologically and physiologically prepared for surgery. Activities are directed toward treating or minimizing preexisting medical conditions and providing information and support to assist the patient through the surgical experience. Nursing activities are planned to achieve positive patient outcomes.
3. Preparations focus on a variety of nursing activities including data collection through patient assessment, patient-family teaching, emotional support, planning care with the patient for the intra- and postoperative periods, and communicating patient information to health care team members.
4. Planning for the achievement of desired patient outcomes begins with a patient assessment. The desired outcome that the patient demonstrate knowledge of the physiological and psychological responses to surgery can be achieved by providing appropriate information and support during the preoperative period. The content of that information and the patient's unique learning needs can only be ascertained through an assessment process.
5. Additional desired patient outcomes such as freedom from infection, freedom from injury, maintained skin integrity, maintained electrolyte balance, and patient participation in the rehabilitation process are planned or based on information obtained from the preoperative assessment. For example, assessment data that reveal a patient has limited range of motion in a shoulder will lead to planned positioning interventions that will prevent further shoulder injury.

PATIENT ADVOCACY

6. The perioperative nurse is the patient's advocate during surgery. The patient, whose protective reflexes are compromised by anesthesia or other requirements for surgery, is dependent on members of the health care team to be his or her advocate. Knowledge of the patient gained through assessment in the preoperative period provides the information that is necessary for advocacy responsibilities.

PREOPERATIVE ASSESSMENT

Overview

7. The perioperative nurse may have the opportunity to perform a complete and thorough assessment of the patient a day or more prior to surgery at the time of preoperative testing; however, the probability is that the perioperative nurse will first encounter the patient in the holding area immediately prior to surgery. Under these conditions there is insufficient opportunity for the perioperative nurse to carry out a comprehensive history and assessment. The perioperative nurse must therefore focus on essential elements that are necessary for desired patient outcomes.

Sources of Patient Information

8. Assessment data may be obtained from a combination of chart review, patient-family interview, patient observation, and communication with other health care providers. The patient's chart may include an assessment and preoperative checklist that was completed prior to transport to the holding area. This document is a valuable resource in patient assessment (see Exhibit 2–1).
9. With the exception of emergency surgery, where life may depend on immediate surgical intervention, a rapid but thorough chart review and patient-family interview can be sufficient to accomplish the essential assessment.

Assessment Parameters

Physiologic

10. Critical physiological assessment data include the following:
    - medical diagnosis, chronic diseases, and treatment
    - medications—especially antibiotics; anticoagulants, including aspirin; and diuretics that deplete potassium
    - surgery to be performed and surgical site
    - previous surgeries and any complications, including anesthesia complications
    - diagnostic and laboratory data—abnormalities
    - age—very young or very old
    - substance abuse—smoking, alcohol, drugs
    - skin condition—color, rashes, lesions
    - allergies
    - nutritional and nothing by mouth (NPO) status
    - sensory impairments—presence of lenses, hearing aids, dentures
    - mobility impairments
    - presence of prosthetic devices—orthopedic implants, pacemaker, vascular prosthesis
    - weight and height—extreme under and over weight, height greater than length of the operating room (OR) table
    - vital signs

Psychosocial

11. Critical psychosocial assessment data include the following:
    - understanding and perception of the procedure to be performed
    - coping ability
    - ability to comprehend
    - readiness to learn
    - anxiety related to surgical intervention or surgical outcome
    - knowledge of perioperative routines
    - cultural or spiritual beliefs relevant to surgical intervention

NURSING DIAGNOSES

12. The perioperative nurse combines unique knowledge of the surgical procedure with patient assessment data and formulates nursing diagnoses that serve as the basis of the patient's plan of care.
13. One hundred thirty-seven nursing diagnoses and more than 400 nursing interventions have been identified through the North American Nursing Diagnosis Association (NANDA; McClosky & Bulechek, 1996, p. 605). These diagnoses and interventions are not mutually exclusive and any one or more may be appropriate for an individual patient.
14. The plan of care is developed as the perioperative nurse identifies nursing actions to be taken based on the patient's nursing diagnoses. Some nursing diagnoses will require interventions in all three phases of the surgical experience. For other nursing diagnoses the interventions will be confined to a single period (see Exhibit 2–2).
15. Each plan of care must be individualized based on specific individual patient needs. There are, however, several nursing diagnoses that are typical of the surgical patient and that require nursing intervention in the preoperative period.
16. The most common nursing diagnoses requiring nursing intervention in the preoperative period are knowledge deficit and anxiety.
17. Knowledge deficit may be related to perioperative routines, surgical interventions, or outcome expectations.

Exhibit 2–1 Preop Visit Assessment Form

OR #: ________

PRE-OP VISIT

PERSONAL PHYSICIAN | SURGEON | ANESTHESIOLOGIST | SEX ☐ M ☐ F | AGE

DATE | TIME | PROCEDURE | NICKNAME

ALLERGIES | ISOLATION PRECAUTIONS ☐ TB ☐ HIV ☐ HEPATITIS

MEDICAL & SURGICAL HISTORY:

HT:
WT:
T:
P:
R:
BP RANGE:
PERIPHERAL PERFUSION:
PULSES:
RR:
LR:
RP:
LP:
SMOKES:
☐ Yes
☐ No
☐ PPD ___
☐ Quit ________

SKIN ASSESSMENT
COLOR:
☐ Pale
☐ Flushed
☐ Dusky
☐ Cyanotic
☐ Jaundice
☐ Normal
☐ Other:
CONDITION:
☐ No Problem
☐ Rash
☐ Boney Area
☐ Redness
☐ Decubiti
☐ Contusions/ Abrasions
☐ Edema
☐ Other:

MENTAL/ EMOTIONAL
☐ Oriented
☐ Disoriented To:
☐ Time
☐ Place
☐ Person
☐ Lethargic
☐ Comatose
☐ Dementia/ Alzheimers
☐ Protective Devices
☐ Calm
☐ Apprehensive
☐ Emotional Disorders
UNITS OF BLOOD:
☐ T & C
Number of Units on Hand:

VISION
☐ Adequate
☐ Decreased
☐ Blind:
☐ Rt ☐ Lt
☐ Glasses
☐ Contacts
HEARING
☐ Adequate
☐ Decreased
☐ Deaf
☐ Rt ☐ Lt
☐ Hearing Aide
COMMUNICATION BARRIERS:
CONSULTING PHYSICIANS/SPECIALTY:

PRE-OP TUBES
☐ Foley
☐ NG
☐ Other:
CHART REQUIREMENTS
☐ Permit
☐ H & P
DENTURES
☐ Upper
☐ Lower
☐ Partial

LABORATORY INFORMATION
☐ BLOOD GLUCOSE MONITORING
SHA / OR / PACU INSTRUCTIONS:
X-RAYS:
SCANS:
EKG:
FAMILY
☐ FWA ☐ ICU FWA ☐ HOME ☐ OTHER:

PRE-OP:
TIME:
ROUTINE MEDS:

COMMENTS:

IVs:
☐ Central
☐ Peripheral
DATE OF INSERTION: ____________

Fluids: ____________
Support Meds: Type____________
Rate________
TPN & Rate:________

☐ OR RN
☐ PACU RN
Signature:

Source: Pilot DRAFT form courtesy of St. Luke's Medical Center, Milwaukee, Wisconsin.

Exhibit 2–2 Perioperative Nursing Diagnosis Flowsheet

PROBLEM	PAT	PRE-OP	INTRA-OP	PACU I	PACU II
DIAGNOSIS #1 DATE: Potential knowledge deficit R/T unknown; the environment and surgical procedures. 1. Assess present knowledge level with patient quote on record. DESIRED OUTCOME 1. Patient will demonstrate understanding of all phases of care by accurately verbalizing knowledge or return demonstration.	____	____	____		
INTERVENTIONS 1. Explain your (nurse) role to patient.					
2. Provide information regarding perioperative nursing.					
3. Clarify previous physician explanations. Refer appropriate personnel for clarification.					
4. Provide written instructions/audiovisual aids.					
DIAGNOSIS #2 DATE: Potential alteration in family and individual coping mechanisms R/T anxiety, fear, and/or inadequate support systems. 1. Assess support person's understanding of patient's perioperative experiences. DESIRED OUTCOME Patient/support person will demonstrate appropriate coping mechanisms.	____	____	____		
INTERVENTIONS 1. Have patient identify support person.					
2. Communicate any specific support needs of family/patient to appropriate personnel.					
3. Keep support person informed.					
DIAGNOSIS #3 DATE: Potential for infection R/T surgical procedures, foreign environment. 1. Assess patient for history and current risk factors. DESIRED OUTCOME Patient will remain free of nosocomial infection.	____	____	____		
INTERVENTIONS 1. Monitor for break in aseptic technique, and take corrective measures.					
2. Monitor and limit excessive travel into/from operating suite.					
3. Proper handwashing.					
4. Use universal precautions.					

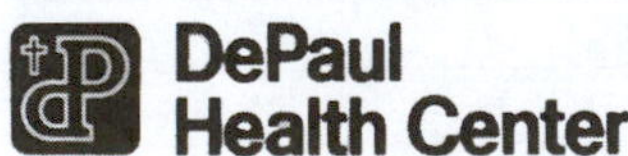

LEGEND
O = Ongoing
O/N = Ongoing, No Intervention
R = Resolved
N/A = Not Applicable

PERIOPERATIVE NURSING DIAGNOSES

FORM NO. 2-417 (REV. 3/93) APPROVED BY MRC 1/93

continues

Exhibit 2–2 continued

PROBLEM	PAT	PRE-OP	INTRA-OP	PACU I	PACU II
DIAGNOSIS #4 DATE: Potential alterations in ventilation and cardiovascular function R/T anesthesia with surgical procedures. 1. Assess patient's current and review past history for potential risk factors. 2. Assess need for O_2 therapy. 3. Assess peripheral circulatory status. DESIRED OUTCOME 1. Patient will maintain or improve pulmonary functions. 2. Patient will maintain or improve cardiovascular functions.	____	____	____ *GEN.		
INTERVENTIONS 1. Respiratory a. Assist with anesthesia induction/assist with O_2 therapy.			*		
b. Observe respiratory function.					
c. Auscultate lung fields.					
d. Elevate HOB.					
e. Deep breathe/cough.					
f. Suction prn.					
g. Monitor ABG/SAO_2.					
2. Cardiovascular a. Monitor heart rhythm.					
b. Implement usage of thermal support.			*		
c. Monitor pulses.					
d. Apply and/or monitor TED/sequential stockings.			*		
3. Monitor skin color.					
4. Teach s/s of alterations expected at home, leg exercises/deep breathing.					
DIAGNOSIS #5 DATE: Potential alterations in fluid/electrolyte balance R/T surgical procedure, blood loss, & NPO status. 1. Assess patient fluid/electrolyte status during perioperative experience. DESIRED OUTCOME 1. Patient will maintain fluid balance.	____	____	____		
INTERVENTIONS 1. Maintain IV fluid therapy.					
2. Notify physician of abnormal lab values.					
3. Monitor blood/fluid loss.					
4. Assist with insertion of invasive hemodynamic monitors.					
5. Monitor for and notify physician of abnormal hemodynamic monitor values.					
6. Teaching of drainage output including amount, frequency, character/follow-up.					

NAME ______________________________ MEDICAL RECORD NO. ____________________

Source: Courtesy of DePaul Health Center, Bridgeton, Missouri.

Knowledge deficit may be the result of impaired communication, a language barrier, a patient's insufficient mental capacity, or a lack of information regarding the surgical procedure. Nursing interventions must be appropriate to the etiology of the patient's knowledge deficit and to the patient's learning needs.

18. Anxiety can range from mild to severe and may have a variety of etiologies. A patient's level of anxiety may be more acute at some periods throughout the surgical experience than at others. For some patients, anxiety is at its height just prior to surgery. For others it is most acute at the time the decision to have surgery is made. Patients who are anxious cannot always identify the exact cause of their anxiety. They may express an uneasiness or nervousness.
19. Anxiety is different from fear (Burden, 1993, p. 178). The patient who is anxious but cannot state the exact cause may manifest anxiety with an increased heart and respiratory rate and an elevated blood pressure. The patient may feel nervous or tense and may not be able to concentrate or retain information. The fearful patient, however, can state the source of fear. Fear is marked by apprehension and dread and may be related to surgical intervention, surgical outcome, anesthesia, impact of surgery on lifestyle, loss of control, pain, death, and so forth. Although some patients will exhibit fear, an anxious state is more common.

NURSING INTERVENTIONS FOR PATIENT PREPARATION

20. The desired outcome related to knowledge deficit is that the patient will demonstrate knowledge of the physiological and psychological responses to surgery.
21. Nursing interventions that address knowledge deficit should include
    - confirmation of the patient's identity
    - verification of the surgical site and procedure
    - verification of consent
    - solicitation of the patient's perception of planned surgery
    - solicitation of questions related to surgery
    - identification of teaching needs, readiness, and ability to learn
    - explanation of surgical routines
    - explanation of procedures that need to be followed postoperatively upon discharge (especially critical for patients who are intended to be discharged on the day of their surgery, therefore limiting the time available for teaching)
    - provision of appropriate information with consideration for patient's level of understanding, ability to comprehend, desired information, culture, and religious beliefs, as well as medical concerns referred to the surgeon
    - solicitation of feedback regarding perioperative procedures
22. The desired outcome related to anxiety is that anxiety and fear will be lessened through gained knowledge and expression of feelings about the surgical intervention.
23. Nursing interventions that address anxiety and fear should include
    - attentive listening
    - provision of information as needed
    - solicitation of patient expressions of anxiety or fear
    - provision of emotional support and reassurance
24. Criteria that may be used to evaluate the achievement of these outcomes are that the patient will (1) confirm the consent, (2) describe the sequence of events, (3) express feelings about the surgical experience, (4) indicate knowledge of expected surgical outcomes, and (5) confirm procedures to be followed upon discharge.

Patient-Family Teaching

25. Patient teaching is ideally begun during a preadmission workup or in the physician's office or clinic where the prospect of surgery is discussed. When possible, the patient's family or support persons should be included in the teaching process. Patient teaching must be appropriate to the patient's and family's ability and readiness to understand and to learn.
26. The patient's age must be considered when patient teaching is implemented.
27. Elderly patients are no less intelligent than younger patients; however, short-term memory may be diminished and additional time and reinforcement may be necessary in order for them to learn and comprehend information. Additional time should be planned for instruction. Instructional materials and voice level should take possible sight and hearing deficits into consideration.
28. Pediatric patients have special needs. The school-age child may view the surgical experience as a threat to recently achieved independence and control. Children under 7 years of age may view illness as a punishment for wrongdoings and surgery may invoke fear of body mutilation and death (Redman, 1993, pp. 90–91). Patient teaching for pediatric patients may include an opportunity for them to handle simple items that they will be faced with in surgery. The ability, for example, to touch

and manipulate an anesthesia mask may provide the child with a needed feeling of control.

29. Patient teaching during a preadmission workup will be more extensive than teaching that is accomplished in the holding area just prior to surgery. Teaching during a preadmission process should include content that is directed toward preparation for surgery and participation in the postoperative rehabilitation process. An example of teaching content in preparation for colon surgery is instruction in bowel cleansing. An example of preoperative teaching directed toward postoperative patient participation in postoperative rehabilitation is crutch walking. Written instructions, pamphlets, and videos related to preparation for surgery and rehabilitation may be provided. Teaching in the preop holding area will be abbreviated and will reinforce previous teaching. Teaching directed toward discharge will be reinforced in the postoperative period prior to discharge.
30. Preoperative teaching content should include at least
    - the procedure, duration, and expected outcome
    - specific instructions such as whether to bathe or shower, to hold or take medications, and whether to maintain NPO
    - an explanation of preoperative events such as diagnostic tests, skin preparation, intravenous (IV) insertion, sedation, and transfer to holding area
    - an explanation of intraoperative events such as function of the circulating nurse or case manager, application of monitoring equipment, administration of anesthesia, maintenance of privacy and dignity, staff communication with family members during the procedure, and transport to the postanesthesia care unit
    - an explanation of postoperative events such as expected length of stay; coughing and deep breathing; turning; presence of lines, drains, and indwelling catheters; pain control; and discharge to a step-down or other unit
31. The nurse who performs an assessment of teaching needs in the holding area may identify that the patient is anxious and unable to recall information presented earlier in preparation for surgery. The anxious patient may have difficulty concentrating or retaining information. Information given earlier about surgical interventions may need to be repeated and information pertaining to discharge and expected recovery will need to be reinforced with both the patient and the family in the postoperative period.
32. In addition to providing information to the patient, the perioperative nurse provides emotional support and reassurance. The perioperative nurse should solicit the patient's expression of feelings and concerns regarding surgery.
33. Anxiety and fear can be alleviated through attentive listening and reassurance as well as through information that is delivered calmly and candidly. An attentive, caring attitude, coupled with appropriate touch, can serve as a source of patient comfort and reassurance. Reduction of anxiety and fear through these interventions may be necessary in order to prepare the patient for teaching.

Communication of Relevant Patient Data

34. Assessment information with relevance to intra- and postoperative care must be communicated to other members of the health care team. Continuity of care and appropriate therapeutic interventions cannot be assured without the communication of information. Documentation of findings and verbal communication of patient data and responses to interventions must be part of the surgical patient's ongoing care.

NOTES

Association of Operating Room Nurses (AORN). (1995). *Standards and recommend practices* (pp. 125–126). Denver, CO: AORN.

Burden, N. (1993). *Ambulatory surgical nursing*. Philadelphia: W.B. Saunders.

McClosky, J., & Bulechek, G. (Eds.). (1996). *Nursing interventions classification* (2nd ed.). St. Louis: Mosby Year Book.

Redman, B. (1993). *The process of patient education*. St. Louis: Mosby Year Book.

ADDITIONAL READING

Bean, M. (1990). Preparation for surgery in an ambulatory surgery unit. *Journal of Post Anesthesia Nursing, 5*(1), 42–47.

Full body assessments contribute to thorough patient screening. (1990, September). *Same Day Surgery*, 125–127.

Knight, C., & Donnelly, M. (1988). Assessing the preoperative adult. *Nurse Practitioner, 13*(1), 6–17.

Longinow, L. (1993). The holding room: A preoperative advantage. *AORN Journal, 57*(4), 914–924.

Lunow, K. (1993). Comprehensive perioperative care: Patient assessment, teaching, documentation. *AORN Journal*, *57*(5), 1167–1177.

Takahashi, J. (1989). Preoperative nursing assessment: A research study. *AORN Journal, 50*(5), 1022–1032.

Appendix 2–A

Chapter 2 Post Test

Instructions: Fill in blanks, mark correct answer(s), or answer the question as appropriate.

1. List four nursing activities the perioperative nurse might perform in the preoperative period to prepare the patient for surgery. (Ref. 3)

 ____
 ____
 ____
 ____

2. The perioperative nurse in the holding area may share responsibility for patient assessment with nurses outside the operating room. (Ref. 7, 8)

 True False

3. Assessment of the patient's understanding and perception of the surgical procedure to be performed should always be included in the assessment process. (Ref. 11)

 True False

4. Before implementing patient teaching the perioperative nurse must assess the patient's (Ref. 11, 19):
 a. knowledge of perioperative routines
 b. understanding of the procedure to be performed
 c. expected cost of services
 d. readiness to learn
 e. anxiety

5. Nursing diagnoses made by the perioperative nurse should not require interventions outside the operating room or postanesthesia care unit. (Ref. 14)

 True False

6. Nursing diagnosis must be individualized and based on patient assessment; however, there are two nursing diagnoses that are typically appropriate for the surgical patient in the preoperative period. These two nursing diagnoses are (Ref. 16, 17, 18):

 ____
 ____

7. Asking the patient if he or she has any questions about the pending surgery is a nursing intervention appropriate to a patient with the nursing diagnosis of knowledge deficit. (Ref. 21)

 True False

8. Soliciting feelings about the patient's pending surgery is a nursing intervention appropriate to a patient with the nursing diagnosis of anxiety. (Ref. 21)

 True False

9. List three criteria to evaluate whether the desired outcome that the patient will demonstrate knowledge of the physiological and psychological response to surgery, has been achieved. (Ref. 24)

____

____

____

10. Elderly patients may have diminished vision; therefore instructional materials should not be printed in very small letters that may be difficult to see. Instructional materials for the elderly should take into consideration the possibility of diminished vision. List two other considerations that should be taken when teaching elderly patients. (Ref. 27)

____

____

11. A 5-year-old child may believe that the pending surgery is a punishment for wrongdoings. (Ref. 28)

    True False

12. Nursing interventions for the school-age child should be directed toward providing the child with a feeling of some control over the pending activities. This may be accomplished by permitting the child to handle items that he or she may come in contact with, such as a blood pressure cuff. (Ref. 28)

    True False

13. Patients who are anxious may need additional reinforcement of teaching because of a reduced ability to concentrate. (Ref. 31)

    True False

Appendix 2–B

Competency Checklist: Preparing the Patient for Surgery

Under observer's initials enter initials upon successful achievement of competency. Enter N/A if competency is not appropriate for institution.

NAME ______________________________

	OBSERVER'S INITIALS	DATE
1. Patient is assessed (or chart reviewed) for:		
a. medical diagnosis	________	________
b. medications	________	________
c. laboratory data	________	________
d. previous surgeries	________	________
e. anesthesia complications	________	________
f. substance abuse	________	________
g. skin condition	________	________
h. allergies	________	________
i. NPO status	________	________
j. sensory impairments	________	________
k. dentures	________	________
l. mobility impairments	________	________
m. presence of prosthesis	________	________
n. weight and height	________	________
o. vital signs	________	________
2. Patient is identified.	________	________
3. Patient is assessed for:		
a. level of understanding	________	________
b. ability to comprehend	________	________
c. information desired	________	________
d. cultural and religious beliefs	________	________
4. Surgical procedure and operative site are verified by the patient.	________	________
5. Operative consent is verified with the patient.	________	________
6. Patient is asked to verbalize understanding of the surgical experience.	________	________
7. Patient is encouraged to ask questions regarding the surgical procedure.	________	________

NAME ______________________________

	OBSERVER'S INITIALS	DATE
8. Patient is encouraged to verbalize concerns about the surgical experience.	________	________
9. Intraoperative routines that the patient should expect are explained.	________	________
10. Postoperative routines are explained to the patient.	________	________
11. The above information is communicated to the surgical team.	________	________

OBSERVER'S SIGNATURE INITIALS

______________________________ __________

ORIENTEE'S SIGNATURE

____

CHAPTER 3

Prevention of Infection—Preparation of Instruments and Items Used in Surgery: Sterilization and Disinfection

Learner Objectives

At the end of Prevention of Infection—Preparation of Instruments and Items Used in Surgery: Sterilization and Disinfection, the learner will

- discuss the relationship of sterilization and disinfection to the prevention of patient infection
- identify the critical factors that determine whether an item must be sterile or whether disinfection is sufficient
- describe four methods used to accomplish sterilization
- discuss critical factors that determine the selection of the sterilization method
- discuss advantages and disadvantages of sterilization methods
- compare and contrast flash and high-vacuum sterilization
- discuss appropriate uses of flash sterilization
- discuss appropriate use of disinfectants
- list hazards associated with sterilization and disinfection processes
- identify methods for monitoring sterilization and disinfection processes

Lesson Outline

I. DESIRED PATIENT OUTCOMES

II. STERILIZATION VERSUS DISINFECTION

- A. Definitions
  1. Sterilization
  2. Spore
  3. Disinfection
- B. Critical and Semicritical Items
  1. Critical Item—Examples
  2. Semicritical Item—Examples

III. METHODS OF STERILIZATION

- A. Overview
- B. Thermal Sterilization—Steam under Pressure: Moist Heat
  1. Advantages
  2. Disadvantages
- C. Steam Sterilizers—Autoclaves
  1. Overview
  2. Gravity Displacement
  3. Prevacuum—Bowie-Dick Test
  4. Pressure-Pulse
- D. Flash Sterilization
- E. Validation of Steam Sterilization Parameters
  1. Mechanical Process Indicators
  2. Chemical Process Indicators
  3. Biological Monitors
- F. Chemical Sterilization—Ethylene Oxide Gas (EO)
  1. Advantages
  2. Disadvantages
- G. Chemical Sterilization—Liquid Peracetic Acid
  1. Advantages
  2. Disadvantages
- H. Low Temperature Hydrogen Peroxide Gas Plasma Sterilization
  1. Advantages
  2. Disadvantages
- I. Mixed Chemical Plasma
  1. Advantages
  2. Disadvantages
- J. Emerging Sterilization Technologies

IV. RECORD KEEPING

V. DISINFECTION

- A. Overview
- B. Levels of Disinfectants—Application
- C. Glutaraldehyde

CHAPTER 3

Prevention of Infection—Preparation of Instruments and Items Used in Surgery: Sterilization and Disinfection

DESIRED PATIENT OUTCOMES

1. Freedom from infection is a critical desired patient outcome.
2. Postoperative wound infection is a complication of surgery with potentially dire consequences for the patient. It can delay recovery, increase patient suffering, and even cause death. Postoperative wound infection contributes to extended hospital stays and higher costs for care.
3. Surgical intervention alters tissue integrity and interrupts skin integrity. Skin is the body's first line of defense against infection. Invasive drains, catheters, and monitors also alter skin integrity. These all put the patient at risk for infection by providing a portal of entry for pathogenic microorganisms.
4. The nursing diagnosis of high risk for infection is applicable to all patients undergoing invasive procedures.
5. Perioperative nursing activities are directed toward prevention of infection with the goal that the patient will be free from infection following the operative procedure.
6. Pathogenic microorganisms are capable of causing disease when they invade human tissue. Contaminated equipment has been reported as a source of nosocomial infection (U.S. Department of Health, 1991, pp. 675–678). Every effort must be made to remove microorganisms from articles and instruments that contact human tissue during surgical intervention.
7. Sterilization and disinfection are two processes used to destroy microorganisms. These processes are the cornerstones of infection control. Prevention of infection requires the perioperative nurse to have an in-depth understanding of principles and practices of sterilization and disinfection.
8. Advances in surgical techniques have resulted in the routine use of a wide variety of complex, sophisticated, and expensive surgical instrumentation. As an example, fiberoptic instruments costing many thousands of dollars are a standard component of many procedures. Cleaning, disinfection, and sterilization procedures appropriate for the simple general line of instruments are not appropriate for much of the new complex instrumentation. The composition and configuration of the instrument and its compatibility with the disinfection and sterilization method must be considered when purchasing and processing decisions are made.
9. The perioperative nurse assumes varying degrees of responsibility for the care and preparation of instruments. Selecting the appropriate method of processing requires a broad knowledge of disinfection and sterilization principles and procedures.
10. Increased acceptance of just-in-time sterilization (sterilizing an item just prior to its use) has required the movement of some sterilization procedures from the central processing department to the point where the instrument is to be used. When disinfection and sterilization are accomplished within the operating room department it is often the perioperative nurse who is responsible for the process.

Section Questions

Q1. Complications of postoperative surgical wound infection affect the patient and impact the cost of health care. Describe two consequences to the patient. (Ref. 2)

____

____

Q2. Explain how a drain that was placed into the wound during surgery can put the patient at risk for infection. (Ref. 3)

____

____

Q3. Explain why the nursing diagnosis of high risk for infection is appropriate for patients undergoing surgery and other invasive procedures. (Ref. 3, 4)

____

____

Q4. Sterilization procedures are carried out primarily by ancillary personnel; however, the perioperative nurse must have an in-depth knowledge of these procedures because (Ref. 7, 8, 9, 10):

a. responsibility for care and preparation of instrumentation is a shared responsibility.
b. the perioperative nurse is responsible for prevention of infection.
c. sterilization of surgical instrumentation usually takes place in the operating room.

Q5. __________ and __________ are two processes used to destroy pathogenic microorganisms. (Ref. 7)

STERILIZATION VERSUS DISINFECTION

Definitions

Sterilization

11. Sterilization may be defined as a process that kills all living microorganisms including spores.

Spore

12. A spore is an inactive or dormant but viable state of a microorganism. Bacteria in their active state are referred to as vegetative.
13. Certain pathogenic bacteria such as *Clostridium tetani*, which produces tetanus, and *Clostridium perfidens*, which results in gas gangrene, are capable of developing spore forms. The environmental conditions that make it possible for spore formation are unknown; however, spores can remain alive for many years. When conditions are favorable for growth, such as when the spore is permitted entry into the body, the spore will germinate to produce a vegetative cell.
14. Spores are resistant, to a greater degree than are other bacteria, to heat, drying, and chemicals. Spores can survive long exposures to these processes. Only the process of sterilization can render an item free of all microorganisms, including spores.
15. The process of sterilization provides the greatest assurance that items are sterile, i.e., free of known and unsuspected pathogenic microorganisms.

Disinfection

16. Disinfection may be defined as the process that kills many or all living microorganisms with the exception of bacterial spores. Disinfection does not provide the same margin of safety that is associated with sterilization. Disinfectants vary in their ability to destroy microorganisms and are classified according to their biocidal activity.

Critical and Semicritical Items

Critical Item—Examples

17. Items that come in contact with sterile tissue or the vascular system, i.e., items introduced below a mucous membrane, are considered critical items. Critical items contaminated with microorganisms present a high risk of infection. Critical items *must* be sterile.
18. Examples of critical items include surgical instruments, orthopedic implants, sutures, and cardiac catheters.

Semicritical Item—Examples

19. Items that contact unbroken mucous membranes and do not penetrate body surfaces are considered semicritical items. Semicritical items may be sterile but *must* be disinfected.
20. Examples of semicritical items include thermometers, cystoscopes, and dental dams.

Section Questions

Q6. Define sterilization. (Ref. 11)

____

____

Q7. Define disinfection. (Ref. 16)

____

____

Q8. Define spore. (Ref. 12)

____

____

Q9. The process that kills all living microorganisms including spores is (Ref. 11):
a. disinfection
b. sterilization

Q10. Once a pathogenic bacterium forms a spore that bacterium is no longer capable of causing an infection. (Ref. 13)

True False

Q11. Spores are ______ resistant to heat than other nonspore forming bacteria. (Ref. 14)
a. more
b. less

Q12. An example of a semicritical item is a laryngoscope. Acceptable infection control practice mandates that this item be sterilized before use. (Ref. 19)

True False

METHODS OF STERILIZATION

Overview

21. There are a number of methods of sterilization. The choice of method is dependent on the compatibility of the item to be sterilized with the sterilization process, configuration of the item, required equipment, cost, availability, safety factors, packaging of the item, and length of time of the sterilization process. Each method has both advantages and disadvantages.
22. Methods of in-house sterilization have traditionally been dominated by steam and ethylene oxide gas. Steam is used for heat- and moisture-stable items. Ethylene oxide sterilization is appropriate for sterilization of items that cannot withstand heat and moisture.
23. Steam and ethylene oxide have been used in hospitals for more than 30 years. Newer sterilization technologies achieving widespread use include peracetic acid and gas plasma. Peracetic acid is used for heat-sensitive items that can be immersed. Gas plasma sterilization is appropriate for both heat- and moisture-sensitive items. Vapor phase hydrogen peroxide and ozone sterilization are emerging technologies that are not yet available in the United States.
24. Two other accepted methods of sterilization are dry heat and ionizing radiation.
25. Dry heat is appropriate for powders, oils, and petroleum products that cannot be penetrated by steam or ethylene oxide or other sterilizing agents. Dry-heat sterilization is rarely used in hospitals today.
26. Because of equipment, safety, and cost considerations, ionizing radiation is confined to industrial settings and is used for bulk sterilization of commercially prepared items.

Thermal Sterilization—Steam under Pressure: Moist Heat

27. Moist heat in the form of saturated steam under pressure is an economical, safe, and effective method of sterilization used for the majority of surgical instruments. It is the most common sterilization method used within health care facilities. Sterilization by this method is accomplished in a steam sterilizer referred to as an autoclave.
28. For sterilization to be achieved, steam must penetrate every fiber of the packaging, contact every surface of the item, and the intended parameters of moisture, temperature, and time must be met.
29. Steam that is saturated (contains the greatest amount of water vapor possible) and is heated to a sufficient temperature is capable of destroying all living microorganisms, including spores, within a relatively short amount of time.
30. Saturated steam destroys microorganisms through a thermal process that causes denaturation and coagulation of protein or the enzyme protein system contained within the microorganism's cell.
31. Steam at atmospheric pressure has a temperature of 212°F (100°C). This temperature is inadequate for sterilization. The addition of pressure to raise the temperature of steam is necessary for the destruction of microorganisms.
32. An increase in pressure of 15 to 17 pounds per square inch will increase steam temperature to 250°F to 254°F (121°C to 123°C). Twenty-seven pounds of pressure per square inch will increase steam temperature to 270°F (132°C).
33. The minimum generally accepted temperature required for sterilization to occur is 250°F (121°C; Perkins, 1969, p. 161). Typical temperatures for the operation of steam sterilizers are 270°F to 275°F (132°C to 135°C), although 250°F (121°C) is also used.
34. Steam sterilization is a function of time and temperature. A temperature of 250°F (121°C) requires more time than a temperature of 270°F (132°C).

Advantages

35. Some of the many advantages to steam sterilization include:
    - Steam is readily available (most often supplied from the health care facility boiler).
    - Steam is economical.
    - Steam is compatible with most in-house packaging materials.
    - Steam leaves no toxic residue and is environmentally safe.
    - Steam sterilization is suitable for a wide range of surgical instrumentation. (Many items used for surgery can withstand repeated steam sterilization without sustaining damage.)
    - Steam sterilization is fast. Destruction of most resistant spores occurs quickly.

Disadvantages

36. Disadvantages associated with steam sterilization include:
    - An increasing number of items used in surgery cannot withstand moist heat at temperatures of 250°F (121°C) or above.
    - Steam sterilization is prone to operator error with regard to preparation of items, setting of parameters, and loading of the autoclave.

- Timing of the sterilization cycle must be adjusted for type of cycle, variances in materials, and size of the load.
- A temperature of 270°F cannot be used for all items. The temperature may need to be reduced from 270°F to 250°F to be compatible with a specific item being sterilized.
- Efficacy depends on attention to detail. Improper preparation of items or improper placement within the autoclave can result in trapped air, which can prevent steam contact with all surfaces and thus prevent sterilization. Items must be disassembled in order for steam to contact all surfaces.

Steam Sterilizers—Autoclaves

Overview

37. An autoclave generally consists of a rectangular metal chamber and a shell. Between the two is an enclosed space referred to as a jacket. When the autoclave is activated, steam and heat fill the jacket and are maintained at a constant pressure, keeping the autoclave in a heated, ready state (see Figures 3–1 and 3–2).
38. Items are placed in the chamber, the door is shut tightly, and the sterilization cycle is initiated. Steam enters the chamber and displaces all the air from the contents of the load. As the pressure rises, steam penetrates the contents and contacts all surfaces. The steam forces the air out through a discharge port outlet at the bottom front of the autoclave (see Figure 3–3).
39. The discharge port outlet is the beginning of a filtered waste line. Beneath the filter is a thermometer. This is the coolest part of the autoclave.
40. Only after the temperature rises and the thermometer senses that the steam has reached the necessary preset temperature does the actual exposure or sterilization time period begin.
41. It is essential that all air be displaced by steam. Air that is trapped will act as an insulator and prevent heating and moisture contact with every surface of every item and the sterilization process will be compromised. For this reason loading of the autoclave is critical. Items must be placed so that steam can circulate freely throughout the chamber and can contact all surfaces.
42. If air is not trapped and parameters of time, moisture, and temperature have been met, microbial destruction will occur.
43. When the exposure time is complete, the steam is exhausted through the outlet port, and if desired, a drying cycle follows. A drying cycle must be used for wrapped items.

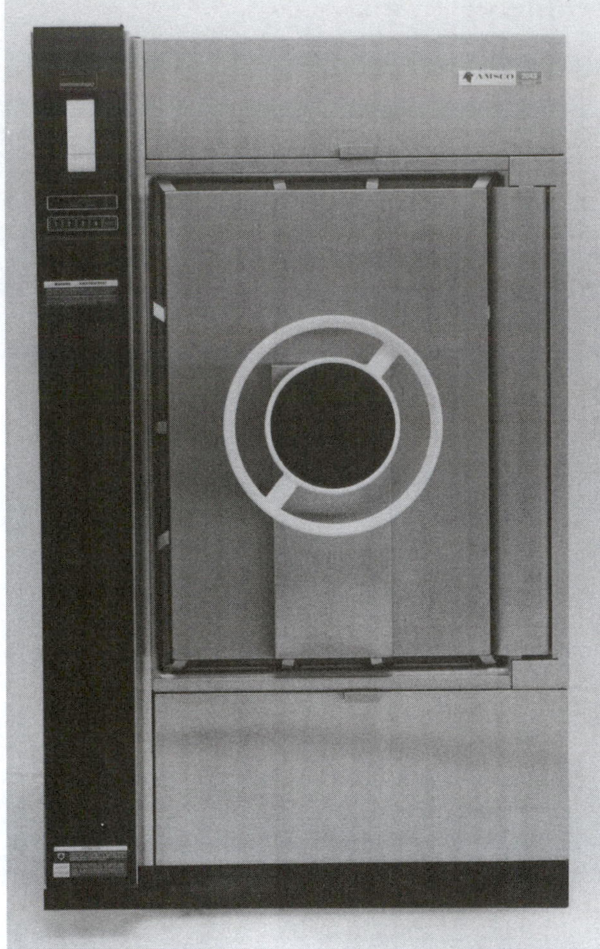

Figure 3–1 Steam Sterilizer. *Source:* Photo courtesy of AMSCO International, Inc.

44. Packages removed from the autoclave are allowed to cool on wire mesh shelves covered with material that will absorb heat and prevent condensation. Warm packages are not placed on cool surfaces because condensate will form, causing the package to become damp.
45. Microorganisms are capable of penetrating wet materials; therefore, moist packages that contact an unsterile surface must be considered contaminated.
46. There are three types of steam sterilizers or autoclaves: (1) gravity displacement, (2) prevacuum or high vacuum, and (3) steam-flush pressure-pulse. These autoclaves differ in how air is removed from the chamber during the sterilization process.

Gravity Displacement

47. In a gravity-displacement autoclave the air in the chamber is displaced by gravity.

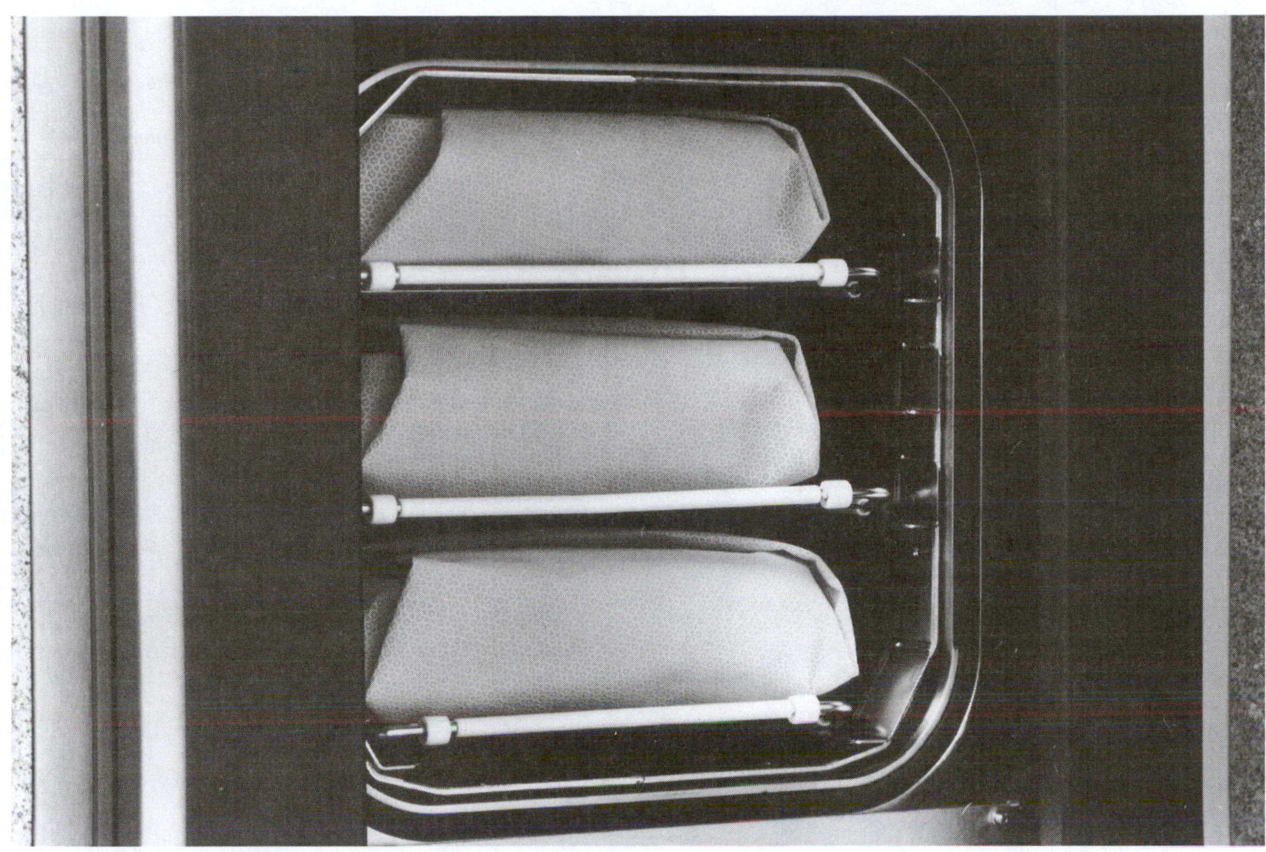

Figure 3–2 Steam Sterilizer Chamber. *Source:* Photo courtesy of AMSCO International, Inc.

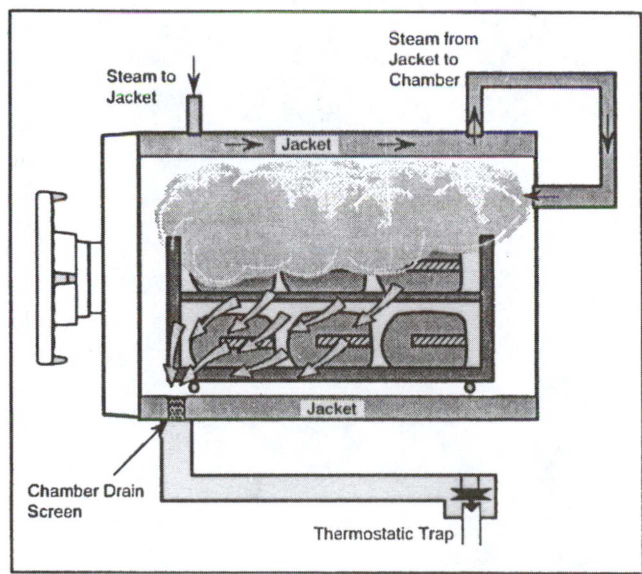

Figure 3–3 Steam Sterilizer—Steam Entry and Air Removal. *Source:* Photo courtesy of AMSCO International, Inc.

48. As steam enters from a port located near the top and rear of the chamber it is deflected upward. Air is heavier than steam and by the force of gravity, the air is forced to the bottom while the steam rides on top of the air. The steam rapidly displaces the air under it and forces the air out through the discharge outlet port.
49. Most gravity displacement autoclaves are commonly operated at temperatures between 250°F and 274°F (121°C to 134°C) and 10- to 30-minute exposure times. Certain powered equipment, however, requires prolonged exposure times of as much as 55 minutes.
50. A higher temperature requires less time than a lower temperature. A temperature of 270°F (132°C) will accomplish sterilization more rapidly than a temperature of 250°F (121°C).
51. The nature of the items and the container in which they are sterilized determine the necessary time and temperature settings. There is no single setting that is appropriate for all items. Manufacturers' guidelines for the items and for the autoclave must be followed. Table 3–1 dem-

onstrates how time and temperature in a gravity displacement autoclave may be varied.

52. The disadvantage of a gravity-displacement process is the length of time required for sterilization and the dependence on gravity to remove air.

Table 3–1 Gravity Displacement Autoclave

	Minimum Exposure Time Required	
	Temperature	
Item	*250°F (121°C)*	*270°F (132°C)*
Unwrapped metal instruments	15 min	3 min
Unwrapped metal instruments with porous items and/or items with a lumen—time required for steam to effectively contact entire lumen	20 min	10 min
Wrapped instruments—additional time required for steam penetration to occur (Atkinson, 1992, p. 136)	30 min	not recommended

Section Questions

Q13. Items that can tolerate moisture and high temperatures are generally sterilized using (Ref. 22, 23):

____

Q14. Dry heat sterilization is the most common sterilization technology used for sterilization within hospitals. (Ref. 25)

True False

Q15. Powders and oils may be sterilized using (Ref 25):

a. steam sterilization
b. dry heat
c. ethylene oxide
d. dry heat and a combination of ethylene oxide

Q16. List five factors that should be considered when selecting the sterilization process to be used. (Ref. 21)

____

____

____

____

____

Q17. A steam sterilizer is referred to as a(n) (Ref. 27)

____

Q18. Common sterilization technologies employed in the health care facility setting include (Ref. 22, 23, 24, 25, 26):

a. steam
b. dry heat
c. ionizing radiation
d. ethylene oxide
e. ozone
f. peracetic acid
g. gas plasma

Q19. Steam at atmospheric pressure can achieve sterilization if exposure time is greatly increased. (Ref. 31)

True False

Q20. The minimum accepted temperature at which steam sterilization may be accomplished is ______°F (______°C). (Ref. 33)

Q21. Steam sterilization is a function of both time and temperature. (Ref. 34)

True False

Q22. Explain why improper preparation of items or placement within the autoclave can prevent sterilization. (Ref. 36, 41)

____

____

Q23. List four advantages of steam sterilization. (Ref. 35)

____

____

____

____

Q24. Actual sterilization in an autoclave begins as soon as the door is closed and the button to begin the cycle is pressed. (Ref. 40)

True False

Q25. Packages removed from the autoclave following sterilization should be immediately placed on a cool surface to reduce the temperature of the items within the package. (Ref. 44, 45)

True False

Q26. Sterilization in a gravity displacement autoclave may be accomplished at a temperature of 250°F (121°C) or 270°F (132°C). (Ref. 50)

True False

Q27. Wrapped items require a _____ exposure time than unwrapped items in a gravity displacement sterilizer. (Ref. 51)
a. longer
b. shorter

Prevacuum

53. The prevacuum autoclave is equipped with a pump that evacuates almost all air from the chamber prior to the injection of steam. The evacuation process takes approximately 8 to 10 minutes and essentially creates a vacuum within the chamber.
54. When the steam enters the chamber, the force of the vacuum causes instant steam contact with all surfaces of the contents. Steam will penetrate almost instantly to every surface without regard to the size of the package or load.
55. Following the prevacuum phase, an exposure time of 3 to 4 minutes at 270°F to 275°F (132°C to 135°C) is the usual recommended time and temperature for accomplishing sterilization (Association for the Advancement of Medical Instrumentation [AAMI], 1994, p. 14).
56. The advantages of a prevacuum sterilization cycle are:
    - Incorrect placement of objects within the chamber will not interfere with air removal.
    - The entire load will heat rapidly and more uniformly than with a gravity displacement autoclave; therefore the exposure time is shorter.
    - The autoclave may be used to a maximum capacity, allowing more supplies to be sterilized within a given time.
57. The disadvantage of a prevacuum sterilizer is that in the event of a leak, such as in the door seal, an air pocket can form and inhibit sterilization.

Bowie-Dick Test.

58. To test whether air is effectively being eliminated from the chamber, prevacuum autoclaves are tested daily with a Bowie-Dick test. A Bowie-Dick test verifies that

air removal is sufficient to achieve steam penetration of a standard load. The Association for the Advancement of Medical Instrumentation recommends this test be performed daily before the first processed load (1994, p. 22).

59. A commercially prepared sheet of paper with various patterns of heat-sensitive ink is used to perform a Bowie-Dick test. The sheet is placed in a specially constructed pack of towels and subjected to sterilization in an otherwise empty autoclave. A uniform color change indicates successful creation of a vacuum.
60. A Daily Air Removal test is another test that may be performed to test for air removal (see Figure 3–4).

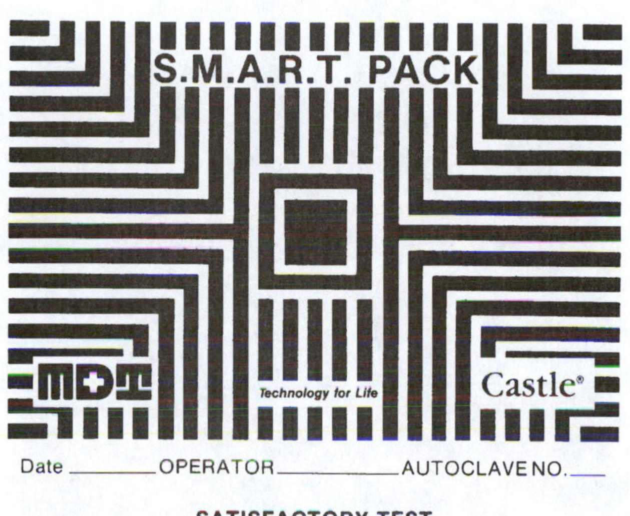

Figure 3–4 Air Removal Test. *Source:* Courtesy of MDT Biologic Company, Rochester, New York.

Pressure-Pulse

61. Instead of a vacuum to remove air from the chamber, a repeated sequence of steam-flush and pressure-pulses above atmospheric pressure are utilized. Because a vacuum is not drawn, a Bowie-Dick test or Daily Air Removal test is not required.
62. A variety of cycle times can be selected based on the nature of the items to be sterilized.
63. The advantage to a pressure-pulse sterilizer is that sterilization is not affected in the event of an air leak into the sterilization chamber.

Flash Sterilization

64. Flash sterilization is a process designed for steam sterilization of a patient care item that is needed immediately and for which there is no replacement immediately available. Items that are flash sterilized are generally unwrapped. Flash sterilization is utilized when there is insufficient time to process an item in the prepackaged method. Flash sterilization should be reserved for instances when an item is needed immediately, for example when an item is dropped during surgery and that item is necessary to complete the surgery.
65. Flash sterilization should not be used for routine sterilization of instruments and should *not* be used to sterilize implants (Association of Operating Room Nurses [AORN], 1995, p. 269).
66. In flash sterilization items are not wrapped and are placed in an open mesh pan that will allow sufficient steam contact. Because there is little or no drying time in the flash cycle the item is wet after processing.
67. Because of immediate need, items prepared for flash sterilization are often cleaned and prepared under less-than-ideal conditions. Items that are not clean may not be rendered sterile.
68. A disadvantage of flash sterilization is that following sterilization, transfer of the item from the autoclave to the sterile field is difficult because of the lack of protective packaging. Special containers designed for use during a flash cycle reduce the risk of recontamination during transfer from the autoclave to the sterile field.
69. Flash sterilization is most often accomplished in a gravity displacement autoclave; however, prevacuum sterilizers are also utilized.
70. Table 3–2 is an example of acceptable time and temperature variation according to items for a flash-cycle sterilization.
71. Exposure times can vary by more than 30 minutes and are determined by factors such as the nature and configuration of the item, the type of sterilizer, and whether

a flash container was utilized. For this reason it is critical that sterilizer, container, and item manufacturer guidelines be followed.

Table 3–2 Time and Temperature for Flash Sterilization

Gravity Displacement Sterilizer	
All metal (nonporous)	3 min at 270°F (132°C)
Porous or metal plus porous items or items with lumen	10 min at 270°F (132°C)
Prevacuum Sterilizer	
All metal (nonporous)	3 min at 270°F (132°C)
Porous and nonporous combined (AAMI, 1992, p. 7)	4 min at 270°F (132°C)

Section Questions

Q28. Explain how the addition of a prevacuum or air removal period prior to sterilization shortens the sterilization cycle. (Ref. 56)

____

____

Q29. Explain the purpose of a Bowie-Dick test. (Ref. 58)

____

____

Q30. The disadvantage to a pressure-pulse sterilizer is that in the event of an air leak into the sterilization chamber, sterilization will be adversely affected. (Ref. 63)

True False

Q31. Describe the most appropriate use of flash sterilization. (Ref. 64)

____

____

Q32. Describe one disadvantage to flash sterilization that increases the risk of contamination of a sterilized item. (Ref. 68)

____

____

Q33. Exposure times in all steam sterilizers should (Ref. 71):

a. be identical for all sterilizers
b. be identical for all items
c. be determined by the type of sterilizer
d. be determined by the item being sterilized
e. be determined according to manufacturer guidelines
f. be determined by the skill of the sterilizer operator

Validation of Steam Sterilization Parameters

72. Before an article can be considered as having been sterilized, certain parameters of time, humidity, pressure, and temperature must have been met. Chemical and mechanical process indicators and biological testing are used to monitor these parameters. Indicators must be checked by the person removing the item from the autoclave.

Mechanical Process Indicators

73. Mechanical indicators are graphs, thermometers, printouts, and gauges that record activities within the chamber during the sterilization cycle.
74. A temperature graph indicates the temperature achieved within the chamber and the length of time that temperature was sustained (see Figure 3–5). A temperature graph also provides information about the time of day

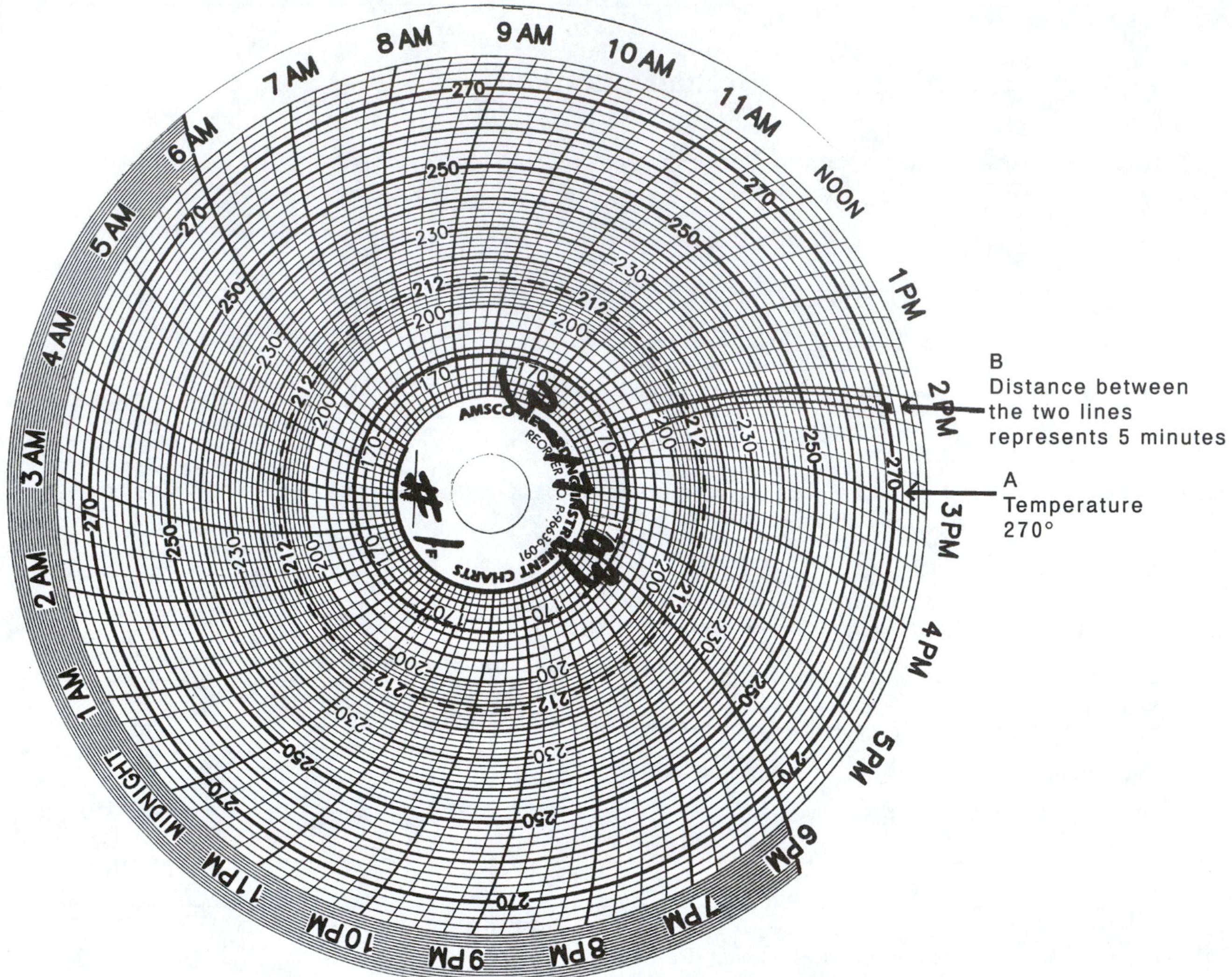

Figure 3–5 Autoclave Graph. The graph is affixed to a 24-hour clock device on the autoclave. The clock device and graph make one complete circle turn in 24 hours. Whenever the sterilization cycle is initiated a marking pen records the temperature achieved (A). The amount of time the temperature remained elevated is calculated by how far the graph turns before the temperature drops during the exhaust phase (B). On the above graph the sterilization cycle was initiated one time at 2:00 PM. The temperature reached slightly above 270°F and the exposure time was 5 minutes long. Note that the date and a number indicating to which autoclave the graph is attached have been written on the graph. *Source:* Courtesy of AMSCO International, Inc. Markings made by author.

that the autoclave was used and the number of cycles run during a 24-hour period. Modern sterilizers employ a printout rather than a temperature graph (see Figure 3–6).

75. A printout record correlates the exact times and temperatures achieved during the conditioning, exposure, and exhaust phases of the sterilization cycle. There are spaces on the printout to enter the items included in the load and to identify the operator.

76. Gauges on the autoclave may register pressure and temperature within the jacket and the chamber.

Chemical Process Indicators

77. Chemical indicators are impregnated with a dye or chemical that develops a visual change when certain conditions have been achieved. Indicators are manufactured as tapes, strips, or labels (see Figure 3–7).

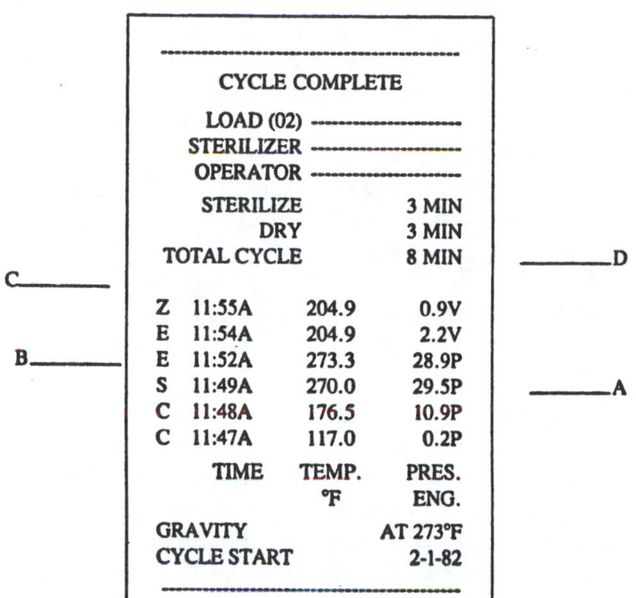

A. At 11:49 AM pressure reached 29.5 pounds per square inch (psi), temperature reached 270.0°F, exposure time began.

B. At 11:52 AM exposure time completed, steam exhausted, and drying time began.

C. At 11:55 AM cycle completed.

D. Sterilization exposure time—3 minutes
Drying time—3 minutes
Total cycle time—8 minutes
Two minutes was necessary for pressure to reach 29.5 psi and temperature to reach 270.0°F.

Figure 3–6 Printout from Gravity Displacement Autoclave. Reading is from bottom to top. *Source:* Courtesy of AMSCO International, Inc.

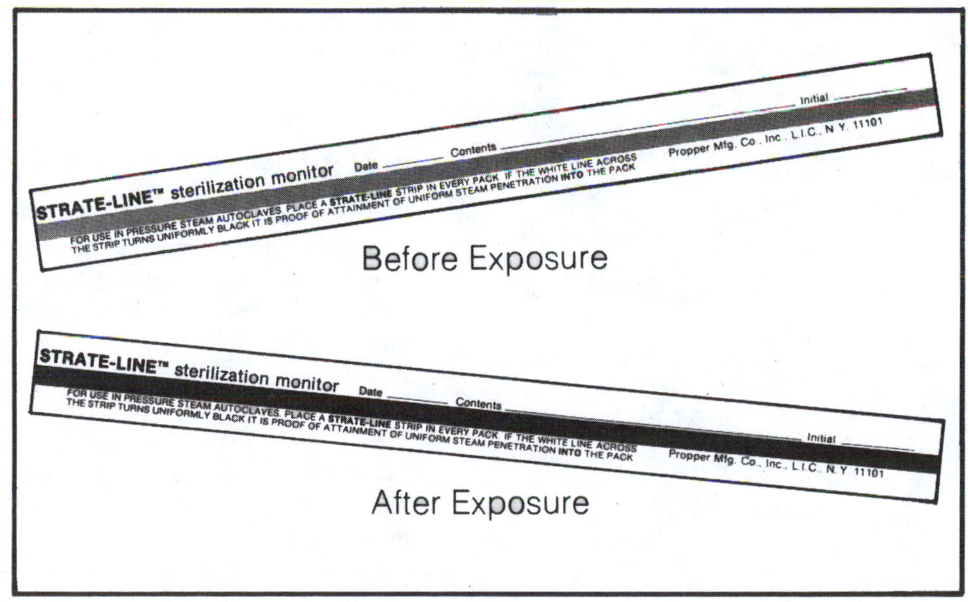

Figure 3–7 Chemical Indicator for Steam Sterilizers. Line turns black upon exposure to steam at 250°F. *Source:* Courtesy of Propper Manufacturing Co., Long Island City, New York.

78. Chemical indicators referred to as integrators provide results that are based on the integration of some or all of the parameters that need to be met.
79. Chemical indicators should be placed inside and outside of all packages. Inspection of these indicators is necessary to show that items have been exposed to one or more of the conditions of the sterilization process.
80. Chemical indicators do not establish sterility. They are tools to determine whether conditions of processing have occurred.

Biological Monitors

81. Biological monitoring is a process used to determine the efficacy of sterilizers. It is the most accurate method of ensuring that the conditions necessary for sterilization have been achieved (see Figure 3–8).

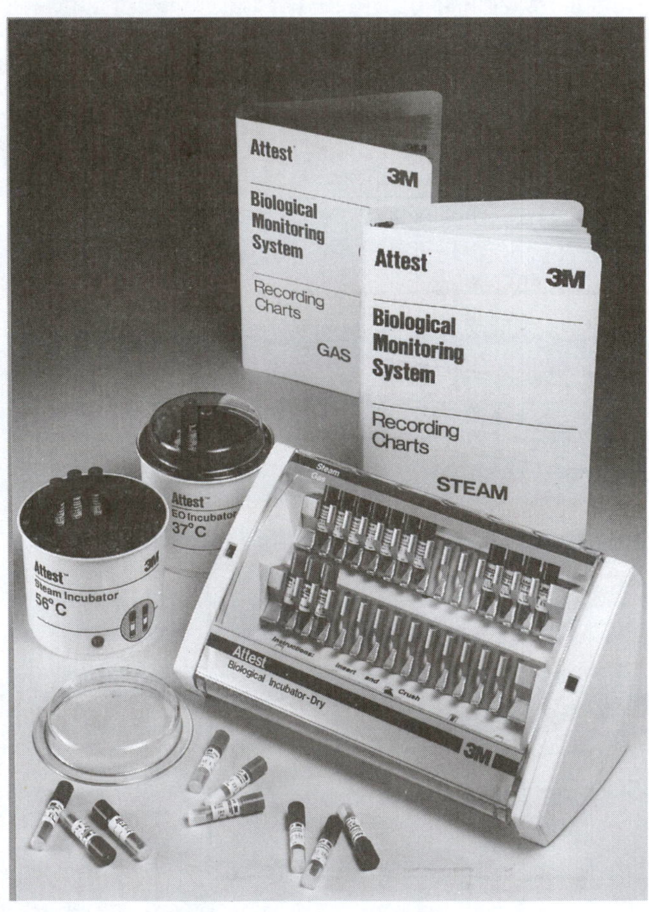

Figure 3–8 Biological Monitor-Capsule Containing a Known Population of Spores. *Source:* Courtesy of 3M Health Care, St. Paul, Minnesota.

82. Strips, ampules, and capsules that contain a known, living, and highly resistant spore population are commercially available for biological monitoring purposes.
83. *Bacillus stearothermophilus* spores are used to test steam autoclaves. *Bacillus stearothermophilus* is a highly resistant microorganism that is nonpathogenic.
84. To test the autoclave, one or two strips, ampules, or capsules containing the spores are placed at a specific location within the chamber or in a special test pack of textiles within the sterilizer according to the manufacturer's instructions, and the autoclave is activated.
85. Incubation of the spores follows completion of the sterilization cycle. Length of incubation varies according to the packaging of the spore product. Incubation times can vary from 1 hour to 48 hours or more.
86. A positive (for growth) reading indicates that sterilizing conditions have not been met and requires that the sterilizer be taken out of service until the problem is corrected and a negative reading is obtained.
87. A positive reading can indicate incorrect packaging of supplies, incorrect placement of items in the autoclave, or that the autoclave is malfunctioning.
88. It is recommended that biological testing of steam autoclaves be conducted daily; with every load of implantables; when evaluating sterilization of new items; and after sterilizer installation, major repair, or relocation (AAMI, 1994, p. 20).
89. Implants should not be implanted until results of biological monitoring are known and are negative for growth.

Chemical Sterilization—Ethylene Oxide Gas (EO)

90. Ethylene oxide is a toxic gas used to sterilize items that cannot tolerate the temperature and moisture of steam sterilization. Ethylene oxide achieves sterilization by interfering with protein metabolism and reproduction of the cell.
91. A wide variety of surgical items cannot withstand moist heat without incurring damage and may be sterilized with ethylene oxide gas. Among the most commonly gas-sterilized items are flexible and rigid endoscopes, plastic goods, electrical instruments, and delicate instruments.
92. The essential parameters of gas sterilization include gas concentration, temperature, humidity, and exposure time.
93. Gas concentration varies with the size of the chamber, the temperature and humidity within the chamber, and the type of gas sterilizer used. Gas sterilizers operate at

temperatures between 85°F (29°C) and 145°F (63°C). Optimum humidity levels are between 30% and 60%. Exposure times generally range from 3 to 7 hours. The sterilizer manufacturer and the item manufacturer recommendations must be followed carefully.

94. Ethylene oxide can be used in 100% concentration. However, because EO is flammable and explosive, it is often mixed with inert gases such as hydrochlorofluorocarbons (HCFC) or carbon dioxide. The use of either 100% EO or a mixture is determined by the sterilizer design.
95. For sterilizers that utilize 100% EO, the gas is supplied in small unit-dose cartridges.
96. In the EO sterilization cycle the air is evacuated from the chamber and its contents, the load is preheated, and humidity is introduced. This phase is termed the preconditioning phase. EO is then released into the chamber where it permeates and penetrates the load. EO sterilization operates under negative pressure. The advantage to this is that if a leak occurs, the EO will be drawn into the chamber rather than to the outside work environment.

Advantages

97. Advantages of EO sterilization are as follows:
    - EO is effective against all types of microorganisms
    - EO does not require high heat
    - EO is noncorrosive
    - EO effectively penetrates large bundles, and permeates all porous items

Disadvantages

98. Ethylene oxide is a toxic gas and the gas sterilization process can be complex and potentially hazardous. Because of the toxic and hazardous nature of ethylene oxide sterilization, items that can tolerate steam sterilization should not be gas sterilized.
99. Other disadvantages are as follows:
    - The sterilization cycle time is lengthy.
    - EO is highly flammable and EO cylinders and cartridges must be carefully handled and stored.
    - The diluent HCFCs used in EO sterilization are subject to strict local, state, and federal regulations and are being phased out because they deplete the ozone layer in the atmosphere.
    - EO sterilization is more expensive than steam sterilization.
    - Toxic byproducts can form under certain conditions. For example, ethylene oxide combined with water yields the toxic byproduct ethylene glycol.
    - Because a variety of materials can absorb EO during the sterilization process, residual EO must be removed from the load contents through an aeration or detoxification process following sterilization. Aeration times in a mechanical aerator may be as short as 8 hours or longer than 24 hours. Length of aeration time is dependent upon the item, packaging, type of sterilization and aeration system, and temperature in the aeration chamber. Items made from materials such as polyvinylchloride require the most lengthy period of aeration.
    - EO is regarded as a human carcinogen by the Occupational Safety and Health Administration (OSHA). It is also recognized as having the potential to cause adverse reproductive effects in humans. In areas where EO is utilized a sign must be posted that reads, "Danger: ethylene oxide, cancer hazard and reproductive hazard. Authorized personnel only. Respirators and protective clothing may be required to be worn in this area."
    - Exposure to EO can cause eye irritation, nausea, dizziness, vomiting, nasal and throat irritation, shortness of breath, tissue burns, and hemolysis.
    - Personnel working with EO must be provided personal protective equipment and instruction in the hazards associated with EO.
    - Concentrations of EO must be identified in the areas where EO sterilization occurs. Monitoring devices that produce an alarm in the event of EO exposure must be in place.
    - The OSHA standard for exposure to EO limits personnel to one part EO per million parts of air averaged over an 8-hour period. OSHA requires a monitoring program to ensure compliance with this standard. Monitors that detect the amount of EO in the work area must be worn periodically by employees to detect EO levels of exposure.
    - EO gas must be vented to the outside to avoid personnel exposure. In addition, some states have abatement requirements that add to the cost. Abators convert waste ethylene oxide into nontoxic gases that are then vented to the outside.
100. Biological monitoring of EO sterilizers is accomplished with the spore *Bacillus subtilis*.
101. It is recommended that EO sterilizers be monitored with each load (AORN, 1995, p. 274).

Chemical Sterilization—Liquid Peracetic Acid

102. Peracetic acid solution contains acetic acid and hydrogen peroxide. Peracetic acid is acetic acid plus an extra oxygen atom. Peracetic acid disrupts protein bands and

cell systems. The extra oxygen inactivates cell systems and causes immediate cell death (Crow, 1993, p. 691).

103. Peracetic acid sterilization may be used for immersible items. It is used primarily for rigid and flexible endoscopes and their accessories. Peracetic acid offers an alternative to gas sterilization.
104. Peracetic acid sterilizers are table-top units. The items to be sterilized are placed within a sterilizer tray and the container is placed into the sterilizer (see Figure 3–9). The sterilant circulates through the tray contacting all surfaces of the items. Items with internal lumens are connected to irrigator adapters to ensure sterilant contact within the lumens.
105. For sterilization to occur, contact time is standardized at 12 minutes at a temperature of 50°C to 55°C. A rinse period follows the contact period. Rinse time depends upon the water temperature and fill time. An entire cycle takes less than 30 minutes.
106. Following sterilization, the circulating nurse lifts the sterilizer tray lid and the sterile scrub person removes the items, which are wet, from the tray and places them on the sterile field. Items that are not delivered to the sterile field are hand dried and stored for later use. Stored items are not considered sterile.

Advantages

107. Advantages of peracetic acid are as follows:
    - The sterilization cycle is less than 30 minutes and offers quick turnaround time.
    - Peracetic acid is combined with anticorrosive and buffering agents that render the sterilant nontoxic to personnel and the environment and noncorrosive to instruments
    - Peracetic acid sterilant is compatible with many materials that cannot withstand steam sterilization.

Disadvantages

108. Disadvantages of peracetic acid sterilization are as follows:
    - The size of the sterilization container does not permit large loads to be sterilized. Only one flexible scope can be processed at a time.
    - Only immersible items fitting into the sterilizer tray may be processed.
    - The items must be used immediately. The nature of the process permits point-of-use sterilization but not sterile storage.
    - As with all sterilizers, there is no method within the health care facility to test whether sterilization occurs within the channels of scopes.
109. Biological monitoring of peracetic acid sterilization is accomplished with a spore strip inoculated with *Bacillus stearothermophilus*. This may be performed daily and should be performed in accordance with manufacturers' recommendations.
110. A diagnostic cycle in which electricity supply, filters, temperature, pressure, and system integrity is checked is run at the beginning of each day.

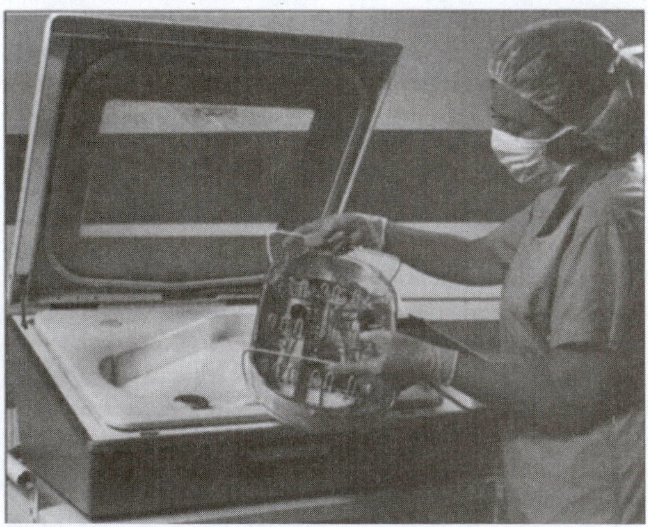

Figure 3–9 Steris Sterilization System. Liquid peracetic acid sterilization. *Source:* Courtesy of STERIS Company, Mentor, Ohio.

Low Temperature Hydrogen Peroxide Gas Plasma Sterilization

111. Plasma is a state of matter that is produced through the action of a strong electric or magnetic field. In low temperature hydrogen peroxide plasma sterilization a plasma state is created by the action of radio-frequency energy upon hydrogen peroxide vapor within a vacuum (see Figure 3–10).
112. Items to be sterilized are placed in a sterilizing chamber, a vacuum is established, and liquid hydrogen peroxide is injected into a cap and enters the chamber in a vaporized or gas form. The hydrogen peroxide gas is charged with radio-frequency or microwave energy that creates a plasma. In the plasma state the hydrogen peroxide is broken apart into reactive species that react with cell membranes, enzymes, or nucleic acids and disrupt the life functions of microorganisms. At the end of the cycle the reactive species recombine to form oxygen and water vapor. The water vapor is in the form of humidity and cannot be felt. Packages are dry at the end of the cycle and may be used immediately or stored for future use.

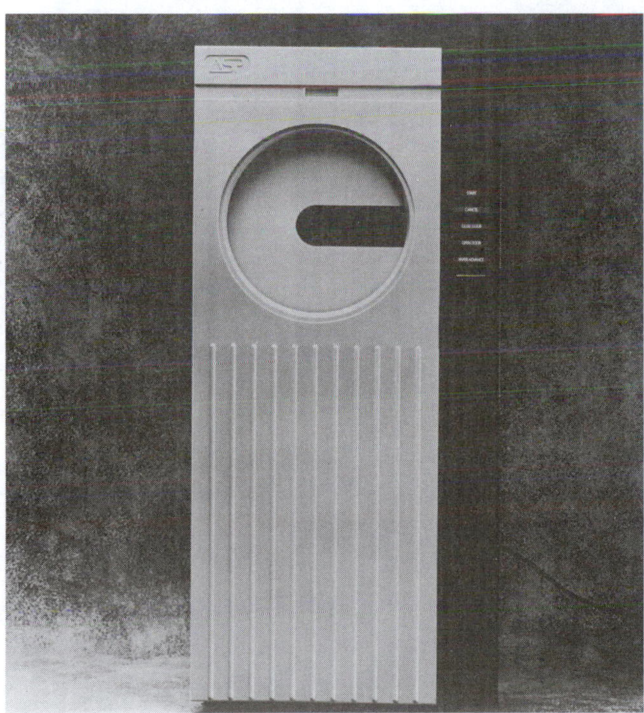

Figure 3–10 STERRAD Hydrogen Peroxide Gas Plasma Sterilizer. *Source:* Courtesy of Advanced Sterilization Products, Irvine, California.

Advantages

113. Advantages of low temperature hydrogen peroxide gas plasma sterilization are as follows:
    - Gas plasma offers a safe alternative to EO sterilization; no toxic chemicals are used and no aeration is required.
    - Because there are no toxic byproducts, personal protective equipment or monitoring of the environment or employees is not required.
    - The sterilization cycle is relatively short (approximately 74 minutes or less).
    - The sterilant is compatible with most metals and plastics.
    - The sterilizer is simple to operate and connects to standard electrical outlets.
    - Cycle time and temperature do not require adjustments to be compatible with various items.

Disadvantages

114. Disadvantages of low temperature hydrogen peroxide gas plasma sterilization are as follows:
    - Gas plasma may not be used with powders, liquids, textiles, and other cellulose-containing items like linen and paper.
    - Packaging materials are limited to nonwoven polypropylene wraps and specialized trays.
    - Lumen restrictions may require reconfiguration of some instrument sets.
115. Biological monitoring of the sterilization process is accomplished with *Bacillus subtilis niger*. Frequency of monitoring should be in accordance with hospital policy.

Mixed Chemical Plasma

116. The mixed chemical plasma sterilization process utilizes a combination of hydrogen peroxide and peracetic acid. A vacuum is drawn and the load is subjected to alternating cycles of peracetic acid and a gas mixture of argon, oxygen, and hydrogen.
117. Biological monitoring of the sterilization process is accomplished with *Bacillus circulans*.

Advantages

118. Advantages to mixed chemical plasma are as follows:
    - Mixed chemical plasma offers a significantly safer alternative to EO sterilization.
    - The cycle time is reduced to 4 hours or less depending on the nature of the load.

Disadvantages

119. Disadvantages to mixed chemical plasma are as follows:
    - A 4 hour-cycle time limits number of cycles that can be run in a day.
    - Use of peracetic acid requires an aeration period.
    - Peracetic acid is a hazardous material and there are safety requirements for changing the bottles of peracetic acid.
    - Items on which it may be utilized are limited.

Section Questions

Q34. Select the correct answer(s) (Ref. 75, 79, 80):
- a. Chemical indicators should be placed on the outside of every package to be sterilized.
- b. Indicator tapes that change color when steam causes a chemical reaction to occur are a guarantee of sterility.
- c. A printout record of the sterilization process displays the exact times and temperatures achieved during conditioning exposure and exhaust times.

Q35. Biological monitoring of steam sterilizers (Ref. 88):
- a. ensures that the autoclave is achieving conditions necessary for sterilization
- b. is accomplished with a known population of spores
- c. should be conducted weekly
- d. should be conducted after major repairs to the sterilizer
- e. should be conducted with every load of implantables

Q36. Explain when ethylene oxide sterilization is appropriate. (Ref. 90, 91)

____

____

Q37. Ethylene oxide sterilizers vary and may employ ethylene oxide (Ref. 94):
- a. in a 100% concentration
- b. mixed with hydrochlorofluorocarbons
- c. mixed with carbon dioxide
- d. mixed with sulfuric acid

Q38. List three advantages of ethylene oxide. (Ref. 97)

____

____

____

Q39. Ethylene oxide is a known carcinogen. List six other disadvantages of ethylene oxide. (Ref. 99)

____

____

____

____

____

____

Q40. What is *Bacillus subtilis* and what is it used for? (Ref. 100)

____

____

Q41. Ethylene oxide sterilizers should be monitored (Ref. 101):
   a. with each load
   b. daily
   c. weekly

Q42. Liquid peracetic acid sterilization (Ref. 103, 105, 106, 108):
   a. is appropriate for flexible endoscopes
   b. results in an unwrapped wet item
   c. results in a wrapped dry item
   d. can only be used for items that are immersible
   e. takes approximately 1½ hours
   f. permits sterile storage of processed items

Q43. Hydrogen peroxide gas plasma is capable of achieving sterilization. (Ref. 112)

True False

Q44. Advantages to hydrogen peroxide gas plasma sterilization include (Ref. 113):
   a. minimal aeration time
   b. relatively short cycle time
   c. monitoring employee exposure to hydrogen peroxide is not required for personnel who operate the sterilizer
   d. no aeration required

Q45. Biological monitoring of hydrogen peroxide plasma sterilization is accomplished with the spore (Ref. 115)

____

Emerging Sterilization Technologies

120. Vapor phase hydrogen peroxide and ozone sterilization are two emerging technologies that offer an alternative to EO sterilization. Vapor phase hydrogen peroxide sterilization is similar to gas plasma technology. Ozone is not widely used and can be highly corrosive to most metals and rubber.

RECORD KEEPING

121. The following records should be filed and kept as a permanent record:
   - results of Bowie-Dick/air evacuation test
   - autoclave graphs and recording charts containing time and temperature and initialed by the operator for verification of cycle parameters
   - results of chemical and biological monitoring
   - records indicating load contents and load control numbers used to designate which sterilizer was used for which items
   - implantable biologic test results
   - sterilizer failure results

DISINFECTION

Overview

122. Disinfection is a process that destroys pathogenic microorganisms through the use of a disinfectant. A disinfectant is an agent that destroys vegetative forms of harmful microorganisms. Disinfectants do not usually kill highly resistant spores.
123. Chemicals used to destroy microorganisms on inanimate objects are identified as disinfectants. Chemicals used to destroy microorganisms on body surfaces are identified as antiseptics.

Levels of Disinfectants—Application

124. Disinfection is used to destroy pathogens on inanimate objects such as walls, tables, small equipment, and instruments. Liquid chemicals are used for disinfection. Disinfectants must be selected according to their intended use. Disinfectants suitable for housekeeping purposes, such as for walls and tables, are not suitable

for disinfection of surgical instruments. Likewise, the most appropriate disinfecting agent for surgical instruments is not the most suitable for housekeeping.

125. Examples of disinfectants include alcohol, chlorine and chlorine compounds, formaldehyde, glutaraldehyde, hydrogen peroxide, iodophors, phenolics, and quaternary ammonium compounds. Disinfectants vary in their ability to destroy microorganisms and they are not interchangeable.
126. Factors that influence the efficacy of a disinfectant include the chemical used, concentration and temperature of the chemical, amount and type of microorganisms present, prior cleaning, configuration of the item to be disinfected, and exposure time.
127. Disinfectants are categorized as high level, intermediate level, and low level.
128. High-level disinfectants kill all microorganisms including vegetative bacteria forms, the tubercle bacilli, fungi, HIV and hepatitis B viruses.
129. Glutaraldehyde, sodium hypochlorite, and hydrogen peroxide are high-level disinfectants.
130. Intermediate disinfectants inactivate the tubercle bacillus and most vegetative bacteria, fungi, and viruses. Low-level disinfectants kill most vegetative bacteria, some fungi, and some viruses. They do not kill the tubercle bacilli.
131. Semicritical items, such as cystoscopes, bronchoscopes, thermometers, and endotracheal tubes, that make direct contact with intact mucous membranes but are not introduced below the skin must be high-level disinfected. (They may also be sterilized.) Most frequently used high-level disinfectants are 2% to 3.2% solutions of alkaline glutaraldehyde.

Glutaraldehyde

132. Glutaraldehyde is a high-level disinfectant that is also capable of sterilization. Because of the lengthy immersion period required for sterilization, glutaraldehyde is rarely used as a sterilizing agent. A 2% solution of glutaraldehyde requires an immersion period of 10 hours for sterilization to be achieved.
133. Glutaraldehyde is irritating to mucous membranes and can irritate skin, eyes, throat, and nasal passages. It should be mixed in a well-ventilated room and stored in a closed container. Protective eye wear, a double set of latex gloves or nitrile gloves, masks, and repellent gowns should be worn when using glutaraldehyde. Exposure varies with the activity. Mixing and discarding the solution and immersing and retrieving items from the solution are activities that pose the greatest risk of exposure.
134. Items disinfected in glutaraldehyde must be thoroughly rinsed prior to use.
135. The current OSHA limits for exposure are 0.2 parts of glutaraldehyde to 1 million parts of air during any part of the work day. Monitoring of the work area and employee exposure is not required by OSHA. Monitoring should be employed when high levels of exposure are suspected.
136. Glutaraldehyde and other disinfectants must be mixed and used according to manufacturer guidelines and standards of practice. Information concerning mixing instructions, use, immersion time (varies from 20 to 45 minutes), toxicity, and length of effectiveness can be found on the package.
137. The strength of the solution should be routinely monitored with indicators designed for this purpose.
138. Date of mixing and length of effectiveness should be indicated on the container in which it is stored. Chemical properties and appropriate hazard warnings should also be indicated.
139. To avoid dilution of the disinfectant and compromise of the disinfection process, all items to be disinfected should be thoroughly cleaned, rinsed, and dried prior to immersion.

Section Questions

Q46. If a sterilizer malfunctions and requires repair it should be biologically monitored before it is put back into service. The results of this monitoring should be kept as a permanent record. (Ref. 121)

True False

Q47. Antiseptics are used on (Ref. 123):
a. inanimate surfaces
b. body surfaces

Q48. The high-level disinfectant, glutaraldehyde, is appropriate for use on (Ref. 124, 131, 132):
a. table tops
b. surgical instruments
c. floors

Q49. All disinfectants can be used for sterilization purposes provided immersion time is sufficient. (Ref. 122, 132)

True False

Q50. Only items that have been thoroughly cleaned, rinsed, and dried should be placed in a disinfectant. (Ref. 139)

True False

NOTES

Advanced Sterilization Products. (1995). *Customer education manual.* Irvine, CA: Author.

Association for the Advancement of Medical Instrumentation. (1992). *Good hospital practice: Flash sterilization—steam sterilization of patient care items for immediate use.* Arlington, VA: Author.

Association for the Advancement of Medical Instrumentation. (1994). *Good hospital practice: Steam sterilization and sterility assurance.* Arlington, VA: Author.

Association of Operating Room Nurses (AORN). (1995). *Standards and recommended practices.* Denver, CO: AORN.

Atkinson, L. (1992). *Berry & Kohn's operating room technique.* St. Louis: Mosby Year Book.

Crow, S. (1993). Sterilization processes: Meeting the demands of today's health care technology. *Nursing Clinics of North America, 28*(3), 687–694.

Perkins, J.J. (1969). *Principles and methods of sterilization.* Springfield, IL: Charles C Thomas.

U.S. Department of Health and Human Services, Centers for Disease Control. (1991). Nosocomial infection and pseudoinfection from contaminated endoscopes and bronchoscopes—Wisconsin and Missouri. *Morbidity and Mortality Weekly Report (MMWR), 40.*

ADDITIONAL READING

Atkinson, L.J. (1992). Sterilization and disinfection. In *Berry & Kohn's Operating Room Technique* (7th ed.). St. Louis: Mosby Year Book.

Lind, N. (1995). Flash sterilization. *Infection Control and Sterilization Technology, 1*(9), 52–53

Lind, N. (1995). High level disinfection. *Infection Control and Sterilization Technology, 1*(8), 46–48.

Reichert, M., & Young, J. (1993). *Sterilization technology for the health care facility.* Gaithersburg, MD: Aspen Publishers, Inc.

Springthorpe, S., & Satter, S. (1995). Understanding chemical disinfection. *Infection Control and Sterilization Technology, 1*(3), 10–20.

Spry, C. (1995). Focus on quality. *Surgical Services Management, 1*(2), 56–59.

Appendix 3–A

Chapter 3 Post Test

Instructions: Fill in the blank(s), mark the correct answer(s), or answer the question as appropriate.

1. Equipment contaminated with pathogenic microorganisms is known to be a source of nosocomial infection. (Ref. 3, 6)

   True False

2. What is the desired outcome for the patient scheduled for an invasive procedure with a nursing diagnosis of high risk for infection? (Ref. 5)

   ____

   ____

3. Sterile means (Ref. 11):
   a. free of all living microorganisms
   b. free of all bacteria
   c. free of all living microorganisms and spores

4. Disinfection means (Ref. 16):
   a. the destruction of all gram-negative bacteria
   b. the destruction of all pathogenic microorganisms except spores
   c. the process used to make skin as clean as possible

5. Semicritical items do not require sterilization. They do require high-level disinfection. Define a semicritical item. (Ref. 19, 20)

   ____

   ____

6. Dry heat sterilization is appropriate for sterilizing (Ref. 25):
   a. linen
   b. powder
   c. rubber items
   d. oils

7. Select the correct answer(s) (Ref. 27, 28, 31):
   a. Steam must be subjected to pressure for it to reach a temperature high enough to accomplish sterilization.
   b. For an item to be rendered sterile, steam must contact every surface of that item.
   c. Steam at a temperature of 212°F (100°C) is sufficient to achieve sterilization.

8. One of the advantages of steam sterilization is that one cycle time is appropriate for all items. (Ref. 35, 36)

   True False

9. If items are improperly prepared or improperly placed within the autoclave air may become trapped and sterilization may fail to occur. Why? (Ref. 36)

   ____

   ____

10. It is appropriate to sterilize a wrapped set of metal instruments for 4 minutes at a temperature of 270°F (132°C) in a prevacuum autoclave. (Ref. 55)

    True False

11. There are four sterilization technologies commonly employed in health care facilities. List three of them. (Ref. 23, 24)

    ____

    ____

    ____

12. Explain why it is inappropriate to place a warm sterilized package on a solid cold surface. (Ref. 44, 45)

    ____

    ____

13. Explain the difference between a gravity displacement autoclave and a prevacuum autoclave. (Ref. 47, 48, 49, 50, 53, 54, 55)

    ____

    ____

    ____

    ____

14. A Bowie-Dick test is a method to biologically monitor prevacuum autoclaves. (Ref. 58, 59)

    True False

15. When a 270°F 3-minute exposure is used on an unwrapped item, it is referred to as a _____ cycle. (Ref. 70)

16. A single unwrapped metal instrument with a lumen requires a cycle time of______ minutes at a temperature of 270°F (132°C) in a gravity displacement sterilizer. (Ref. 70)

17. What information can be obtained from reading an autoclave printout? (Ref. 75)

    ____

    ____

18. Chemical indicators (Ref. 77, 78, 79, 80):
    a. are not a guarantee of sterility
    b. are used to show that parameters of sterilization have been met
    c. should be visible on the outside of every package
    d. include *Bacillus subtilis* and *Bacillus stearothermophilus*

19. Match the technology with the biological monitor. (Ref. 83, 100, 115)

_____ Hydrogen peroxide gas plasma	a. *Bacillus subtilis*
_____ Ethylene oxide	b. *Bacillus stearothermophilus*
_____ Steam	c. *Bacillus subtilis niger*

20. Steam sterilizer monitoring should be conducted (Ref. 88):
    a. weekly
    b. daily
    c. with every load
    d. with every implantable
    e. after major repair

21. Ethylene oxide sterilizers should be biologically monitored (Ref. 101):
    a. weekly
    b. daily
    c. with every load

22. Ethylene oxide sterilization is appropriate for (Ref. 90, 91):
    a. endoscopes
    b. lensed instruments
    c. linen
    d. leather
    e. electrical instruments

23. Ethylene oxide is toxic and exposure can cause vomiting, headache, and irritation of the eyes and respiratory passages. Therefore, all porous items sterilized in ethylene oxide must go through a final aeration process. When a mechanical aerator is used this process requires a minimum of (Ref. 99):
    a. 15 minutes
    b. 1 hour
    c. 8 hours

24. The OSHA standard for exposure to ethylene oxide limits personnel to one part of ethylene oxide to _____ parts of air averaged over an 8-hour time period. (Ref. 99)

25. Peracetic acid sterilization (Ref. 103, 105, 106):
    a. may be used with immersible items only
    b. is used for flexible and rigid endoscopes
    c. results in a wet item that does not permit sterile storage
    d. requires a 1-hour cycle time

26. Hydrogen peroxide gas plasma sterilization (Ref. 113, 114):
    a. leaves no toxic residue and requires no aeration
    b. offers an alternative to ethylene oxide for sterilization of heat- and moisture-sensitive items
    c. is appropriate for linen and paper goods
    d. requires a lengthy cycle time
    e. is biologically monitored with *Bacillus subtilis niger*
    f. results in a dry package at the end of the cycle that can be stored for future use

27. Cycle time in mixed chemical plasma is _____ than in ethylene oxide. (Ref. 118, 119)
    a. shorter
    b. longer

28. Results of biological monitoring, sterilizer failure records, and records indicating load contents and load control numbers that designate which sterilizer was used for which item should be kept as a permanent record. (Ref. 121)

    True False

29. Low-level disinfectants are capable of destroying the tubercle bacillus. (Ref. 130)

    True False

30. Glutaraldehyde is a high-level disinfectant that (Ref. 132, 133, 136):
    a. is suitable for disinfection of cystoscopes
    b. can achieve sterilization in 45 minutes immersion time
    c. is irritating to mucous membranes
    d. requires the user to don protective eye wear, mask, repellent gown, and double latex or nitrile gloves during use

31. Although OSHA does not require monitoring of worker exposure to glutaraldehyde the exposure limits are _____ parts of glutaraldehyde to 1 million parts of air during any part of the work day. (Ref. 135)

32. Items disinfected in glutaraldehyde must be (Ref. 136, 139):
    a. cleaned and rinsed before immersion
    b. dried before immersion
    c. immersed for 1 hour for disinfection to occur
    d. rinsed prior to use

Appendix 3–B

Competency Checklist: Sterilization and Disinfection

Under observer's initials enter initials upon successful achievement of competency. Enter N/A if competency is not appropriate for institution.

NAME ____________________________________

	OBSERVER'S INITIALS	DATE
1. Identifies appropriate method of sterilization for item to be sterilized.	________	________
2. Steam sterilization		
a. sets appropriate cycle	________	________
b. sets appropriate time	________	________
c. sets appropriate temperature	________	________
d. includes chemical process indicator or integrator	________	________
e. selects tray compatible with sterilization method	________	________
f. packages correctly	________	________
g. moistens lumens	________	________
h. loads correctly	________	________
i. operates according to manufacturer's instructions	________	________
j. observes graph/printout/indicator for parameters	________	________
k. (flash) transports without contamination following sterilization	________	________
l. (wrapped) allows package to cool before removing from autoclave	________	________
3. Biological monitor—steam		
a. selects appropriate monitor	________	________
b. documents date, autoclave, and operator	________	________
c. places within chamber correctly	________	________
d. sets appropriate time and temperature	________	________
e. incubates processed biological monitor and control according to manufacturer's instructions	________	________
4. Peracetic acid sterilization		
a. runs diagnostic cycle	________	________
b. loads properly	________	________
c. operates in accordance with manufacturer's instructions	________	________
d. transports without contamination	________	________
e. performs biological monitor according to manufacturer's instructions	________	________

NAME ______________________________

	OBSERVER'S INITIALS	DATE
5. Hydrogen peroxide gas plasma sterilization		
a. includes chemical process indicator	________	________
b. selects tray appropriate for sterilization process	________	________
c. packages correctly	________	________
d. loads correctly	________	________
e. operates sterilizer according to manufacturer's instructions	________	________
6. Biological monitor—hydrogen peroxide gas plasma		
a. selects appropriate monitor	________	________
b. documents date, sterilizer, and operator	________	________
c. places within chamber correctly	________	________
d. incubates processed biological monitor and control according to manufacturer's instructions	________	________
7. Identifies items appropriate for high-level disinfection.	________	________
8. Prepares disinfectant according to manufacturer's instructions.	________	________
9. Wears appropriate personal protective equipment during preparation of disinfectant and use.	________	________
10. Items are:		
a. washed and dried before use	________	________
b. rinsed after use	________	________
c. handled so as to prevent contamination	________	________

OBSERVER'S SIGNATURE INITIALS

______________________________ ________

ORIENTEE'S SIGNATURE

____

CHAPTER 4

Prevention of Infection—Preparation, Packaging, and Storage of Sterile Supplies

Learner Objectives

At the end of Prevention of Infection—Preparation, Packaging, and Storage of Sterile Supplies, the learner will

- discuss the relationship of preparation, packaging, and storage of sterile supplies to patient outcomes of freedom from infection and freedom from injury
- describe the responsibilities of the registered nurse in relation to preparation, packaging, and storage of sterile supplies
- discuss the decontamination process for surgical instruments
- explain the role of ultrasonic cleaning in instrument decontamination
- list six criteria for packaging materials
- describe four principles of packaging
- describe three packaging materials, use, and advantages and disadvantages of each
- define and discuss shelf life

Lesson Outline

I. **NURSING DIAGNOSIS**

II. **DESIRED PATIENT OUTCOMES**

III. **NURSING RESPONSIBILITIES**

IV. **DEFINITIONS**
   - A. Contaminated
   - B. Decontamination

V. **PREPARATION OF ITEMS AND INSTRUMENTS FOR STERILIZATION/ CLEANING**
   - A. Intraoperative Cleaning
   - B. Postoperative Cleaning
   - C. Manual and Mechanical Cleaning
   - D. Ultrasonic Cleaning
   - E. Lubrication
   - F. Inspection

VI. **PRINCIPLES OF PACKAGING—STEAM**
   - A. Instruments
   - B. Other Items
     1. Basins, Bowls, Cups
     2. Rubber Goods, Tubing, Items with a Lumen, Wood
     3. Cloth

VII. **PACKAGING FOR ALTERNATE METHODS OF STERILIZATION**

VIII. **CHEMICAL INDICATORS**

IX. **PACKAGING MATERIALS—BARRIERS**
   - A. Selection Criteria
   - B. Types of Packaging
     1. Woven Fabric
     2. Nonwoven Materials
   - C. Plastic, Paper, Tyvek®
   - D. Rigid Containers
   - E. Sealing

X. **PACKAGE INFORMATION AND IDENTIFICATION**
   - A. Chemical Indicators
   - B. Labels

XI. **SHELF LIFE**
   - A. Storage Considerations
   - B. Determining Factors

Chapter 4

Prevention of Infection—Preparation, Packaging, and Storage of Sterile Supplies

NURSING DIAGNOSIS

1. The nursing diagnoses high risk for infection and high risk for injury are applicable to patients who undergo invasive procedures. Infection may result from contact with contaminated instruments and injury can result when instrumentation fails to function properly.

DESIRED PATIENT OUTCOMES

2. Perioperative nursing activities are directed toward the prevention of infection and injury with the goal that the patient will be free from infection and free from injury following the operation. Many perioperative nursing activities contribute to the achievement of these outcomes. Among these are adequate preparation and proper packaging and storage of sterile supplies, items, and instruments.

NURSING RESPONSIBILITIES

3. The perioperative nurse assumes varying levels of responsibility for preparation, packaging, and storage of sterile supplies. There is no single preparation or packaging process that is appropriate for all supplies. The processes involved require judgment based on a solid knowledge of principles of preparation, packaging, and storage of sterile supplies.
4. Although the perioperative nurse may not provide a hands-on contribution to these processes, the nurse must be a resource for those who do. More importantly, the perioperative nurse must be able to identify that specified requirements of preparation, packaging, and storage of supplies or instruments has occurred. The perioperative nurse makes the final decision as to whether an item is fit to be entered into the sterile field for use on a patient.
5. As an advocate for the patient, with the goals of freedom from infection and freedom from injury, the perioperative nurse must be able to ensure that all supplies, primarily instruments, used in surgery that are intended to be sterile are indeed sterile and are in working order. Desired patient outcomes may not be achieved when improperly prepared supplies harbor microorganisms that can cause infection and when instruments fail to function as intended and have the potential to cause injury.

DEFINITIONS

Contaminated

6. In the operating room environment the term *contaminated* refers to items that are not sterile. Items soiled or infected with microorganisms are considered to be contaminated. Items that were opened for surgery, whether or not they were actually used during surgery, and whether or not they are known to contain microorganisms, are also considered to be contaminated.

Decontamination

7. Contaminated items have the potential to cause or contribute to nosocomial postoperative wound infection. To

achieve freedom from infection and to prevent surgical wound infection, instruments and supplies used in surgery must be free of contamination at the time that they are used. Effective disinfection or sterilization to rid items of contamination are critical factors in the prevention of postoperative wound infection.

8. Effective disinfection and sterilization are dependent on proper decontamination.
9. Decontamination is the process that renders a contaminated item safe for handling. Decontamination includes a cleaning process and a biocidal process.
10. Cleaning may be achieved manually through a mechanical washer and/or through ultrasonic cleaning.
11. The biocidal process is referred to as *terminal disinfection* or sterilization. Terminal disinfection or sterilization is usually achieved in a washer-decontaminator, through a sterilization cycle of a washer-sterilizer, through processing in a steam sterilizer, or through the use of a liquid chemical agent or some other disinfection or sterilization process.
12. Following decontamination, terminally disinfected or sterilized items or instruments are inspected, assembled into sets, arranged within containers or wrapped, and put through a final sterilization process in preparation for storage for future use.

PREPARATION OF ITEMS AND INSTRUMENTS FOR STERILIZATION/CLEANING

Intraoperative Cleaning

13. Contaminated instruments, including all instruments opened and/or used for a surgical procedure, should be washed as soon as possible after use to prevent blood and other debris from drying in crevices or on instrument surfaces. Dried-on debris can interfere with the sterilization process by preventing the sterilizing agent from contacting every surface of every item to be sterilized.
14. During the surgical procedure, instruments and items should be wiped and rinsed with a wet sponge or immersed in sterile water to remove large particles and to prevent debris from lodging in serrations and other crevices. Instrument lumens should be kept free of debris by irrigating the channels. Only sterile water should be used for cleaning items during surgery.

Postoperative Cleaning

15. At the end of surgery, instruments should be covered and transported to a dedicated decontamination area where they are prerinsed by submerging them in an enzymatic detergent solution for a minimum of 2 minutes (Association of Operating Room Nurses [AORN,] 1995a, p. 198). A detergent-germicide should be selected that provides maximal destruction of microorganisms without damage to the instruments that are being cleaned.
16. Powered surgical instruments and some specialty items are cleaned separately according to the manufacturer's written guidelines and generally are not submersed.
17. After soaking, instruments are rinsed in water. Heavily soiled instruments may need additional hand washing or brushing. Hand washing or brushing should be done below the surface of the water to prevent splashing, aerosolation, and the spread of airborne contaminants.
18. Personnel who wash contaminated instruments should be attired in heavy-duty rubber gloves, a waterproof coverup, cap, mask, and protective eye wear. Rubber boots offer further protection (AORN, 1991, p. 144).

Manual and Mechanical Cleaning

19. After soaking and rinsing, instruments are manually or mechanically cleaned. Heat-sensitive instruments are removed and washed and rinsed by hand. Delicate instruments may also be washed by hand.
20. The remainder are disassembled, opened, and placed in trays with a wire open-mesh bottom. Scissors, lighter weight instruments, and microsurgical instruments are placed on top. Heavy retractors and other heavy instruments should be placed in a separate tray (AORN, 1995a, p. 198). Trays are then placed in a washer-sterilizer or washer-decontaminator where mechanical cleaning occurs.
21. Washer-sterilizers and decontaminators employ water and detergent to clean instruments. In a washer-sterilizer, cold water enters the chamber and mixes with detergent. Steam and air are automatically injected into the chamber to generate turbulence and agitation. The water heats, and as the chamber fills, blood and debris are loosened and lifted from the instruments. The water is flushed out through a bottom drain. Steam under pressure then enters the chamber and the items are subjected to a sterilization cycle. Washer-sterilizers have a tendency to bake organic debris onto instruments and for this reason decontamination is usually accomplished in a washer-decontaminator.
22. Washer-decontaminators clean through a pressurized spray action. A cold water prewash is followed by a detergent bath that is delivered under pressure. A rinse cycle is followed by steam, heat, and hot-air drying.

23. Instruments that have been processed through a washer-sterilizer or washer-decontaminator or are hand washed are considered safe to handle but are *not* ready for immediate use and are not considered sterile.

Ultrasonic Cleaning

24. Following initial manual or mechanical washing, instruments should be processed in an ultrasonic cleaner. Ultrasonic cleaning is not microbiocidal and is not a substitute for sterilization or disinfection.
25. The purpose of ultrasonic cleaning is to remove and dislodge tenacious debris. Sound waves generate tiny bubbles that expand until they collapse or implode. Implosion creates a negative pressure on the surfaces of the instruments that dislodges soil that may have remained in hard-to-reach crevices. Ultrasonic cleaning is especially beneficial for items with box locks, serrations, and interstices.
26. Instrument manufacturer guidelines should be followed to determine whether ultrasonic cleaning is compatible with the instrument. When instruments of dissimilar metal are combined in the ultrasonic cleaner, etching and pitting may occur when ion transfer is caused by the cleaning process.

Lubrication

27. Instruments are rinsed after ultrasonic cleaning and those with movable parts should be lubricated with an antimicrobial, water-soluble lubricant that protects against rusting and staining. The lubricant must be water soluble to allow penetration of the sterilizing agent. Oils must not be used because they prevent penetration of the sterilant.

Inspection

28. Instruments are inspected for cleanliness, integrity, and function. Noncritical instruments and items intended to be disinfected immediately prior to use are dried and stored in a clean dry area. Items that do not function as intended are removed. This is a critical requirement. The opportunity to check an instrument for functioning immediately prior to an emergency surgery situation is limited. It is imperative that careful inspection and checking for function occur prior to packaging. The difference between whether an instrument functioned properly or failed in surgery can be the determining factor regarding patient injury.

Section Questions

Q1. The perioperative nurse must have a solid knowledge of principles of preparation, packaging, and storage of sterile supplies because (Ref. 2, 3, 4):
a. the perioperative nurse must be able to identify whether items may be permitted to be placed within the sterile field
b. the perioperative nurse is usually responsible for actual wrapping of supplies in preparation for sterilization
c. infection control measures are dependent upon proper preparation and packaging of supplies

Q2. Sterile items that were opened during a surgical procedure but were not used or handled are considered contaminated. (Ref. 6)

True False

Q3. The decontamination process (Ref. 9, 23):
a. sterilizes instruments in preparation for surgery
b. renders items safe for handling
c. may be accomplished by hand or by machine

Q4. The instrument cleaning process may begin during surgery when instruments that are used are rinsed and wiped. (Ref. 14)

True False

Q5. List four items of protective attire that should be worn by personnel who are responsible for the decontamination of instruments. (Ref. 18)

____

____

____

____

Q6. Not all instruments can be put through a mechanical cleaner such as a washer-decontaminator or washer-sterilizer. Some must be washed by hand. Give an example of a type instrument that must be washed by hand. (Ref. 16, 19)

____

Q7. An ultrasonic cleaner (Ref. 24, 25):
a. cleans by destroying microorganisms
b. may be substituted for a washer-sterilizer
c. removes microorganisms by implosion
d. is used after the washer-sterilizer

Q8. Instruments with movable parts should be lubricated with oil prior to sterilization. (Ref. 27)

True False

PRINCIPLES OF PACKAGING—STEAM

Instruments

29. Critical instruments and items intended for sterilization are placed in trays or containers that are compatible with the intended sterilization process and that will maintain items in a sterile state until the point of use.
30. Instruments and items are arranged in sets and are placed in a tray with a perforated or mesh bottom or other specially designed container that permits the sterilant to penetrate and also prevents air from being trapped. A towel may be placed in the bottom of the tray that is intended for steam sterilization to help absorb condensate that is formed during sterilization and to help speed the drying process.
31. A critical factor in arranging instruments and items is that they are placed so that all surfaces of each item will be exposed to the sterilant.
32. Joints and hinges of instruments must be opened and detachable parts disassembled. Racks, pins, or stringers may be used to assist in arranging instruments and to secure them in an open position.
33. Instruments are not held together with rubber bands. Rubber bands can prevent the sterilizing agent from coming in contact with all surfaces of an item.
34. To prevent damage, heavy instruments are placed on the bottom of the tray, and delicate instruments are placed on top.
35. To facilitate the achievement of necessary temperature and adequate drying, the weight of the instrument set should be determined by the container and the manufacturer's instructions. Instrument sets that are too heavy may concentrate too much metal mass and prevent the achievement of sufficient temperature during steam sterilization processes for sterilization to occur.

Other Items

Basins, Bowls, Cups

36. Basins, bowls, and cups can be nested one inside the other if they are separated by a porous material such as gauze or an absorbent towel. The porous material permits entry of the sterilant, contact of the sterilant with all surfaces, and exit of the sterilant.
37. Nested items should be placed in the same direction. This prevents air pockets, allows circulation of the steam, and permits condensate to drain out.

Rubber Goods, Tubing, Items with a Lumen, Wood Items

38. Rubber sheeting or other impervious material is not folded on itself. It is covered with a porous material, such as gauze, of the same size, loosely rolled, and then wrapped. This allows steam contact with the entire surface of the rubber or other impervious material.
39. Items with a lumen such as ventricular and irrigation needles and rubber catheters must be cleaned and the lumen rinsed with distilled water. During steam sterilization the moisture in the lumen will become steam as the temperature rises, and it will displace the air in the lumen. Sterilization of the lumen can then be achieved.
40. Few items made of wood are used in surgery today; however, they deserve special mention as resin can be forced out of wood during steam sterilization and condense onto other items and cause a tissue reaction when contacted by a mucous membrane. Therefore, wood items should be individually wrapped and not included in sets with other instruments.

Cloth

41. Prior to sterilization, linen must be hydrated by laundering and must be stored at a humidity level of 35% to 75%. Linen that is not laundered or stored under these conditions may be dehydrated and subject to superheating during the steam-sterilization process. Superheating occurs when the temperature of the fabric exceeds the temperature of the surrounding steam. Superheating destroys cloth fibers and causes linen to deteriorate.
42. To facilitate steam penetration, linen items such as drapes and gown packs are fan folded or loosely rolled and alternate layers crossed. Recommended maximum size is 12 × 12 × 20 inches and maximum recommended weight is 12 pounds (Association for the Advancement of Medical Instrumentation [AAMI], 1989, p. 182).
43. Cloth wrappers have a limited life and after repeated use will lose their barrier qualities. For this reason the wrapper should not be utilized beyond its intended life. A tracking or marking system to indicate the number of uses should be in place where reusable wrappers are utilized.

Section Questions

Q9. To prevent loss, instruments must remain assembled and in a closed position during sterilization. (Ref. 32)

True False

Q10. Explain why it is necessary to separate nested items with a porous material. (Ref. 36)

____

____

Q11. Prior to steam sterilization, items with a lumen must have their lumen (Ref. 39):
a. flushed with water
b. blown dry

Q12. When instruments sets are too heavy, sterilization may not occur when processed in steam because (Ref. 35):
a. there may be too many instruments in the set
b. the metal mass may not permit achievement of adequate temperature

Q13. Why must linen be laundered prior to sterilization? (Ref. 41)

____

____

Q14. To facilitate steam penetration, linen packs are limited in size to 12 × 12 × 20 inches and weigh no more than ________ pounds. (Ref. 42)

PACKAGING FOR ALTERNATE METHODS OF STERILIZATION

44. Cleaning and packaging for ethylene oxide (EO) sterilization is the same as for steam sterilization, with some exceptions.
45. Items prepared for gas sterilization must be dry. Ethylene oxide in contact with water forms ethylene glycol. This is a toxic acid residue that can be avoided if items are dry before being EO sterilized. To ensure drying, items with a lumen should be blown dry.
46. Oil-based lubricants must be removed. Ethylene oxide cannot penetrate the film left by these lubricants.
47. For hydrogen peroxide gas plasma, all items must be thoroughly dry. Gauze, linen, or towels may not be included within the load. Polypropylene wrap must be used to wrap sets. Paper and cloth may not be used.

CHEMICAL INDICATORS

48. Chemical or process indicators should be placed in all packages, either in the center or in the area most difficult to sterilize. Regulatory and standard setting agencies differ in their requirement for internal indicators. The Association of Operating Room Nurses recommends only that a monitoring device be used on each package to be sterilized and that when the device is not visible from the outside of the package, a separate process indicator be used on the outside of the package (AORN, 1995a, p. 275).
49. Chemical indicators measure parameters that are necessary for sterilization to occur. For steam sterilization these include time, temperature, and moisture. For EO sterilization these include time, temperature, gas concentration, and relative humidity. The parameters for

hydrogen peroxide gas plasma are concentration, pressure, time, and temperature. All indicators do not measure all parameters.

50. Chemical indicators do not guarantee sterility. They demonstrate only that the items have been exposed to the physical conditions within the chamber that are monitored by the indicator.
51. The perioperative nurse must understand the nature of indicator used and be able to immediately interpret the reading to determine whether or not an item has been subjected to the requirements for sterilization.

PACKAGING MATERIALS—BARRIERS

Selection Criteria

52. Packaging material must be selected that is compatible with the sterilization process and the manufacturer's recommendations. Certain materials are not compatible with every process; however, all materials must meet certain standard criteria as follows. Packaging must
    - cover items completely
    - permit penetration of the sterilant
    - allow for adequate air removal
    - permit removal of the sterilant
    - resist tears and punctures and be capable of maintaining items in a sterile state following the sterilization process
    - be impervious to the penetration of microorganisms, dust, and moisture
    - be visually tamper proof with a secure seal
    - allow for aseptic delivery of contents to the sterile field
    - permit labeling to identify contents
    - permit display of evidence that the items have been subjected to the sterilization process

Types of Packaging

Woven Fabric

53. Muslin was the standard woven reusable wrapping material for many years. Muslin is a reusable cotton suitable for steam and EO sterilization. To prevent the penetration of dust and airborne microorganisms, muslin wrappers with a minimum of 140 threads per square inch and consisting of two double layers (four thicknesses) was used. Although muslin permits entry and exit of the sterilant, it does not provide a tortuous path for microorganisms and does not provide a protective barrier against moisture. For this reason muslin has almost entirely been replaced by cotton and polyester blend fabrics that have been treated to be water repellent.
54. Packages are traditionally wrapped in two layers. The two wrappers are folded sequentially to create a package within a package. The purpose of this technique is to provide a tortuous path to prevent microorganisms from migrating through and penetrating the material. Newer wrappers have been developed that provide a sufficient tortuous path and barrier without double sequential wrapping. The policy for wrapping must be driven by the ability of the wrap to maintain items in a sterile state. Institutional policy may or not require double sequential wrapping.
55. Packages are secured with pressure-sensitive tape that also serves as a chemical indicator. Chemical indicator tape must be selected that is specific to the intended sterilization method.
56. Woven wrappers do not exhibit "memory," a characteristic that causes a material to return to the state in which was originally folded or placed.
57. Woven fabrics should be laundered between use to prevent superheating and deterioration of the fabric. Reusable fabrics must be inspected between uses for pinholes and tears that must be repaired with heat-sealed patches. Woven fabrics may produce lint. They lose their water repellency over time and must be retreated or discarded.

Nonwoven Materials

58. Nonwoven wrappers are made of a combination of cellulose and/or other synthetic materials. Nonwoven wrappers are single use; disposable; almost entirely lint free; resist tearing; and provide an excellent barrier against dust, airborne microorganisms, and moisture.
59. Items wrapped in nonwoven material are wrapped according to manufacturer recommendations. Some nonwoven wraps require two layers and sequential wrap. Others require a single wrap only. The deciding factor of whether one or two layers or sequential wrapping is required is the degree of barrier provided by the wrapper.
60. Nonwoven wrappers eliminate the need for washing, inspecting, and patching. Quality is consistent because wrappers are used only once and are then discarded.
61. Nonwoven cellulose-based wrappers are not compatible with hydrogen peroxide gas plasma sterilization. Polypropylene wrappers must be used instead.
62. Nonwoven wrappers may display undesirable memory as wrapper edges try to return to their original fold when packages are opened. This creates the potential for contamination of package contents.

63. A disadvantage of nonwoven materials is that steam condensate may not be completely evaporated during drying. This can result in a damp or wet package that is not noticed until the package is opened. The placement of an absorbent towel in the bottom and underneath the instrument tray during packaging will help absorb moisture during the sterilization process and alleviate this problem. Packages wrapped in nonwoven materials that display droplets or puddles inside are considered contaminated and must be rejected.
64. Some nonwoven packaging materials may require a longer sterilization time than woven packaging materials. This information must be supplied by the manufacturer.

Plastic, Paper, Tyvek®

65. Combination plastic and paper and plastic and Tyvek® (material made from high-density polyethylene fibers) pouches or peel packs may be used to wrap items in preparation for sterilization. The plastic-paper combination is appropriate for steam or EO sterilization. Tyvek® plastic is used with EO and hydrogen peroxide gas plasma sterilization. With both types of pouches the plastic film is fused to the paper or Tyvek® so that one side is clear and the other opaque.
66. Advantages of combination plastic and paper, or Tyvek® wrappers are that they are inexpensive, permit visualization of the contents, are lint free, provide an effective barrier against airborne microorganisms, and are suitable for packaging a limited number of small items.
67. Disadvantages are a tendency to display memory and the paper and plastic combination provides little resistance to punctures.
68. Items packaged in pouches are single or double pouched depending on manufacturer guidelines and individual institutional policies. Where double pouching is used, the inner pouch should fit into the outer pouch without being folded (AORN, 1995b, p. 607).
69. The paper portions should be placed together to ensure penetration of sterilant, air, and moisture. The sterilant penetrates the paper portion of the pouch while the plastic portion allows the item to be viewed (AAMI, 1989, p. 131; AORN, 1995a, p. 223).
70. Pouch packages should be processed in a vertical position.
71. Items, such as bulb syringes, that can trap air and interfere with the sterilization process should not be packaged in pouches.

Rigid Containers

72. Rigid containers are rectangular receptacles made from aluminum, stainless steel, heat-resistant plastics, or a combination. The lid and bottom contain perforations that are sealed with a bacterial filter. The filters allow entry and exit of the sterilant. The lid and base are held together by a latch or a lock and key.
73. Advantages of rigid containers are that they are durable and more resistant than other packaging materials to contamination during storage. Containers eliminate the necessity for a wrapper.
74. Disadvantages include weight and potential for residual condensation. Containers weigh 4 to 10 pounds. Recondensation on the inner or outer surfaces following steam sterilization sometimes occurs.
75. Containers must be washed prior to filling. The gaskets, valves, and filters should be checked and changed according to the manufacturer's recommendation.
76. Information on how to arrange and package items within containers, as well as information on how to seal and label the containers, must be obtained from the manufacturer. In addition, the manufacturer should be requested to supply data that support shelf-life claims.

Sealing

77. All items intended for sterilization must be securely sealed.
78. Pressure-sensitive tape is used for woven and nonwoven wrappers. Plastic and paper and plastic and Tyvek® pouches may be either heat sealed or sealed with pressure-sensitive tape.
79. To prevent damage or loss of package integrity, heat seals must be such that they do not permit resealing once opened.

PACKAGE INFORMATION AND IDENTIFICATION

Chemical Indicators

80. Chemical indicators should be visible from the outside of all packages intended for sterilization. A piece of heat-sensitive tape, an indicator strip, or heat-sensitive labels may be used.
81. The indicator should be placed where it is easily visualized. Where there is no visible indicator the package must be considered contaminated.

82. Pouch packaging often includes an external indicator as part of the pouch.

Labels

83. Items packaged for sterilization should be clearly labeled with the contents, initials of the package assembler, and lot control number. The lot control number indicates the sterilization date, the expiration date (unless no expiration date is required), which sterilizer was used, and the cycle or load number.
84. Indelible, nonbleeding, felt-tip ink pens or very soft lead pencils may be used to mark packages (AAMI, 1990, p. 134; AORN, 1995a, p. 223).
85. The sterilization date may be indicated according to the Julian calendar, which numbers days from 001 to 365. The expiration date may be indicated according to the Gregorian calendar (i.e., 22 May 96). Accordingly, an item labeled 024/24 Feb. 96 indicates that the item was sterilized on January 24, that is, the 24th day of the year, and will expire 1 month later at midnight on February 24, 1996.
86. The lot control number facilitates identification of items. Lot control numbers assist in retrieval of items in the event of sterilization failure or malfunction, inventory control, and rotation of stock (AAMI, 1989, p. 17).

SHELF LIFE

Storage Considerations

87. Sterilized items should be stored in a well-ventilated, limited-access area with controlled temperature and humidity (AORN, 1995a, p. 273). Dust particles and aerosols should be controlled.
88. Sterile items should be stored in an area separate from clean items.
89. To reduce dust accumulation, wire mesh shelving is preferable to closed shelving.
90. Cabinets and shelves should permit adequate cleaning and air circulation. Storage cabinets and shelves should be far enough away from floors, ceiling fixtures, vents, sprinklers, and lights to prevent contamination.

Determining Factors

91. Shelf life is the amount of time an item may be considered sterile. Theoretically, if an item is not contaminated during storage it will remain sterile indefinitely. Shelf life is related to the events that can occur that will cause an item to become contaminated. Many institutions have policies that require that an expiration date be placed on stored items after which time the item is no longer considered sterile and must be reprocessed. The expiration date is only a guideline to indicate how long the package has been on the shelf. Contamination may occur long before the expiration date. Actual shelf life is event related, not time related. Events are what determine shelf life. Only proper packaging, handling, and storage can prevent contamination. The more a package is handled, and the longer it is stored, the greater the possibility is for contamination.
92. Some institutions have eliminated the use of expiration dates. This is appropriate only when designated parameters related to shelf life have been identified and achieved.
93. Shelf life is determined by many factors. These include the following:
    - Type and configuration of packaging material—items packaged in rigid containers may have a longer shelf life than items packaged with woven and nonwoven materials.
    - Use of dust covers—dust covers can extend shelf life.
    - Conditions of storage—dust, temperature, humidity, and traffic can affect shelf life.
    - Number of times a package is handled before use—the more handling the greater the risk of contamination.
    - Whether stored on open or closed shelves—closed cabinets can extend shelf life.
94. Commercially prepared items may not indicate an expiration date and are usually considered sterile provided the package is intact. Expiration dates on commercially prepared items may indicate that the integrity of the device or material will be compromised after the indicated date and the item should not be used once this date has been reached.

Section Questions

Q15. Water in combination with ethylene oxide forms ______________________________ which is toxic. Therefore items to be sterilized in ethylene oxide must be dried. (Ref. 45)

Q16. Packaging for hydrogen peroxide gas plasma sterilization may be (Ref. 47):
- a. cloth
- b. paper
- c. polypropylene

Q17. Chemical indicators placed in the center of packages determine whether sterilization has occurred. (Ref. 50)

True False

Q18. Packaging materials (Ref. 52, 53):
- a. must be compatible with the sterilization process
- b. must resist tears and punctures
- c. used for steam sterilization must not permit air removal
- d. must be impervious to penetration of microorganisms
- e. must be made of muslin

Q19. Select the correct statements. (Ref. 53, 54, 56, 58, 59)
- a. Muslin wrap is rarely used today.
- b. Wrappers may be either single or double provided they provide a barrier to the passage of microorganisms.
- c. Woven wrappers exhibit memory.
- d. Woven wrappers must be laundered between use.
- e. Nonwoven wrappers are single use items.

Q20. Describe one method to reduce the possibility of a wet pack. (Ref. 63)

____

____

Q21. List three advantages of paper and plastic or Tyvek® and plastic wrappers. (Ref. 66)

____

____

____

Q22. Containers (Ref. 73, 74, 75):
- a. must be wrapped in polypropylene
- b. are more resistant to contamination than other packaging materials
- c. can permit recondensation on their inner surface following steam sterilization
- d. must be washed between use

Q23. If a chemical indicator is not visible on the outside of the package a reading may be taken from the indicator inside the package. (Ref. 81)

True False

Q24. List three pieces of information that should be indicated on packages prepared for sterilization. (Ref. 83)

____

____

____

Q25. Shelf life is determined by factors such as (Ref. 91, 93):

a. the method of sterilization used
b. the packaging material used
c. conditions of storage
d. number of times a package is handled

NOTES

Association for the Advancement of Medical Instrumentation (AAMI). (1989). *Good hospital practice: Steam sterilization and sterility assurance* (Vol. 2). Chicago, IL: American Hospital Publishing.

Association for the Advancement of Medical Instrumentation (AAMI). (1989). *Good hospital practice: Steam sterilization and sterility assurance* (Vol. 2. p. 131). Chicago, IL: American Hospital Publishing. In Association of Operating Room Nurses. (1995). *Standards and recommended practices* (p. 223). Denver, CO: AORN.

Association for the Advancement of Medical Instrumentation (AAMI). (1990). *Good hospital practice: Guidelines for the selection and use of reusable rigid container systems.* In Association of Operating Room Nurses (1995). *Standards and recommended practices* (p. 223). Denver, CO: AORN.

Association of Operating Room Nurses (AORN). (1991). *Standards and recommended practices.* Denver, CO: AORN.

Association of Operating Room Nurses (AORN). (1995a). *Standards and recommended practices.* Denver, CO: AORN.

Association of Operating Room Nurses (AORN). (1995b). Proposed recommended practices for selection and use of packaging systems. *AORN Journal*, *61*, 605–611.

ADDITIONAL READING

Groah, L. (1996). *Perioperative nursing* (3rd ed.). Stamford, CT: Appleton & Lange.

Reichert, M., & Young, J. (1993). *Sterilization technology for the health care facility.* Gaithersburg, MD: Aspen Publishers, Inc.

Appendix 4–A

Chapter 4 Post Test

1. Preparation of instrumentation can impact whether or not the patient sustains an injury or infection during surgery. (Ref. 5)

   True False

2. Contaminated instruments and items include (Ref. 6):
   a. items opened and used during surgery
   b. visibly soiled items
   c. items opened for surgery, not used, and no visible debris

3. If an instrument is insufficiently cleaned, sterility may not be achieved during the sterilization process. (Ref. 13, 14, 15)

   True False

4. Instruments that are heavily soiled may need to be washed or brushed by hand. Washing and brushing should be done beneath the surface of the water to prevent (Ref. 17):

   ____

   ____

5. Instruments are not considered safe to handle until they are decontaminated. (Ref. 9)

   True False

6. Ultrasonic cleaning (Ref. 24, 25, 26):
   a. kills microorganisms
   b. may be used in place of disinfection
   c. removes debris from instruments
   d. may be used for all instruments

7. Instrument lubrication must be water soluble. (Ref. 27)

   True False

8. Items that may be nested, such as medicine cups and basins, should all be packaged in the same direction to (Ref. 37):
   a. prevent damage
   b. permit circulation of the sterilizing agent
   c. prevent air pockets
   d. allow condensate to drain out

9. Explain why rubber sheeting or other impervious material is covered with a porous material and loosely rolled in preparation for sterilization. (Ref. 38)

   ____

   ____

   ____

10. What must be done to linen to prevent superheating during the sterilization cycle? (Ref. 41)

____

____

11. Explain why the number of times a cloth wrapper is used should be tracked. (Ref. 43)

____

____

12. Chemical indicators should be visible on the outside of the package to check whether certain parameters necessary for sterilization have been met. (Ref. 48)

True False

13. Packaging materials should be compatible with the sterilization process. List five additional considerations when selecting packaging materials. (Ref. 52)

____

____

____

____

____

14. Muslin, water-repellent cotton and polyester, and nonwoven packaging material are equally effective barriers against passage of microorganisms. (Ref. 53, 54, 58, 59, 61, 63, 64)

True False

15. Prior to ethylene oxide sterilization items with a lumen must have the lumen (Ref. 39, 45):
    a. moistened with water
    b. blown dry

    Explain why.

____

____

16. Pouch packages should be processed in a vertical position. (Ref. 70)

True False

17. The date of sterilization may be indicated according to the Julian calendar. If the date indicated is "32", what day would that be according to the Gregorian calendar? (Ref. 85)
    a. March 2
    b. February 1
    c. January 31

18. Shelf life is a guarantee that items will remain sterile until the expiration date. (Ref. 91)

    True False

19. Tyvek® plastic pouches may be used in (Ref. 65)
    a. steam
    b. ethylene oxide
    c. hydrogen peroxide gas plasma

Appendix 4–B

Competency Checklist: Preparation, Packaging, and Storage of Sterile Supplies

Under observer's initials enter initials upon successful achievement of competency. Enter N/A if competency is not appropriate for institution.

NAME ______________________________

	OBSERVER'S INITIALS	DATE
1. Items are rinsed/wiped/irrigated during procedure.	________	________
2. Contaminated instruments are covered during transportation or are transported in designated carts.	________	________
3. Instruments that can be immersed are placed in designated solution for soaking.	________	________
4. Personal protective equipment is worn during washing procedures.	________	________
5. Hand washing is accomplished below the surface of the water.	________	________
6. Decontamination equipment is operated according to manufacturer's instructions.	________	________
7. Instruments are processed in ultrasonic cleaner following decontamination.	________	________
8. Ultrasonic cleaner is operated according to manufacturer's instructions.	________	________
9. Instruments are lubricated with water-soluble lubricant.	________	________
10. Instruments are inspected for		
a. cleanliness	________	________
b. function	________	________
11. Instruments are packaged appropriately:		
a. appropriate tray/container	________	________
b. disassembled	________	________
c. opened	________	________
d. delicate on top of heavy	________	________
e. nested items separated with porous material and placed facing same direction	________	________
f. lumens rinsed for steam	________	________
g. lumens dried for ethylene and gas plasma	________	________
h. chemical process indicator/integrator included	________	________
i. appropriate wrapping material selected	________	________

NAME ______________________________

	OBSERVER'S INITIALS	DATE
j. wrapped/packaged according to wrapper/pouch manufacturer guidelines	________	________
k. labeled and dated	________	________
12. Container washed before placement of instruments for sterilization.	________	________
13. Gaskets, valves, filters checked prior to placement of instruments for sterilization.	________	________
14. Items packaged in container system according to manufacturer's guidelines.	________	________

OBSERVER'S SIGNATURE INITIALS

______________________________ ________

ORIENTEE'S SIGNATURE

____

CHAPTER 5

Prevention of Infection—Asepsis: Aseptic Technique, Prepping, Attire, Scrubbing, Gowning and Gloving, Draping, and Sanitation

Learner Objectives

At the end of Prevention of Infection—Asepsis: Aseptic Technique, Prepping, Attire, Scrubbing, Gowning and Gloving, Draping, and Sanitation, the learner will

- describe the impact of a surgical wound infection
- discuss the relationship of asepsis to the prevention of infection
- list three criteria to evaluate the achievement of the desired patient outcome of freedom from infection
- identify the perioperative nurse's responsibility with regard to aseptic practice
- define restricted, semirestricted, and unrestricted areas of the operating room
- describe appropriate attire within restricted, semirestricted, and unrestricted areas
- discuss principles of aseptic technique
- define and discuss "surgical conscience"
- list the desired characteristics of topical antimicrobial agents
- describe the purpose and technique of a surgical prep
- discuss six guidelines for draping
- list the desired characteristics of surgical gowns and drapes
- describe open and closed gloving techniques
- describe the purpose and process of a surgical scrub
- identify four sources of infection
- explain the concept of universal precautions and its application in the operating room
- discuss procedures and practices to control patient, personnel, and environmental sources of infection

Lesson Outline

I. **NURSING DIAGNOSES**
II. **DESIRED PATIENT OUTCOME/CRITERIA**
III. **OVERVIEW**
IV. **NURSING RESPONSIBILITIES**
V. **PATHOGENIC MICROORGANISMS**
VI. **SOURCES OF INFECTION (ENDOGENOUS)**
   A. Patients
   B. Personnel
   C. Environment
   D. Equipment
VII. **UNIVERSAL PRECAUTIONS**
VIII. **CONTROL OF SOURCES OF INFECTION**
   A. Aseptic Technique
   B. Control of Patient Sources of Infection—Skin Prep
   C. Control of Personnel Sources of Infection
      1. Attire
      2. Scrubbing, Gowning, and Gloving
         a. Scrub Procedure
         b. Gowning and Gloving Procedure
         c. Assisting Others to Gown and Glove
   D. Creating a Sterile Field—Draping
      1. Draping Guidelines
      2. Standard Drapes
   E. Control of Environmental Sources of Infection
      1. Operating Room Environment
      2. Traffic Patterns
      3. Operating Room Sanitation
      4. Additional Considerations—Cleaning and Scheduling

CHAPTER 5

Prevention of Infection—Asepsis: Aseptic Technique, Prepping, Attire, Scrubbing, Gowning and Gloving, Draping, and Sanitation

NURSING DIAGNOSES

1. A common nursing diagnosis for the patient undergoing surgical intervention is high risk for wound infection. A surgical incision creates an opportunity for microorganisms to enter and for infection to result.
2. Risk of wound infection is related to the implementation of proper practices of asepsis. Attire, aseptic technique, gowning, gloving, prepping, draping, and sanitation of the suite if not performed in accordance with accepted principles may increase the patient's risk of developing a wound infection.

DESIRED PATIENT OUTCOME/CRITERIA

3. The desired patient outcome for the patient who undergoes surgery is freedom from wound infection following the operative procedure.
4. Infection may be evidenced by fever, erythema, cellulitis, abscess, or dehiscence and is often not noted until after the patient has left the health care facility. The patient should exhibit none of the above signs or symptoms.

OVERVIEW

5. The patient who develops a postoperative wound infection may experience delayed wound healing, discomfort, and pain. Postoperative wound infection may even lead to death. It is a major cause of extended hospitalization and can add 7.4 to 10.1 days to a patient's hospitalization stay (Cardo, Falk, & Mayhall, 1993, p. 212).
6. A nosocomial infection is an infection acquired during hospitalization. Surgical wound infection is the second most common nosocomial infection (Cardo, Falk, & Mayhall, 1993, p. 212). If a wound infection develops within 3 to 8 days postoperatively it is probable that the infection was acquired during hospitalization (Meeker & Rothrock, 1995, p. 37). Nosocomial infections are not always identified before the patient leaves the hospital. The rise in the number of ambulatory surgeries has made it more difficult to track numbers and source of wound infections.

NURSING RESPONSIBILITIES

7. *Asepsis* refers to the absence of pathogenic organisms. Asepsis in the operating room, also referred to as aseptic technique, refers to the practices by which contamination with microorganisms is prevented. Although it is impossible to eliminate all microorganisms in the surgical environment, strict adherence to aseptic technique is the most important measure in preventing the patient and staff from acquiring an infection.
8. The perioperative nurse is responsible for creating and maintaining a sterile field and for monitoring aseptic practice of all members of the surgical team. Appropriate implementation of this responsibility requires an understanding of infection sources, transmission modes, and the methods to reduce or eliminate microorganisms in the surgical setting. The perioperative nurse must have in-depth knowledge of principles and practices associated with attire, aseptic technique, gowning and

gloving, prepping, draping, and operating room sanitation.

9. The responsibility for reducing the number of microorganisms in the operating room to the lowest level possible is shared by all members of the surgical team and personnel employed in the department. However, the perioperative nurse assumes major responsibility for ensuring that each patient is provided with as aseptic an environment as possible and that risk for wound infection is reduced to its lowest potential.

PATHOGENIC MICROORGANISMS

10. Pathogenic microorganisms are microorganisms that cause disease. There are four pathogenic microorganisms frequently associated with nosocomial infections.
    1. Gram-positive microorganisms are those that stain blue under specific laboratory testing such as *Streptococcus* and *Staphylococcus*.
    2. Gram-negative microorganisms are those that do not stain under specific laboratory testing such as *Pseudomonas*, *Escherichia coli*, and *Mycobacterium tuberculosis*.
    3. Fungi microorganisms are those such as *Candida albicans* and *Aspergillus*.
    4. Virus microorganisms are those such as herpesvirus, human immunodeficiency virus (HIV), and hepatitis

SOURCES OF INFECTION (ENDOGENOUS)

Patients

11. Endogenous sources of infection arise from within the body. The patient is a source of endogenous infection because of the large number of microorganisms normally found in and on the body. If these microorganisms remain in their normal environment and if their numbers are not altered by external factors, no infection will develop.
12. The skin is the first line of defense against the entry of microorganisms into the body. By incising the skin, a portal of entry for pathogenic microorganisms is created and the patient is immediately exposed to the risk of infection. In addition, certain factors or conditions, if present, may significantly impact a patient's risk for developing a postoperative wound infection. These include old age; poor nutritional status; obesity; a compromised immune system; preexisting disease, especially diabetes; presence of preexisting infection; burns; and a smoking history.
13. Length of surgery, type of procedure, surgical technique, and an extended preoperative hospital stay can also increase risk of postoperative wound infection.
14. Geriatric and neonate patients have an increased risk of postoperative wound infection. Impaired healing in the aged is often related to inadequate circulation due to atherosclerosis or the presence of coexisting disease. Delayed healing increases the opportunity for wound infection. The premature infant has increased susceptibility to infection due to immature globulin synthesis, antibody formation, and cellular defense. The smaller the neonate the less resistance there is to infection. Invasive procedures increase the risk of infection.
15. Poor nutritional status, such as frequently accompanies drug or alcohol addiction, can delay wound healing and increase risk for infection. Obesity is a risk factor because less blood is supplied to fatty tissue and avascular tissue is susceptible to infection.
16. Defense mechanisms are impaired in the immunocompromised patient. Patients receiving radiation therapy, chemotherapy, corticosteroids, or who have AIDS are immunocompromised. Additional stress is placed on the immune system of patients with chronic conditions such as diabetes, cancer, and cardiac and respiratory diseases.
17. The presence of infection anywhere in the body is always a contraindication for elective surgery.
18. The first line of defense is the patient's skin. When it is destroyed the patient is susceptible to infection.
19. Smoking decreases the delivery of oxygen to the tissues and wound healing is delayed, which may cause an infection to occur.
20. The risk of infection increases with the length of exposure of internal tissues to the environment, the presence of implants, and the amount of ischemic tissue present. Although necessary, catheters and drains may increase the risk of infection because they provide a pathway for pathogenic microorganism migration. The longer these are left in place the greater is the risk for infection.
21. There are multiple sources for infection; however, for an infection to occur there must be
    - pathogens of sufficient virulence
    - a sufficient quantity of pathogens
    - a susceptible host
    - a portal of entry
    - a mode of transmission

Personnel

22. Exogenous sources of infection are from outside the body and include the environment and personnel.

23. Personnel are a major source of microorganisms in the operating room. The higher the number of personnel in the operating room, the higher the number of microorganisms.
24. The skin of all persons in the area is a potential source of infection. Cells and surface organisms are constantly being shed from skin surfaces. Certain body areas such as the head, neck, axilla, hands, groin, legs, and feet harbor an especially large number of microorganisms. Hair is a major source of *Staphylococcus*. The number of microorganisms present in hair is related to its length and cleanliness.
25. Talking, coughing, and breathing release numerous organisms into the environment.
26. Jewelry, artificial nails, cracks in nail polish, and cosmetic detritus may harbor millions of microorganisms (Pottinger, Burns, & Manske, 1989, p. 340). The effect of nail polish on the number of microorganisms found on the fingernails of personnel after a surgical hand scrub has been questioned and one study found no significant difference between polished, unpolished, damaged, or undamaged nails in the number of microorganisms found on fingernails (Baumgardner, Maragos, Walz, & Larson, 1993, p. 87).

Environment

27. The operating room is not a sterile area; therefore organisms are present in the air, on dust particles, and on dirt in the environment.
28. The walls, floors, overhead lights, light tracks, cabinets, and other stationery fixtures in the operating room may harbor microorganisms and are therefore potential sources of infection.

Equipment

29. All instruments, supplies, and equipment that come in contact with air and personnel become potential sources for infection because personnel transfer organisms to whatever instruments, supplies, or equipment they touch.
30. Whenever dust particles in the air settle on instruments or supplies, the organisms on those dust particles are also deposited on those items.

UNIVERSAL PRECAUTIONS

31. Universal precautions is a method of infection control that requires that blood and body fluid of all humans (patients and personnel) be considered infectious and that the same safety precautions be taken whether or not the patient is known to have a bloodborne infectious disease. The practice of universal precautions is a method of infection control that protects both the patient and operating room personnel.
32. In 1992 the Occupational Safety and Health Administration established mandatory universal precautions practice standards. The three critical components of universal precaution standards are (1) use of personal protective barriers, (2) proper hand washing, and (3) precautions in handling sharps.
33. The standards include but are not limited to the following (Johnson & Johnson, 1992, pp. 4–10):
    - Employers must list job classifications, tasks, and procedures in which employees have occupational exposure to blood or other potentially infectious body fluids.
    - Gloves must be worn when direct contact with blood or other potentially infectious body fluids is expected to occur.
    - Masks with face shields or protective eye wear with side shields must be worn when splashes, splattering, or aerosolation of blood and body fluids is anticipated.
    - Gowns, appropriate to the procedure being performed, must be worn when aerosolation or splattering of blood or other body fluids is anticipated. Gowns must not permit passage of blood or body fluids.
    - Personal protective equipment (gloves, masks, face shields, gowns, and so forth) is provided by the employer at no cost to the employee.
    - Hands and other skin surfaces must be washed as soon as feasible if contaminated with blood or body fluids.
    - Contaminated needles are not recapped or removed unless required by a specific procedure. If recapping or removal is required, it must be accomplished with a mechanical device.
    - Sharps are deposited in rigid, leakprook, puncture-resistant containers that must be readily accessible.
    - A written schedule of cleaning and appropriate disinfection of equipment and the environment must be implemented and maintained.
    - Contaminated laundry is placed in labeled or color-coded laundry bags that prevent leakage.
    - Infectious waste containers must be closable, prevent leakage, and be labeled or color coded as potentially infectious.
    - The employer must provide a hepatitis B vaccination and a postexposure follow-up program. A pre-exposure vaccine must be offered free of charge.
    - Training and education programs must be made available to all employees who may be exposed to blood or other body fluids that are potentially contaminated with hepatitis B virus (HBV) or HIV.

Section Questions

Q1. Postoperative wound infection (Ref. 3, 4, 5, 6, 7):
a. is related to implementation of proper aseptic technique
b. is a major cause of extended hospital stay
c. frequently results in death
d. that occurs 8 to 10 days after surgery was probably acquired in the hospital
e. may be evidenced by dehiscence

Q2. A compromised immune system can influence the risk of postoperative wound infection. List five additional endogenous factors that can influence and increase the risk of postoperative wound infection. (Ref. 12, 13, 14, 15, 16, 17, 18, 19)

____

____

____

____

____

Q3. Operating room personnel represent an exogenous source of infection. (Ref. 23)

True False

Q4. Hair is a potential source of infection and is a major source of *Streptococcus*. (Ref. 24)

True False

Q5. Talking is a source of contamination. (Ref. 25)

True False

Q6. Polished nails are known to harbor more bacteria than unpolished nails following a surgical scrub. (Ref. 26)

True False

Q7. Universal precautions (Ref. 31, 32):
a. protects patients
b. protects personnel
c. should be practiced for all patients
d. includes hand washing
e. includes precautions in handling sharps
f. is mandated by OSHA

Q8. List four articles of personal protective attire worn to be in compliance with universal precautions in the presence of infectious fluids. (Ref. 33)

____

____

____

____

CONTROL OF SOURCES OF INFECTION

34. Infection prevention in the operating room includes practices of aseptic technique, requirements for surgical attire, sterilization of instruments and equipment, staff and patient skin preparation, creation and maintenance of a sterile field, and control of the environment. A major responsibility of the perioperative nurse is to implement and ensure practices that are designed to prevent infection.
35. Some aseptic practices are mandated by regulatory bodies such as the Occupational Safety and Health Administration. Others are derived from standard-setting bodies such as the Association of Operating Room Nurses (AORN) and the Association for Advancement of Medical Instrumentation (AAMI).
36. Regardless of the source of the aseptic practices, they are only as good as the surgical conscience of the individual practitioner. A surgical conscience is an inner commitment to adhere strictly to aseptic practice, to report any break in aseptic technique, and to correct any violation whether or not anyone else is present or observes the violation. A surgical conscience mandates a commitment to aseptic practice *at all times*.

Aseptic Technique

37. Aseptic technique, also referred to as aseptic practice, is the method used to prevent contamination from microorganisms. The Association of Operating Room Nurses has identified recommended practices of aseptic technique. The purpose of these practices is to prevent contamination of the open wound and to create and maintain a sterile field that is isolated from the surrounding unsterile area. Adherence to these practices contributes to providing a safe environment for the patient that minimizes potential for wound infection. The AORN recommended practices are critical components of infection control and are addressed throughout this chapter. They are:
38. a. *Scrubbed personnel function within a sterile field* (AORN, 1995, p. 211).

    Sterile gowns and gloves should be used within the sterile field. Surgical gowns and gloves establish a barrier that minimizes the passage of microorganisms between nonsterile and sterile areas. Once donned, the gown is considered sterile in front from the chest to the level of the sterile field. The sleeves are considered sterile from 2 inches above the elbow down to the top edge of the cuff. The neckline, shoulders, axilla, and cuffed portion of the sleeves may become contaminated by perspiration and therefore are not considered sterile. The back is considered unsterile because it cannot be under constant observation by the scrubbed person. The cuffs are considered contaminated once the hands have passed through them.

    b. *Sterile drapes should be used to establish a sterile field* (AORN, 1995, p. 136).

    To create a sterile field, sterile drapes are placed on the patient and on all furniture and equipment that will be part of the sterile field. Sterile drapes are a barrier to the passage of microorganisms, isolate the sterile field from the surrounding environment, and minimize passage of microorganisms between sterile and nonsterile areas.

    c. *Items used within a sterile field should be sterile* (AORN, 1995, p. 136).

    Items used during surgery are wrapped and sterilized prior to surgery. On occasion, unwrapped items may be taken directly from the autoclave following sterilization and dispensed to the sterile field.

    Sterility of items must be ensured by the person dispensing them to the sterile field and by the person accepting them. For wrapped items, the integrity of the wrapper, expiration date (if there is one), and the color of the indicator tape need to be checked. The chemical indicator or integrator inside the package is checked by the scrub person to ensure that parameters of sterilization were attained during the sterilization process. If an item is taken directly from the autoclave, the circulating nurse must ensure that the proper technique is used to transfer items to the sterile field.

    Whenever the integrity of a sterile barrier is broken, the contents must be considered unsterile. Wrappers, gowns, gloves, and drapes are all examples of sterile barriers. Examples of sterile barriers that have been permeated are a tear or hole in a wrapper or glove; a wet, scorched, or stained wrapper; or a barrier that looks questionable.

    The contents of wet or stained wrappers may have been subject to strike-through, which occurs when liquids soak through a barrier from a sterile to an unsterile area and vice versa. Strike-through provides for passage of microorganisms through the barrier and therefore the contents must be considered contaminated. When strike-through occurs, it may not be noticed initially and the item may dry. Therefore, items contained in wrappers that are stained should be considered contaminated. If the sterility of any item is in doubt, it is considered contaminated and is discarded.

    Items that become contaminated must not be permitted on the sterile field. Items, such as suction and cautery, that remain on the drapes during the procedure are secured to prevent them from sliding below the level of the sterile field.

d. *Items introduced to a sterile field should be opened, dispensed, and transferred by methods that maintain sterility and integrity* (AORN, 1995, p. 137).

Several techniques may be used by unscrubbed personnel to dispense sterile items onto the sterile field while maintaining the sterility of the field.

When dispensing an item to the sterile field, the unscrubbed person should open the wrapper flap that is furthest away first and the wrapper flap that is closest last. All wrapper edges should be secured to prevent accidental contamination of the scrub person or sterile field with a wrapper edge. If an item cannot be carefully placed or flipped onto the field, the scrub person must lift the item straight up out of the package (see Figure 5–1). Sterile gowns and drapes and other similar items may be placed onto the sterile field providing that the portion of the unscrubbed person's hand that may extend over the sterile field is covered by the sterile wrapper.

Heavy, awkward, or sharp items should not be tossed onto the sterile field because they may roll off the edge of the sterile field, displace other items from the sterile field, or penetrate the sterile barrier. These items should be received directly by the scrub person (see Figure 5–2).

Sterile basins into which sterile solutions will be poured are placed at the edge of the table or are held by the scrub person. This decreases both the risk of splashing the sterile field and creating the potential for strike-through. Because the edge of the bottle cap as well as the opening of the bottle are considered contaminated, once the cap is removed, it cannot be replaced. To do so

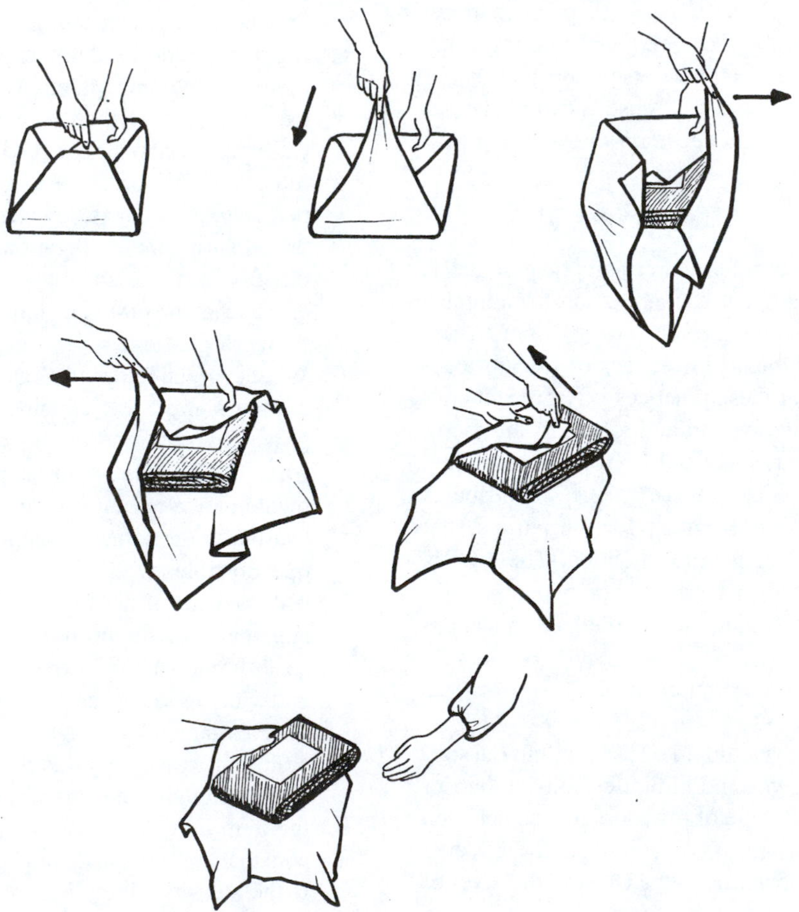

Figure 5–1 Opening a Package. Circulating nurse passes sterile item to scrub person by opening package and bringing wrapper back over hand to form a protective barrier.

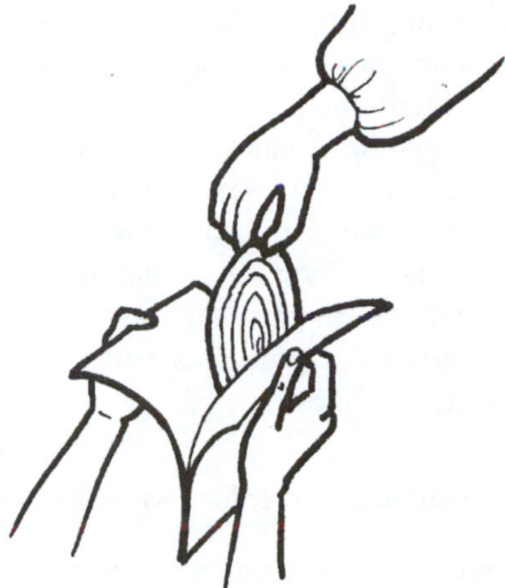

Figure 5–2 Retrieving an Item. Large or awkward items are presented directly to the scrub person, who is careful not to touch the wrapper.

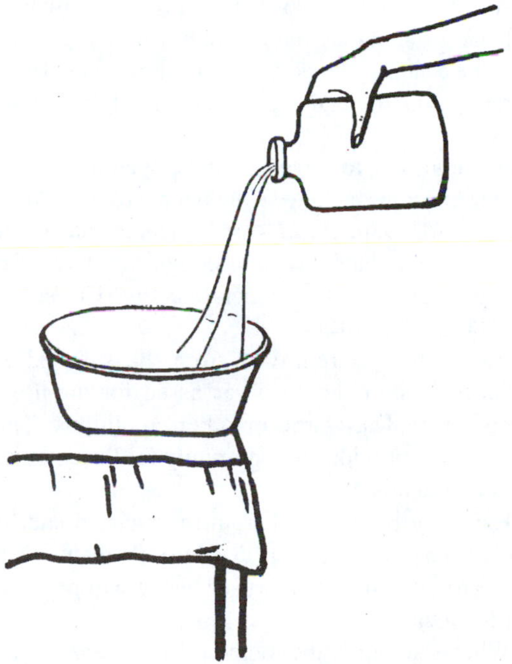

Figure 5–3 Pouring Liquid. Sterile basin is placed at edge of table allowing only sterile lip of bottle to extend over the edge of basin while solution is poured.

would risk contamination of the bottle contents. Therefore the entire contents of the bottle should be poured into the receptacle (see Figure 5–3).

Boundaries between sterile and unsterile are not always clearly defined, and good judgment and keen observation are needed to ensure that only sterile items are introduced to the sterile field.

e. *A sterile field should be maintained and monitored continuously* (AORN, 1995, p. 214).

A sterile field should be set up as close to the time of surgery as possible. The longer sterile items are open to the environment the greater opportunity there is for contamination to occur.

A sterile field should not be covered because it is difficult to remove the cover without causing contamination to occur. Uncovering requires that a portion of the cover that has been below the level of the sterile field be drawn up over the top of the sterile field. This can cause contamination. Some institutional policies may permit covering using two drapes. Each drape is positioned to cover half of the sterile field and to meet in the middle where an everted cuff is formed from each drape. Using the cuffs, each drape is removed from the center outward rather than up and over the field. This is not an AORN recommended practice, however, and where it is practiced strict guidelines should be provided on application and technique.

Once a sterile field has been created it should be monitored by all team members for possible contamination. For this reason the sterile field should not be left unattended.

f. *All personnel moving within or around a sterile field should do so in a manner that will maintain the sterile field* (AORN, 1996, p. 215).

The surgical team must be aware of sterile and unsterile items within the operating room and move in a manner that does not cause sterile items or fields to become contaminated.

Scrubbed persons touch only sterile items and areas. Scrubbed persons remain as close to the sterile field as possible and do not wander about or leave the room. Scrubbed persons face the sterile field. When scrubbed persons move or change places with each other they do so face to face or back to back and maintain a safe distance apart (see Figure 5–4).

The scrubbed person should not change levels from standing to sitting and the reverse. Changing levels can cause the lower portion of the gown, which is considered contaminated, to be drawn close to or in contact with the sterile field and increases the risk of sterile-field contamination. The only time scrubbed persons should sit is when the entire procedure is performed at this level.

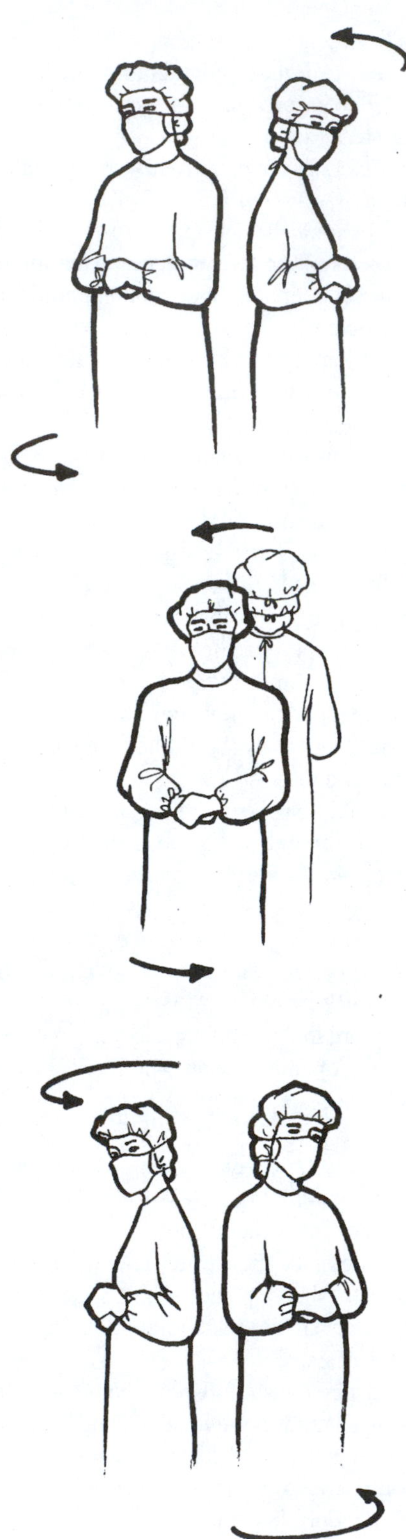

Figure 5–4 Back to Back. Two gowned persons shown passing each other back to back.

The patient is the center of the sterile field. All additional sterile equipment is grouped around the patient within view of the scrub person.

Unscrubbed persons contact only unsterile items. Unscrubbed persons keep a safe distance from the sterile field to prevent accidental contamination. Determining a safe distance requires astute judgment. Unscrubbed persons who approach the sterile field do so by facing the sterile field. Unscrubbed persons do not walk between two sterile fields.

Control of Patient Sources of Infection—Skin Prep

39. Efforts to reduce patient sources of infection are aimed at lowering the number of bacteria on the skin prior to surgery and reducing potential bacterial contamination from within the patient during surgery. Although the skin cannot be sterilized, the incision site and the area immediately surrounding it should be as free of microorganisms as possible prior to surgery.
40. Aseptic practices to reduce microorganisms on the patient's skin may include removal of hair and does include cleaning the skin with an antimicrobial agent. Hair removal and cleansing are commonly referred to as a skin prep.
41. It is advisable to leave hair at the operative site unless its presence interferes with the intended procedure (Cruise & Foord, 1980, pp. 27–40). The incidence of wound infection is reduced by omission of the shave if minimal hair is present at the operative site (Cruise & Foord, 1980, pp. 27–40).
42. Before hair is removed from the surgical site, the patient's skin should be assessed for the presence of rashes, moles, warts, or other conditions. Trauma to these can provide an opportunity for the colonization of microorganisms.
43. Hair may be removed from the incision site by razor, electric clippers, or a depilatory cream. Depilatory creams are infrequently used because of potential irritation to the skin.
44. When shaving is the method used to remove hair, it is performed wet and as close as possible to the time of surgery to prevent microorganism growth in nicks and scratches that can be left by the razor. The incidence of postoperative wound infection increases in relation to the length of time before surgery that the shave is performed (Olsen, MacCallum, & McQuerrie, 1986, p. 182).
45. To prevent airborne dispersal of hair and possible contamination of the sterile field, hair removal should be performed outside the room where surgery will be performed.

46. Clippers decrease the potential for nicks and scratches in the skin and are the preferred method of hair removal.
47. The operative site and the immediate surrounding area is cleaned and disinfected prior to surgery. In some instances the patient may be instructed to shower with an antimicrobial soap just prior to surgery.
48. The objective of skin cleansing is to remove dirt and skin oils, to reduce the number of microorganisms on the skin to a minimum, and to prevent further microbial growth throughout the procedure.
49. The patient may be instructed to shower with an antimicrobial agent the night before or morning of surgery. Whether or not this is done, the patient's skin will be cleaned again with an antimicrobial agent just prior to surgery.
50. The choice of antimicrobial agent depends on the condition of the skin, patient allergies, incision site, and surgeon and hospital preference.
51. Acceptable antimicrobial products should have the following properties:
    - cleanses effectively
    - reduces microbial count rapidly
    - has a broad spectrum of activity
    - is easy to apply
    - is nonirritating and nontoxic
    - provides residual protection
52. The most common antimicrobial agents include iodophors, chlorhexidine gluconate, and alcohol preparations in concentrations of 60%–90%.
53. The duration of the prep should be based on the manufacturer's recommendation and studies on the effectiveness of the antimicrobial agents.
54. Prior to the skin prep, the patient should be assessed for allergies or sensitivities to prep solutions. An alternate antimicrobial solution is chosen if allergies or sensitivities are known.
55. The area prepped should include the incision site and a substantial area surrounding it. Anticipated additional incision sites and potential drain sites must also be prepped. (See Figures 5–5 through 5–11.)
56. The following guidelines should be adhered to when performing the skin prep:
    - If the patient is awake an explanation should be given regarding the prep.
    - Unnecessary exposure of the patient is avoided. To retain patient dignity and to prevent unnecessary heat loss, only the area to be prepped is exposed.
    - The prep is performed using mechanical friction. The prep begins at the incision site and continues outwardly to the periphery. A widening circular motion is preferable to a back and forth motion. A back and forth motion can cause bacteria to be dragged from the unprepped areas back to the clean center portion of the prepped area. The process is repeated several times. The length of the skin scrub may vary from 1 minute for an alcohol wipe, to a 5-minute or longer scrub with an iodophor soap. The area is blotted with a sterile towel and an antiseptic paint solution may be applied.
    - A sponge used to prep an area is never reapplied to an area previously prepped. The sponge should be discarded once the periphery is reached so that bacteria from adjacent nonprepped areas are not inadvertently transferred to the prepped area.
    - Prep solutions are not allowed to pool under the patient or flow under a tourniquet cuff or electrocautery dispersive electrode. Prep solutions that are allowed to pool have the potential to cause chemical burn. Folded towels should be placed at the periphery area to absorb excess fluid and prevent pooling.
    - The dirtiest areas are prepped last. Movement in all areas is from clean to dirty. In cases where skin is intact, and open wounds and body orifices are not part of the area to be prepped, the prep begins at the proposed line of incision. In cases where potentially contaminated areas are included in the prep area, the prep begins at the surrounding skin area. The umbilicus is cleaned separately with cotton-tip applicators. A colostomy or stoma is covered until the surrounding area is prepped and then prepped with a separate sponge. In a perineal prep the vagina and/or anus is prepped last with a separate sponge (see Figure 5–7). In a shoulder prep the axilla is prepped last.
    - For unusual wounds or incision sites when it may be difficult to know where to begin, nursing judgment must be used to decide upon the prep process that will result in reducing the number of microorganisms at the incision site to the lowest level possible.
57. In addition to the previous guidelines, the following considerations should be noted:
    - Eyes are washed with cotton balls with a nonirritating solution. The prep is begun at the nose and continues toward the cheeks. Warm sterile water may be used to rinse off the solution. The solution should not be allowed to pool on the patient's eyes.
    - For traumatic wounds, large amounts of irrigating solution may be used prior and in addition to the prep to remove dirt and debris.
    - When it is necessary to prep a limb, an additional person or apparatus is needed to hold the limb securely so the entire circumference can be prepped adequately and safely.

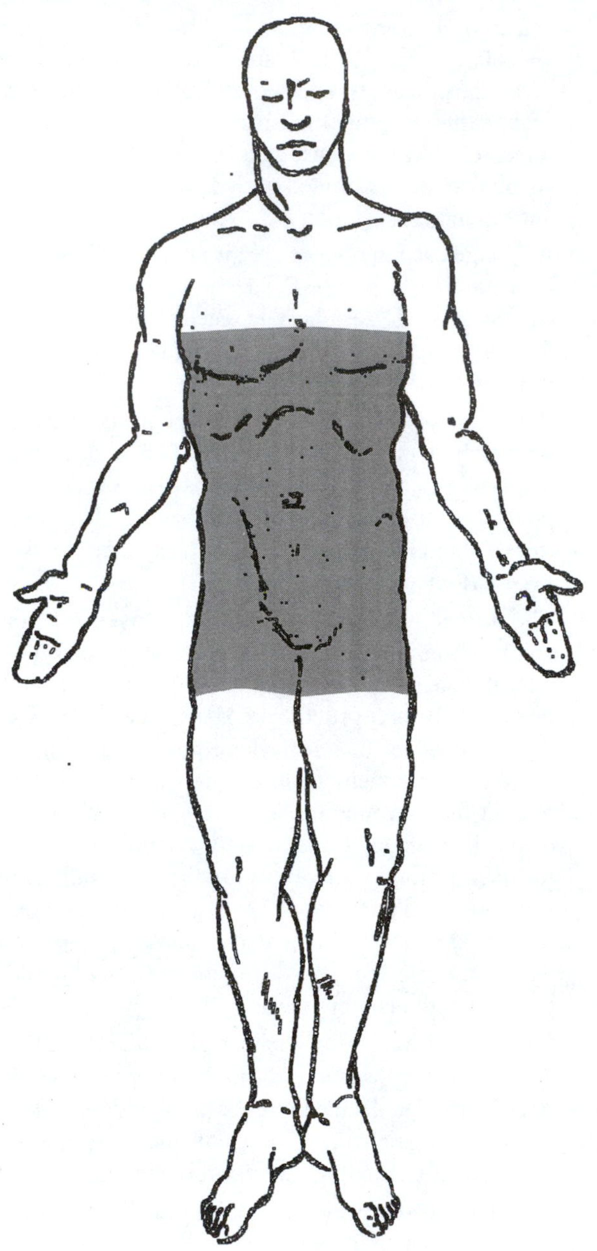

Figure 5–5 Abdomen Prep

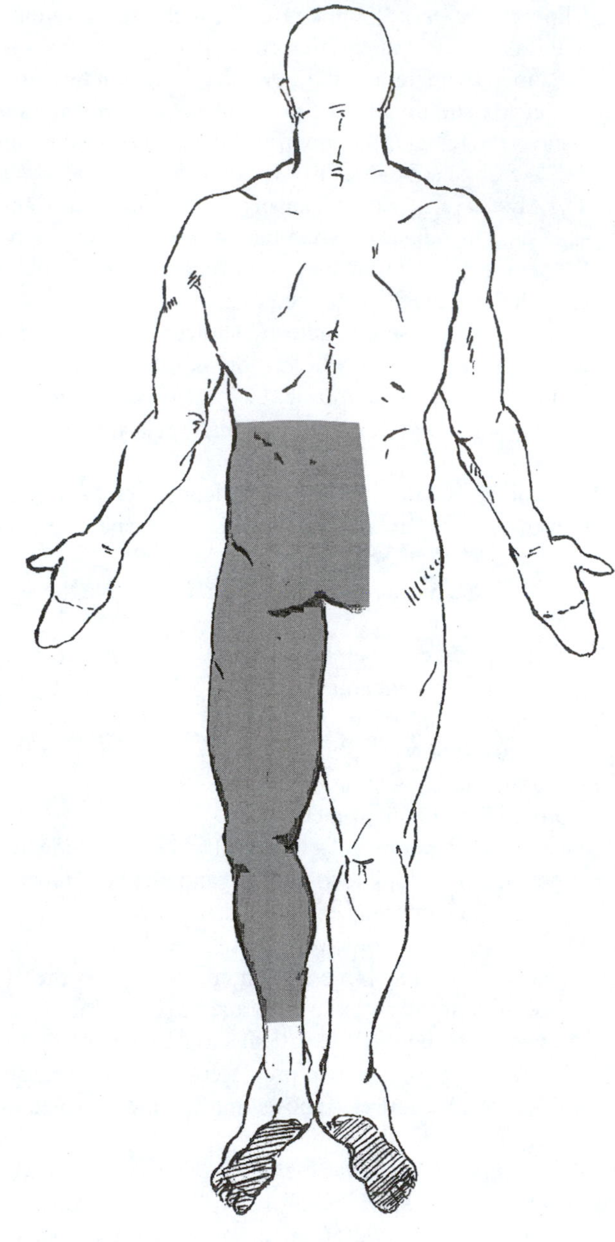

Figure 5–6 Hip Prep

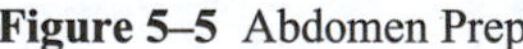

- A scrub brush may be useful for areas such as hands and feet. Care must be taken when using a scrub brush to avoid irritating tender skin or creating scratches and a portal of entry for bacteria.
- Warm prep solutions are preferable. They may help maintain body temperature and are more pleasing to the awake patient. Care must be taken not to overheat and possibly compromise the efficacy of the prep solution.
- During certain preps, such as for a malignant breast tumor, prepping must be gentle to prevent potential spread of cancer cells.
- If volatile prep solutions must be used, the surgery should not begin until the solution on the patient has

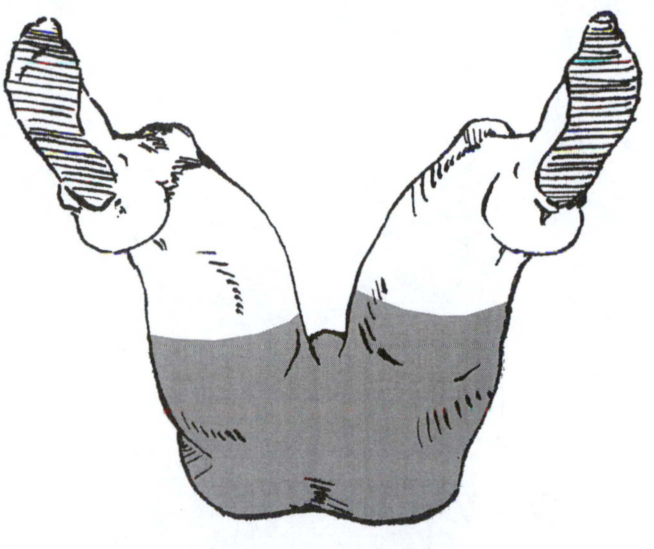

Figure 5–7 Perineum Prep

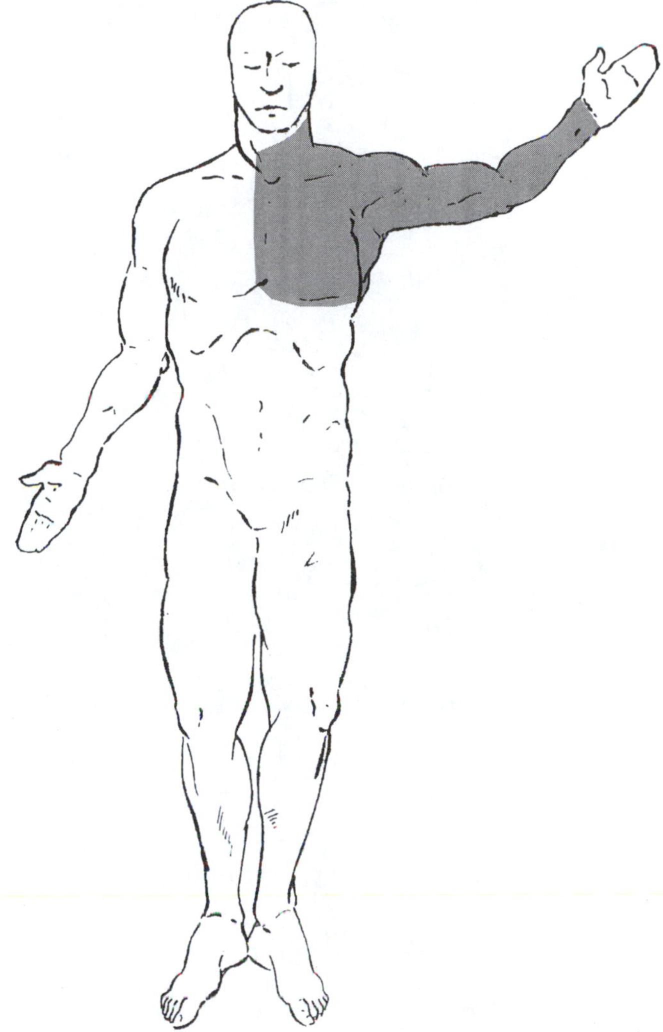

Figure 5–8 Shoulder Prep

dried. Equipment used in surgery may produce a spark with the potential to ignite volatile prep solutions.

58. Documentation of the skin prep should include the following:
    - assessment of the skin at the operative site
    - hair removal, if performed, including area, method, time, and person who removed hair
    - patient skin allergies or sensitivities
    - prep agents or solution
    - name of person performing the prep
    - patient response to prep, i.e., allergic reaction

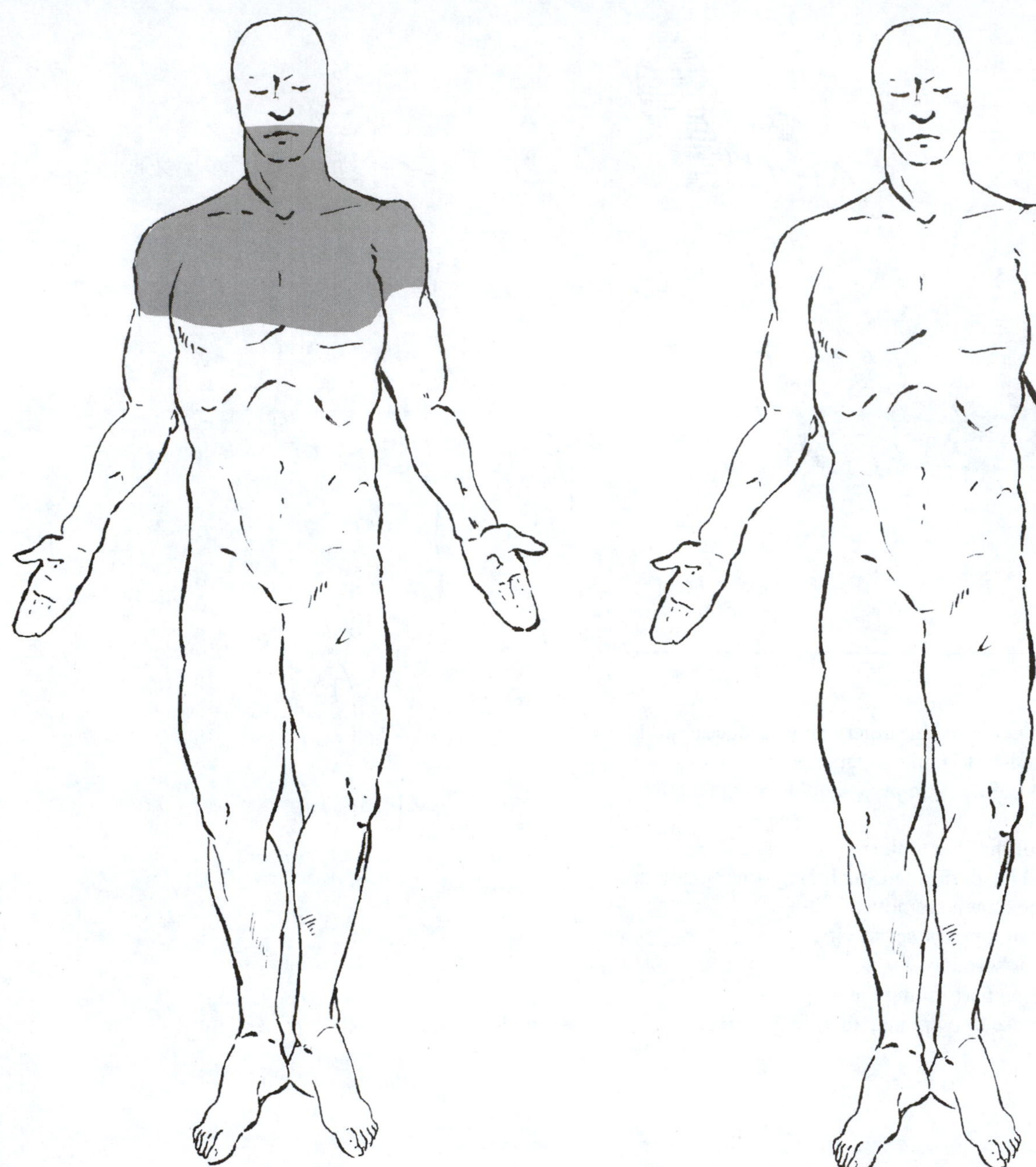

Figure 5–9 Head and Neck Prep

Figure 5–10 Hand Prep

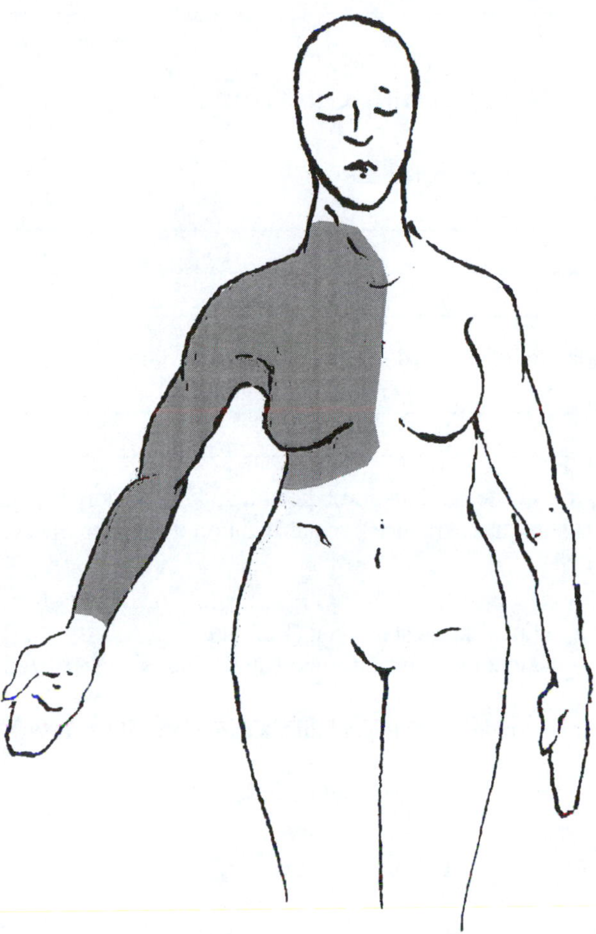

Figure 5–11 Breast Prep

Section Questions

Q9. Define what is meant by surgical conscience. (Ref. 36)

____

____

____

Q10. The parts of the sterile gown that are considered sterile include (Ref. 38a):

____

____

Q11. Before an item is dispensed to the sterile field the scrub person and the person dispensing the item are responsible for checking the item to ensure that parameters of sterilization have been met. (Ref. 38c)

True False

Q12. If the wrapper of a sterile packaged item has a stain on it (Ref. 38c):

a. and the wrapper is intact and the chemical indicator indicates it has been sterilized, the item may be dispensed to the sterile field
b. and the wrapper is dry and intact and the chemical indicator indicates it has been sterilized, the item may be dispensed to the field
c. it is considered contaminated and not dispensed to the sterile field

Q13. Define strike-through. (Ref. 38c)

____

____

Q14. It is proper aseptic technique for two scrubbed persons to pass each other back to front. (Ref. 38f)

True False

Q15. Sterile setups should be (Ref. 38e):

a. covered if surgery is delayed
b. monitored for possible contamination
c. prepared as close to the time of surgery as possible

Q16. Explain why it is important that shaving of the operative site, if it must be done, be performed as close to the time of surgery as possible. (Ref. 44)

____

____

Q17. List four desirable properties of an antimicrobial product used for a skin prep. (Ref. 51)

____

____

____

____

Q18. The surgical prep (Ref. 56, 57)
  a. is begun at the dirtiest area and progresses toward the incision
  b. begins at the incision and progresses toward the periphery
  c. must last at least 10 minutes
  d. should always be performed vigorously

Control of Personnel Sources of Infection

Attire

59. Personnel who work in the surgical suite are required to change into special operating room or surgical attire designed to interfere with the passage of microorganisms from personnel to the patient and the environment and from patient to personnel.
60. Appropriate surgical attire in the operating room suite includes hats or hoods, scrub outfits (commonly referred to as scrubs), and shoe covers (optional).
61. Hats or hoods are worn so that head and facial hair is completely covered. Hair is a gross contaminant and major source of bacteria. It attracts and sheds bacteria in proportion to its length, oiliness, and curliness. To prevent contamination of scrubs from hair or dandruff, a hat or hood should be the first item of apparel donned. Hair should not be combed once scrubs are donned. A hat or hood should be worn in areas where supplies are processed and stored. Hats are usually disposable. Reusable hats should be laundered when soiled and between each wearing. Hats should be removed and deposited in a designated receptacle before leaving the operating room suite.
62. Scrubs are either a one-piece coverup, such as a dress, or a two-piece shirt and pants set. Pants may be designed with stockinette cuffs to prevent shedding. Bacterial shedding is greater with a dress; therefore shirt and pants are preferable. To prevent shedding, the shirt must fit close to the body or be tucked into the pants. Scrubs may be made of a tightly woven reusable fabric that minimizes shedding or they may be disposable. Reusable scrubs should be freshly laundered under monitored laundry conditions, such as a hospital laundry where load mix, detergent, cycle time, and water temperature are controlled.
63. In addition to scrubs, unscrubbed or nonsterile team members should wear a warm-up jacket with long sleeves to prevent shedding from bare arms. Operating rooms are cool and warm-up jackets also serve to keep personnel warm. Warm-up jackets should be snapped or buttoned to prevent the edges from inadvertently coming into contact with and contaminating sterile supplies. Warm-up jackets may be reusable or disposable.
64. Hospital policy dictates whether scrubs are to be removed when leaving the operating room suite and fresh ones donned upon reentry or if cover gowns or lab coats must be worn over scrubs outside the operating room. There is insufficient research to determine whether changing of scrubs or use of cover gowns impacts surgical wound infection rates (AORN, 1995, p. 142). Surgical attire should be changed or removed when it becomes visibly soiled or wet. Fresh scrub attire should be worn each day.
65. High-filtration masks are worn in areas specifically designated according to hospital policy and should be worn in the presence of open sterile supplies (AORN, 1995, p. 142). Masks contain droplets expelled from the mouth and nasopharynx during talking, sneezing, and coughing. Masks should have a microbial filtration efficiency of 95% or greater against particles of 0.1 μm in size. Whether masks reduce risk of infection when worn by personnel who are not scrubbed and who are in forced ventilation systems is not clear and requires further research. For this reason policies on wearing of masks may vary.
66. Masks should cover the nose and mouth completely and securely. The mask contains a small malleable metal strip that should be pinched to conform to the nose to provide a secure, proper fit. The mask should be tied securely at the back of the head. Ties should not be crossed in order to prevent a gap from forming at the side of the mask that will allow unfiltered exhaled air to escape from the sides.
67. Masks with face shields or splash guards, or masks worn with protective eye wear, are worn whenever splashes, sprays, or aerosols of potentially infectious agents, such as blood, are anticipated.
68. Masks are either on or off and should not be left to dangle from the neck or folded and placed in a pocket for future use. Masks should be removed and discarded frequently and when they become wet. Masks should be removed and discarded by handling only the ties. Masks that have been worn are contaminated with droplet nu-

clei. Handling of the face portion of the mask after use can transfer microorganisms from the mask to the hands; therefore only the ties should be handled. Masks should be disposed of in a designated receptacle. Hands should be washed after mask removal.

69. Shoe covers are optional and have not been shown to contribute to reducing wound infection rates. The primary reason for their use is to facilitate sanitation (Groah, 1990, pp. 156–157). Shoe covers may be worn to protect personnel footwear from becoming soiled. Various length high-top shoe covers that cover the shoe and lower leg are appropriate when contact with copious or potentially infectious fluids is anticipated to occur on the legs and shoes of personnel.
70. Shoe covers should be removed and deposited in a designated receptacle before leaving the operating room suite. Removal of shoe covers can permit transfer of microorganisms from the shoe covers to the hands. Hands should be washed after shoe cover removal.
71. Although the impact of wearing jewelry on wound infection rates is unknown, jewelry easily harbors bacteria and therefore should be confined or removed. Confinement of jewelry also reduces the potential for it to fall onto the sterile field.
72. Nails should be short, clean, and free of chipped polish. Artificial nails should not be worn. Long nails may puncture protective gloves or scratch a patient during transfer. Artificial nails harbor greater numbers of bacteria than do natural nails (AORN, 1995, p. 143). Available data suggest that chipped nail polish, or polish worn more than 4 days, harbors greater numbers of bacteria than natural nails or freshly polished nails (Pottinger, Burns, & Manske, 1989, p. 340).
73. Other attire worn to protect personnel from infectious agents includes gloves, liquid-resistant aprons, and gowns.
74. Personnel who scrub for surgery are referred to as members of the sterile team or scrubbed persons. In addition to wearing appropriate operating-room attire, scrubbed persons must scrub their hands and arms with an antimicrobial detergent and don sterile gowns and gloves prior to surgery.

Scrubbing, Gowning, and Gloving

75. The surgical scrub is an activity performed immediately prior to gowning and gloving in preparation for surgery. The purpose of the surgical hand scrub is to remove dirt, skin oils, and transient microorganisms; to reduce the amount of resident microorganisms on the nails, hands, and lower arms to as low a level as possible; and to prevent growth of microorganisms for as long as possible. This is accomplished through mechanical washing and chemical antisepsis.
76. Mechanical washing is the removal of dirt, oils, and microorganisms by means of friction. Antisepsis is the prevention of sepsis by the exclusion, destruction, or inhibition of growth or multiplication of microorganisms from body tissues and fluids.
77. The purpose of the surgical scrub is to prevent the transfer of microorganisms from personnel to patients and from patients to personnel in the event of glove tears or gown penetration.
78. Prior to scrubbing, all jewelry must be removed from hands and arms. All other jewelry must also be removed or be completely contained. Hands and arms should be examined for cuts and other lesions that could ooze serum, which is a medium for microbial growth and serves as a potential means of transmission of microorganisms into the patient. Persons with cuts and abrasions should not scrub.
79. Personnel with respiratory infections should not scrub.
80. An antimicrobial soap or detergent with the following properties should be used for the surgical scrub:
    - broad spectrum of activity (effective against gram-negative and gram-positive organisms)
    - rapid acting
    - nontoxic or nonabrasive to skin
    - not dependent on cumulative action (the first application is as effective as subsequent applications)
    - rapid growth of microorganisms inhibited
81. Commonly accepted antimicrobial scrub agents are providone-iodine, chlorhexidine gluconate, and triclosan. Parachlorometaxylenol (PCMX) and a nonmedicated soap scrub followed by application of an alcohol-based cleanser is appropriate for persons who are sensitive to providone-iodine and chlorhexidine gluconate (AORN, 1995, p. 187).

Scrub Procedure.

82. The surgical scrub should be performed according to hospital policy, which should specify the agent and the method to be used. Manufacturer's recommendations and supporting literature regarding use of the agent should be incorporated into policy.
83. Most scrub policies call for an anatomical scrub or a timed scrub. In either method, the scrub should include cleaning and scrubbing of all surfaces of each nail, finger, hand, and arm to 2 inches above the elbow.
84. Anatomical scrubs may indicate the number of strokes to be applied to each area to be scrubbed. The entire surface to be scrubbed is broken into specified areas with a specified number of strokes for each area. For example,

each finger has four surfaces each of which is scrubbed a specified number of times.

85. Timed scrubs specify the length of time a scrub should last and may specify how long the scrub should last on each specified surface. The number of strokes and time may both be incorporated into a scrub policy.
86. Scrub policies have traditionally called for a 5-minute or longer scrub.
87. The Association of Operating Room Nurses does not specify the length of time that a scrub should last.
88. The American College of Surgeons states that a 120-second scrub is adequate.
89. The Association for Practitioners in Infection Control (APIC) has recently published surgical scrub guidelines that "recommend applying an antimicrobial agent to wet hands and forearm with friction for at least 120 seconds" (APIC, 1995, p. 13).
90. Basic steps included in all scrub procedures include the following:
    - The faucet is turned on with water set at a comfortable temperature.
    - Hands are washed with a surgical scrub agent and rinsed.
    - The packaged scrub brush (if used) containing nail cleaner is opened.
    - Nail cleaner and brush are removed from the package.
    - The brush is held in one hand and under running water, the nail cleaner is used to clean nails and subungual spaces on the other hand.
    - The process is repeated with the opposite hand.
    - The nail cleaner is discarded.
    - Nails and hands are rinsed.
    - The brush, if it is impregnated with antimicrobial soap, is moistened. If the brush is not impregnated with antimicrobial soap, an antimicrobial soap is added to the hands, usually from a foot-pump container.
    - The arms are held in a flexed position with the fingertips pointing upward. Throughout the scrub, the hands are held up and away from the body. The elbows are flexed and the hands held higher than the elbows. Water and cleanser flow from the fingertips (the cleanest area) to the elbow and into the sink.
    - Using circular motion and pressure adequate to remove microorganisms but not sufficient to abrade skin, the nails, fingers, hands, and arms are methodically scrubbed beginning with the fingertips and continuing to 2 inches above the elbow. Care is taken not to splash water onto surgical attire. Wet surgical attire can cause the transfer of microorganisms from personnel to the sterile gown worn during surgery.
    - The scrub brush is discarded.
    - The hands and arms are rinsed. Arms are flexed with hands above elbows as the scrubbed person enters the operating room.

Gowning and Gloving Procedure.

91. A gown package containing a sterile towel and sterile gown is opened on a small table, separate from the instrument or back table, within the operating room. The gown and towel are packaged so that when it is opened the towel is on top of the gown. The gown is folded inside out and from bottom to top in such a manner that the top inside portion of the gown is directly beneath the towel. The towel and gown may be reusable or disposable.
92. After scrubbing, the hands and arms must be thoroughly dried before the gown is donned. If the hands and arms are not thoroughly dried, contamination of the gown may occur by strike-through from organisms contained in moisture on the skin.
93. The scrub person grasps the sterile towel and lifts it straight up and away from the gown without dripping water on the gown or the sterile field. The scrub person steps away from the sterile field and allows the towel to unfold without contacting the scrub attire. If the towel contacts an unsterile surface, the towel is considered contaminated and a new one is used.
94. The top half of the towel is held in one hand while the opposite hand and forearm are dried. To decrease the risk of contamination, a rotating motion beginning at the hand and working toward the elbow is used for drying. When the first hand and forearm are dry, the lower half of the towel that is unused is grasped with the dry hand, and the opposite hand and forearm are then dried. Care is taken not to return to an area that is already dried.
95. Sterile gowns may be reusable or disposable. The gown should be constructed of a material that provides a barrier to prevent the passage of microorganisms from the surgical team to the patient and from the patient to the surgical team.
96. Gowns should be fire retardant, as lint free as possible, free from tears or holes, and fluid resistant or fluid proof. Fluid *proof* gowns are coated or laminated with an impervious film that does not permit penetration of fluids. Fluid *resistant* gowns provide an effective barrier and do not permit ready penetration of liquids. Fluid-resistant gowns should be worn whenever splashes or spraying of blood or other infectious fluids is anticipated. Where large amounts of fluid are anticipated fluid-proof gowns should be worn.
97. Reusable gowns eventually lose their barrier qualities with repeated laundering. Quality monitoring should be

in place to ensure that only gowns of appropriate quality are used.

98. The forearms and portions of the gown above the waist are made with a water-repellent material. The cuffs are stockinette and fit tight to the wrist. Gowns may or may not be wraparound style and are held closed with cotton tapes, snaps, or Velcro fasteners.
99. Using the following procedure, the scrubbed person dons the sterile gown:
    - The sterile gown is grasped by the inside neckline and lifted away from the gown wrapper.
    - Holding the gown by the neck edge, the scrub person moves away from areas of possible contamination and lets the gown unfold downward.
    - The scrub person locates the armholes, and both arms are simultaneously inserted into the sleeves. If a closed-gloving technique is intended to be utilized, the arms are inserted into the gown only until the hands reach the proximal edge of the cuff. If an open-gloving technique is intended, the arms are inserted into the gown until the hands advance through the cuffs.
    - The gown is fastened in the back at the neckline and the waist by a nonsterile team member.
    - Gloves are donned.
    - After gloving is completed, the scrubbed person extends a paper tab, attached to one of the gown ties, to another team member (sterile or unsterile). The scrub person then pivots away from the other team member, causing the gown to wrap around the scrub person. The scrub person then grasps the tie and pulls it, releasing it from the paper tab. The scrub person then ties the gown securely in front. If a tab is not included with the gown, the scrub person may attach a sterile instrument to the end of one tie and hand it to another unsterile team member who utilizes the instrument in the same manner as a paper tab (see Figure 5–12).
100. Sterile gloves are a barrier that is intended to prevent passage of microorganisms from the scrubbed person to the patient and from the patient to the scrubbed person.
101. Gloves should be selected according to desired strength, durability, and compatibility. Extra-strength specialty gloves are available for procedures, such as bone and joint surgeries, where risk of percutaneous blood exposure is high.
102. Latex-free gloves must be used where personnel or the patient have latex allergies. Hypoallergenic and powder-free gloves should be chosen for personnel sensitive to glove chemicals and powders.
103. Sterile gloves should be rinsed or wiped with sterile water or sterile saline prior to the surgical incision in order to remove glove powders that can incite an inflammatory response and delay healing if introduced into the patient (Ellis, 1990).
104. Closed gloving is a method of donning sterile gloves whereby the scrubbed hands remain inside the gown sleeve until the glove cuff is secured over the gown cuff.
105. Closed gloving is begun with the hands inside the sleeves. Using the right hand that is still inside the right cuff, the scrub person grasps the left glove by the glove's everted cuff.
106. The left forearm is extended with the palm facing up and the hand still inside the sleeve. The left glove is then placed palm side down on the upturned left sleeve, palm to palm, thumb to thumb, with the fingers of the glove pointing toward the scrubbed person's body. Using the left thumb and index finger, the glove cuff is grasped through the stockinette cuff and the glove is held in place. The fingers of the left hand must not extend beyond the stockinette cuff to grasp the glove. With the use of the sleeve-covered right hand, the cuff of the left glove is then stretched over the open end of the left sleeve. The glove should totally encompass the stockinette portion of the sleeve. The sleeve-covered right hand is then used to exert an even pull on the left sleeve of the gown, causing the left hand to slide into the glove.
107. To glove the right hand, the right glove is grasped with the already gloved left hand and placed on the right sleeve, palm to palm, thumb to thumb, with glove fingers pointing toward the scrub person's body. With the use of the right thumb and index finger, the right glove cuff is grasped through the stockinette cuff and held in place. The fingers of the right hand must not extend beyond the stockinette cuff to hold the glove in place. With the gloved left hand, the right glove is stretched over the open end of the right sleeve. The left hand is then used to pull lightly and evenly on the right sleeve, causing the right hand to slide into the right glove (see Figure 5–13).
108. In the open-glove technique the scrub person extends the hands through the stockinette cuff of the sleeves when donning the gown. During gloving, the surgically clean hand touches only the inside of the sterile glove and never contacts the exterior of the glove.
109. The gloves are opened by a nonscrubbed person on a clean, dry surface. Using the right hand, the scrub person grasps the everted cuff of the left glove and slides the fingers and thumb of the left hand into the glove, leaving the everted cuff of the glove over the hand and below the cuff of the gown sleeve. The scrub person

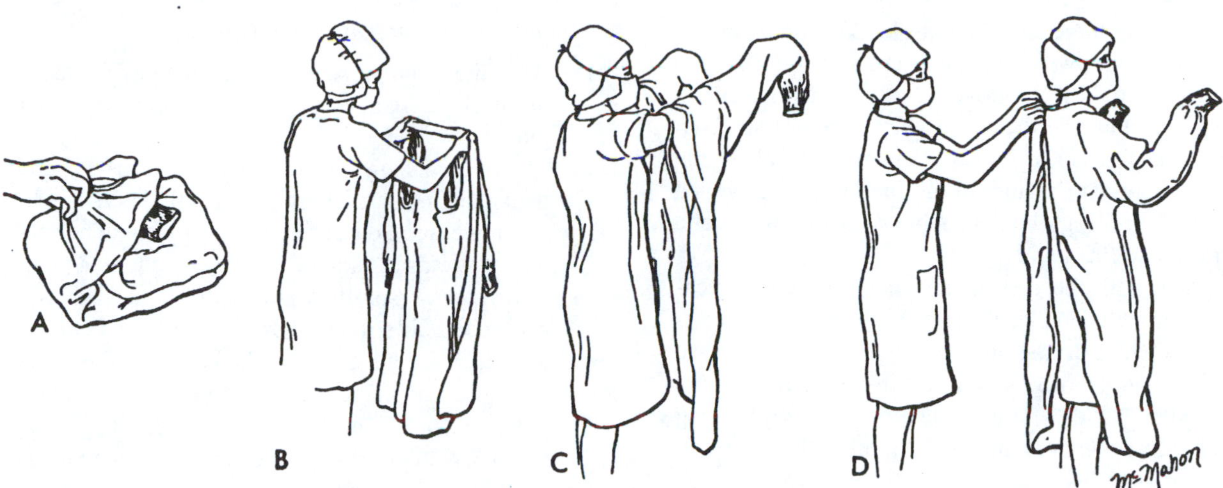

Figure 5–12 Gowning Self. Technique for gowning oneself. **A**, Grasp the gown firmly and bring it away from the table. It has been folded so that the outside faces away. **B**, Holding the gown at the shoulders, allow it to unfold gently. Do not shake the gown. **C**, Place hands inside the armholes and guide each arm through the sleeves by raising and spreading the arms. Do not allow hands to slide outside cuff of gown. **D**, The circulator will assist by pulling the gown up over the shoulders and tying it. *Source:* Reprinted with permission from J.R. Fuller, *Surgical Technology: Principles and Practice*, 2nd ed., p. 45, © 1986, W.B. Saunders Company.

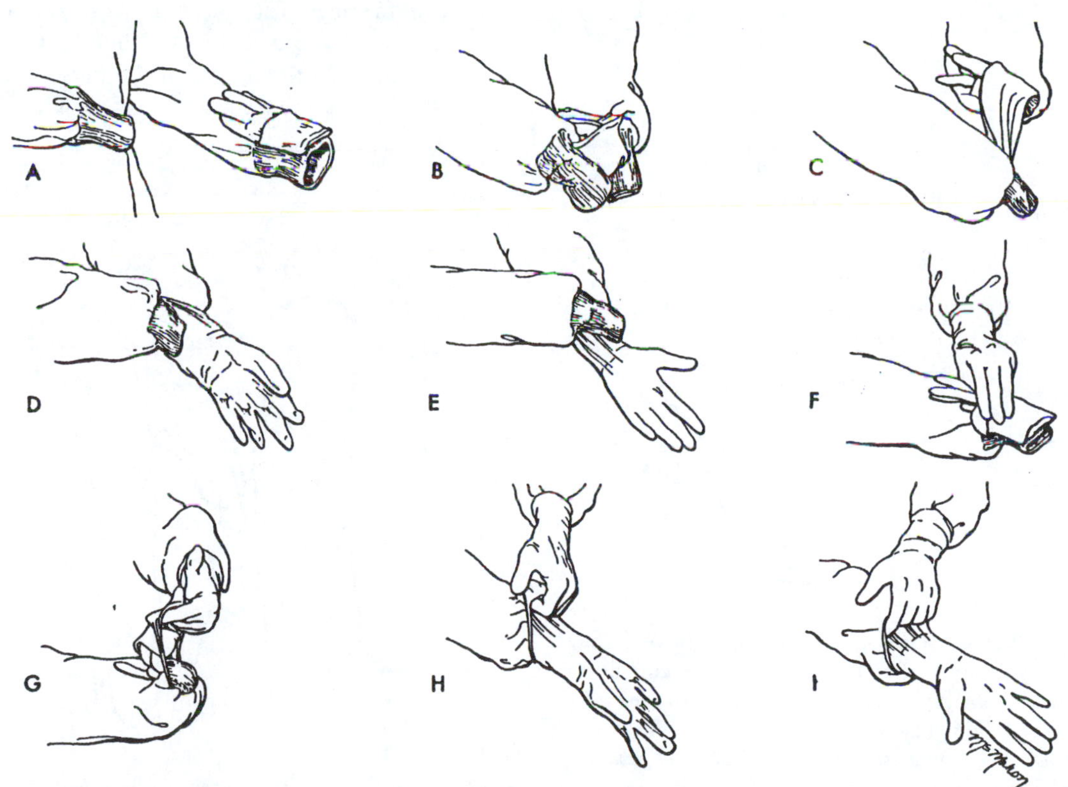

Figure 5–13 Closed Gloving. Gloving self—closed technique. **A**, Lay the glove palm down over the cuff of the gown. The fingers of the glove face toward you. **B** and **C**, Working through the gown sleeve, grasp the cuff of the glove and bring it over the open cuff of the sleeve. **D** and **E**, Unroll the glove cuff so that it covers the sleeve cuff. **F**, **G**, **H**, and **I**, Proceed with the opposite hand, using the same technique. Never allow the bare hand to contact the gown cuff edge or outside of glove. *Source:* Reprinted with permission from J.R. Fuller, *Surgical Technology: Principles and Practice*, 2nd ed., p. 46, © 1986, W.B. Saunders Company.

then slips the fingers of the left gloved hand under the everted cuff of the right glove and slides the fingers and hand into the right glove. The everted glove cuff is brought up and over the cuff of the gown. Care is taken to prevent the sterile gloved hand from touching the skin of the wrist or hand. In the final step, the everted cuff of the right glove is brought over the stockinette cuff of the right sleeve.

110. Although both the closed- and the open-glove techniques are acceptable, the closed-glove technique is often preferred. In the open-glove technique there is a greater chance of the scrub person's bare hands contacting the outside of the sterile glove, thereby causing it to become contaminated (see Figure 5–14).

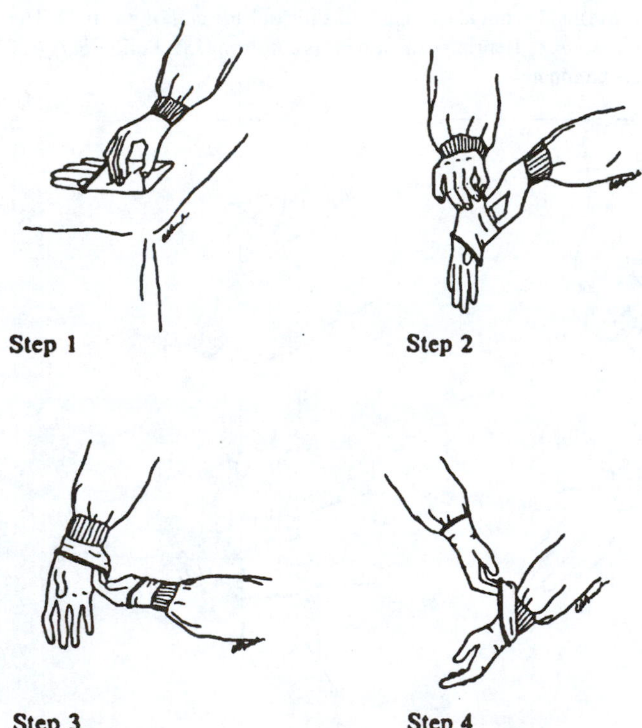

Figure 5–14 Open Gloving. Open-glove technique. Step 1, The glove is picked up by the top surface of the folded-down cuff. Step 2, The glove is held by the inner surface and pulled onto the left hand. Step 3, The right glove is picked up by grasping the glove under the folded-down cuff with the gloved left hand. The glove is pulled onto the hand and the cuff of the glove flipped up and over the cuff of the gown. Step 4, With the gloved right hand the turned-down cuff of the left glove is flipped up and over the cuff of the gown. *Source:* Reprinted with permission from L.C. Crooks (Ed.), *Operating Room Technologies for the Surgical Team*, p. 19, © 1979, Little, Brown & Company.

Assisting Others to Gown and Glove.

111. After the scrub person has donned a gown and gloves, he or she assists other team members to gown and glove.
112. The scrub person extends a towel to a newly scrubbed person, being careful not to touch that person's hands. The towel should be presented by placing one end over the outstretched hand of the newly scrubbed person.
113. The scrub person then grasps the folded gown at the neck edge, lifts it away from the sterile field, and allows it to unfold. Keeping the hands on the outside of the gown and using the neck and shoulder area of the gown to form a protective cuff over the gloves, the scrub person offers the inside of the gown to the newly scrubbed team member.
114. The newly scrubbed person will don the gown by inserting the arms into the sleeves and extending the hands through the stockinette cuff of the gown. A nonsterile team member will then secure the gown at the neck and waist area (see Figure 5–15).
115. The scrub person will then glove the newly scrubbed team member. The sterile glove is grasped under the everted edge and held so the thumb of the glove is in opposition to the thumb of the person being gloved. The cuff is then stretched open wide. The newly

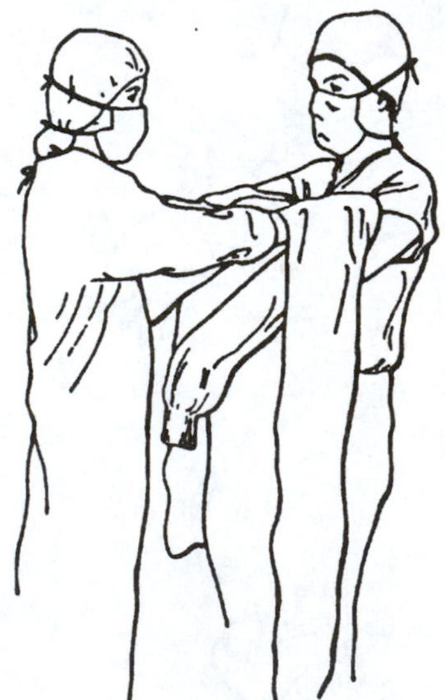

Figure 5–15 Gowning Others. Using the outside of the gown neck and shoulder area to form a protective cuff over her gloves the scrub person offers a gown to the newly scrubbed team member. *Source:* Reprinted with permission from J.R. Fuller, *Surgical Technology: Principles and Practice,* 2nd ed., p. 48, © 1986, W.B. Saunders Company.

gowned person then advances a hand into the glove. The cuff of the glove must be stretched wide enough and high enough to cover the stockinette gown cuff entirely. This procedure is repeated to glove the other hand.

116. Double gloving may be indicated for certain surgical procedures where risk of percutaneous exposure to bloodborne pathogens is high. Individual institutional policies, sound judgment, and knowledge of surgical procedures should influence the decision of whether to wear two pairs of gloves.
117. If a team member's glove becomes contaminated, that person steps back from the sterile field and extends the contaminated hand to a nonsterile team member who dons protective gloves and removes the sterile team member's contaminated glove by grasping the outside of the glove approximately 2 inches below the top of the glove and pulling the glove off inside out. Care must be taken that the gown cuff not be pulled down or slip down over the hand because the gown cuff is considered contaminated once the original gloves are donned. The scrub person may reglove the team member in the same manner as previously performed, or the open-glove technique can be used to reglove without assistance.
118. If a team member's gown becomes contaminated, a nonsterile team member dons protective gloves and unfastens the gown at the neck and waist, grasps it at the shoulders, and pulls it forward and off over the scrubbed person's hands, which are still gloved. The gown should come off inside out. The nonsterile team member then removes the sterile team member's gloves and the scrub person regowns and regloves the team member. The contaminated gown should always be removed *before* the gloves are removed. This prevents microorganisms and debris that may be found on the gown from being dragged across unprotected, ungloved hands.
119. The closed-glove technique is not acceptable for changing a contaminated glove. During initial gowning and gloving, the scrubbed, but not sterile, ungloved hand passes through the gown cuff, causing the cuff to be considered contaminated. In the closed-glove technique the cuff contacts the sterile glove; therefore the new sterile glove would be contaminated by the contaminated cuff.
120. At the completion of surgery, the gown and gloves are removed. The gown is removed first. It is grasped near the neck and sleeve and brought forward over the gloved hands, inverting the gloves as it is removed. The gown is folded so the contaminated outside surface is on the inside. It is deposited in a designated linen basket or waste receptacle.
121. Gloves are removed so that bare skin does not contact the contaminated external glove. The gloved fingers of one hand are placed under the everted glove cuff of the opposite hand and pulled off. The fold on the remaining glove is grasped with the bare fingers of the opposite hand and the glove is pulled off. This technique must be performed carefully to prevent bare skin from contacting the contaminated glove surface. Gloves are deposited in a designated waste receptacle.
122. After gloves are removed, the hands are washed with an approved detergent. Hand washing lessens the chance of contamination of the hands that may have occurred from an invisible hole or tear in the glove.
123. Gown and gloves are not worn outside the operating room.

Creating a Sterile Field—Draping

124. Drapes serve as a barrier to prevent the passage of microorganisms between sterile and nonsterile areas. Sterile drapes are used to create a sterile surface around the incision site that may be used for sterile supplies and equipment. This area is referred to as the sterile field.
125. The sterile field includes the patient, furniture, and other equipment that is covered with sterile drapes (see Figure 5–16). The sterile field is isolated from unsterile surfaces and items. Only sterile items are placed on a sterile field.
126. Sterile drapes are positioned over the patient in such a way that only a minimum area of skin around the incision site is exposed.
127. Frequently draped furniture includes instrument tables, Mayo stands (see Figure 5–17), and the instrument or "back" tables.
128. Drapes may be reusable or disposable. Criteria for drapes are that they be
    - resistant to blood and liquid penetration and provide an effective barrier to prevent passage of microorganisms from nonsterile to sterile areas
    - lint free to reduce airborne contamination or shedding into the operative site—microorganisms and dust particles may settle on airborne lint and shed into the operative site
    - flame resistant—meet the standards of the National Fire Prevention Association
    - memory free—easily conform to body and equipment contours
    - comfortable

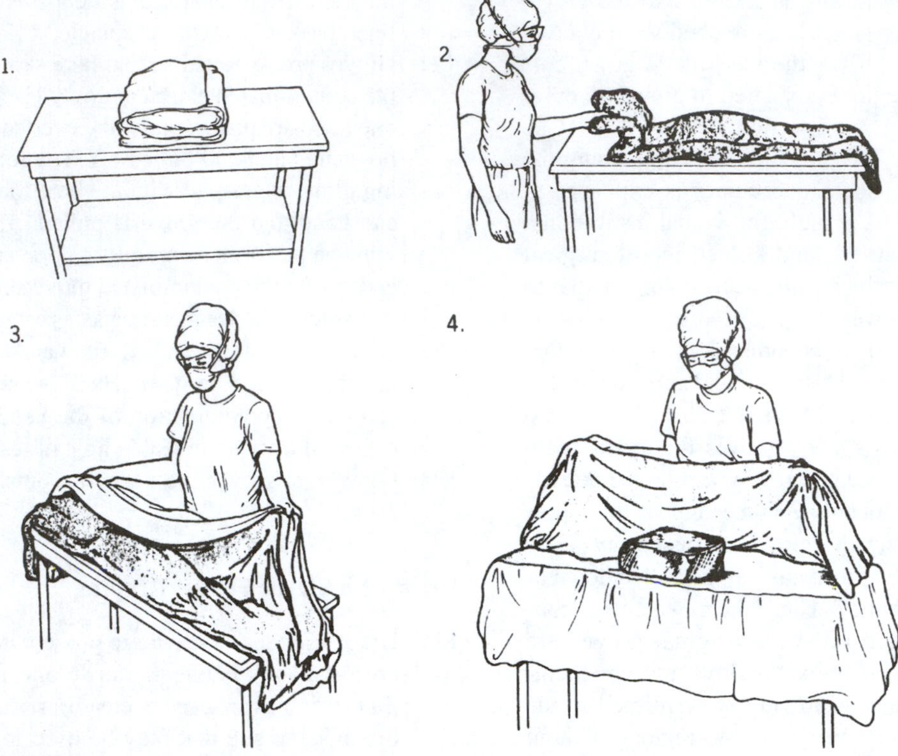

Figure 5–16 Draping a Table. *Source:* Reprinted with permission from S.S. Fairchild, *Perioperative Nursing: Principles and Practice,* pp. 235–236, © 1993, Little, Brown & Company.

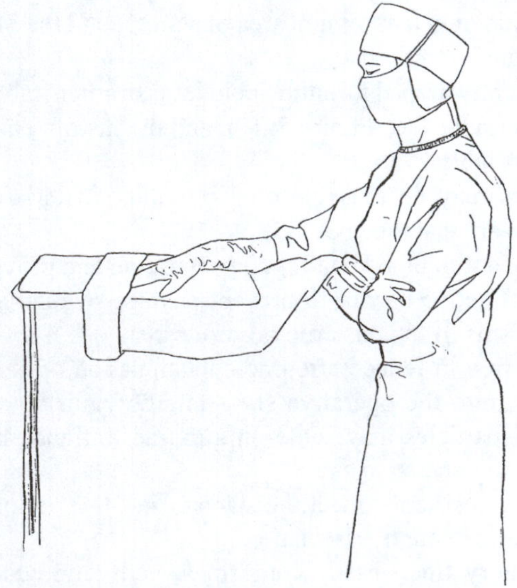

Figure 5–17 Draping the Mayo Stand

129. As with gowns, drapes may be fluid resistant or fluid proof. Materials that are liquid resistant have varying degrees of resistance.
130. Both reusable and disposable drapes are used. Reusable drapes are manufactured in a variety of fabrics with varying degrees of barrier effectiveness. All reusable drapes will, however, over time, lose their barrier qualities with repeated laundering and sterilizations. Laundering and steam sterilization swells fibers and drying shrinks them. This reduces the tightness of the fibers and causes ultimate loss of barrier effectiveness. The number of times a drape has been laundered should be tracked. Some reusable drapes contain a grid for this purpose. All reusable drapes, however, must be routinely inspected for tears and punctures.
131. Disposable drapes are composed of nonwoven natural and synthetic materials also manufactured with varying degrees of barrier effectiveness. These fabrics include a fluid-proof polyethylene film laminated be-

tween the fabric layers at strategic locations of the drape, usually around the drape fenestration. Nonwoven drapes are available in a variety of configurations and are commercially packaged and sterilized. They are designed for one-time use and are not resterilized.

132. Clear plastic drapes with or without adhesive backings are available in various sizes. They are available plain or impregnated with iodophor. These are applied directly over the skin over the operative site. They may be partially applied over the drapes, in which case they assist in keeping the drapes in place without the use of towel clips. The incision is made through the plastic drape.
133. These drapes are particularly useful for draping irregular body areas such as joints and ears. Plastic drapes may be used to seal off a contaminated area such as a stoma.
134. Excess use of plastic drapes may cause retention of heat and raise the patient's body temperature (Belkin, 1992, p. 1522).
135. Impervious polyvinyl drapes are available for equipment and specialty needs such as sealing off the perineal area, to cover a tourniquet, or to contain body fluids and irrigation.

Draping Guidelines

136. The following guidelines should be followed during draping:
    - Only sterile drapes that are intact are used for draping. All defects must have been patched with a vulcanized heat seal patch.
    - Drapes should be handled as little as possible.
    - Drapes are carried folded to the operating table and are not allowed to drop below the waist of the scrubbed person carrying the drapes. The area below the level of the waist is considered contaminated and drapes that fall below this level are discarded.
    - Draping is done from the operative site to the periphery.
    - One must not reach across the unsterile area of the operating table to drape the opposite side. All draping is done from the appropriate side.
    - Once a drape is placed, it is not moved or repositioned. Drapes that are incorrectly placed are removed by an unscrubbed person.
    - When draping, a cuff is formed from the drape to protect sterile gloved hands.
    - A towel clip that has been positioned through a drape has its points contaminated and must not be removed until completion of the procedure.
    - Drapes are gently placed. They are not flipped or shaken. Shaking and flipping causes air currents that are a vehicle for dust, lint, and droplet nuclei.
    - Whenever the sterility of a drape is in doubt it is considered contaminated and is not used (see Figure 5–18).

Standard Drapes

137. The amount, type, and size of drapes that are selected for a procedure require careful planning. Selection factors will include the type of procedure to be performed, the amount of area around the incision that should be included in the sterile field, and furniture and equipment that will be draped. Cost considerations require that variety and amount of drapes be kept to a minimum.
138. Standard drapes include
    - flat sheets used to drape instrument tables and areas of the patient
    - Mayo stand covers
    - towels used to drape the operative site
    - fenestrated drapes with openings of various sizes and configurations to drape for specific procedures (typical types include abdominal laparotomy, chest/breast, head and neck, and extremity); fenestrations are generally reinforced with an impervious barrier; the fenestrated drape is large enough to cover the entire patient and the operating table with sufficient material to extend over the foot of the table, the ether screen at the head of the table, and the arm boards.
    - aperture drape—a small clear fenestrated plastic drape frequently used in eye and ear procedures
    - equipment drapes—clear plastic drapes that cover x-ray, microscopic, and other equipment
    - stockinette drape used to drape feet and hands
    - leggings—part of drape set intended for surgery with the patient in the lithotomy position

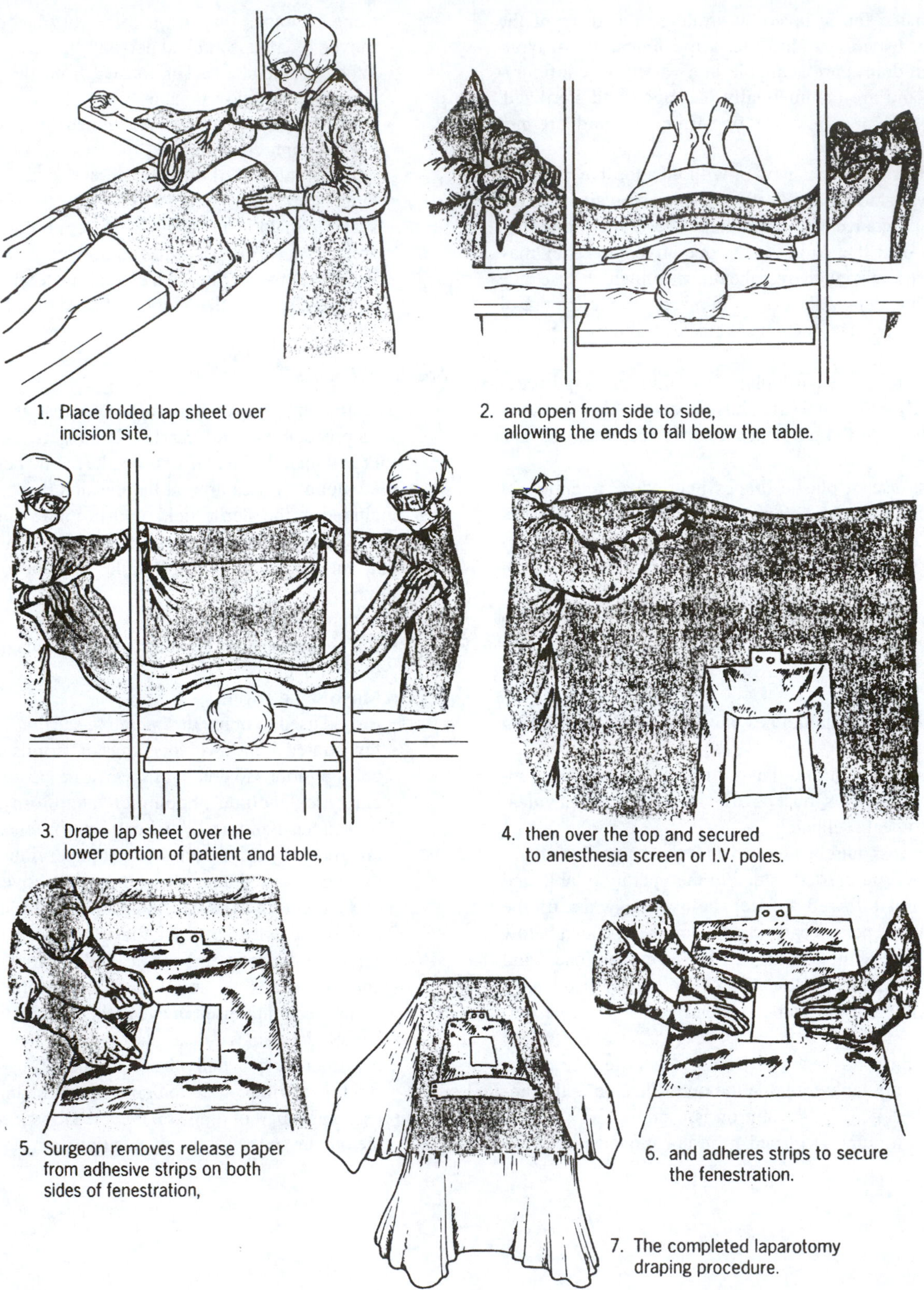

Figure 5–18 Draping the Patient. *Source:* Reprinted with permission from S.S. Fairchild, *Perioperative Nursing: Principles and Practice*, p. 248, © 1993, Little, Brown & Company.

Section Questions

Q19. Scrub attire (Ref. 62, 64):
- a. should be changed when it becomes wet
- b. should be laundered between wearings
- c. may be laundered either at home or a hospital laundry

Q20. Explain why mask ties should not be crossed before being tied at the back of the head. (Ref. 66)

____

____

Q21. Shoe covers (Ref. 69):
- a. decrease risk of infection
- b. protect personnel footwear

Q22. The purpose of the surgical scrub is (Ref. 75):
- a. to sterilize the hands of the scrubbed person
- b. to remove dirt and skin oils
- c. to remove transient microorganisms
- d. to reduce the number of resident microorganisms
- e. to prevent growth of microorganisms for as long as possible

Q23. The surgical scrub (Ref. 83, 84, 85):
- a. may be timed or anatomical
- b. should include the nails, fingers, hands, and arms to 2 inches below the elbow
- c. should always last 6 minutes or more

Q24. During the surgical scrub the hands are held away from the body and higher than the elbows. (Ref. 90)

True False

Q25. Repeated laundering will cause a fluid-proof gown to lose its barrier qualities over time. (Ref. 97)

True False

Q26. Explain why it is good practice for the scrub person to wipe his/her sterile gloves with sterile water prior to the surgical incision. (Ref. 103)

____

____

Q27. Regarding gloving (Ref. 110, 116, 119, 120):
- a. During initial gloving the open- and closed-gloving techniques are both acceptable.
- b. When a glove becomes contaminated and a new one is donned, the closed-glove technique is preferable.
- c. Wearing two pairs of gloves is acceptable practice.
- d. At the completion of surgery the sterile team members should remove their gloves only after they remove their gowns.

Q28. Explain how drapes assist in the creation of a sterile field. (Ref. 124)

___

___

Q29. Explain why it is important for drapes to be as lint free as possible. (Ref. 128)

___

___

Q30. If a drape is incorrectly placed on the patient it must be carefully repositioned by the scrub person. (Ref. 136)

True False

Q31. Explain why a towel clip that has been positioned through a sterile drape is not removed until after surgery. (Ref. 136)

___

___

Control of Environmental Sources of Infection

Operating Room Environment

139. The operating room is considered a clean environment. The design of the operating room, its location within the health care facility, limited access, traffic patterns, and policies and procedures for control and cleaning of the environment help to maintain its cleanliness.
140. The operating room has a separate ventilation and air filtration system. Filters are designed to remove dust and aerosol particles from the air. Air flow is from ceiling to floor.
141. Air is directed into the operating room under positive pressure. The air pressure is higher in each operating room than in the hallways so that the more contaminated hallway air is not pulled into the room. (The exception to positive-pressure air flow is for rooms specifically designed for procedures that should be performed in a negative-pressure environment.) Because of this pressure difference, doors to each operating room must be kept closed to prevent disruption of the air flow.
142. To maintain the cleanest air possible, a majority of operating rooms adhere to the standards identified in Guidelines for Construction and Equipment of Hospitals and Medical Facilities, which require an air flow rapid enough to change the total volume of air in each operating room a minimum of 15 times per hour with at least three exchanges of outside air (Bartley, 1993, p. 13). Although the minimum is 15 air exchanges, most conventional operating rooms are ventilated with 20 to 25 changes per hour. Ventilation systems must comply with local, state, and national regulations, which may vary in the requirement for the number of air exchanges per hour, whether the air can be recirculated, or if it must be fresh.
143. Laminar air-flow systems may be found in some operating rooms. A laminar air-flow system is an unidirectional ventilation system in which filtered, bacteria-free air is circulated over the patient from a filtered outlet and returned through a receiving air inlet. Only sterile items are permitted within the area across which the filtered air flows. The value of such systems is a subject of disagreement (Pittet & Ducel, 1994, p. 459).
144. Room temperature is maintained between 70°F and 75°F. This is comfortable enough for the surgical team yet will inhibit bacterial growth. Relative humidity that is maintained at 50% to 60% slows bacterial growth and also reduces the potential for static electricity (Bartley, 1993, p. 15).

Traffic Patterns

145. To reduce potential contamination from outside sources, the operating-room suite is usually located away from major traffic areas within the facility.

146. The operating room itself is divided into three areas that are defined by the activities that occur within each area. These areas are restricted, semirestricted, and unrestricted.
147. The restricted area is where surgical procedures are performed and sterile supplies are unwrapped and sterilized. This area includes the operating rooms, scrub-sink areas, and the clean core. Hats, scrubs, and masks are required in this area. Although individual institutional policy may not require masks to be worn in this area unless sterile supplies are open, masks are recommended by the Association of Operating Room Nurses (AORN, 1995, p. 283).
148. The semirestricted area includes storage and instrument-processing areas and corridors leading to restricted areas. Depending on the design of the suite, lounges may be included in the semirestricted area. Hats and scrubs are required in the semirestricted area. Only authorized personnel and patients are permitted in this area.
149. The unrestricted area is where operating room personnel interface with outside departmental personnel, locker rooms, patient reception areas, and areas where supplies are received. Street clothes are permitted in the unrestricted area.
150. Movement from unrestricted to restricted areas should be through a transition zone such as a locker room, office, or holding area.
151. Numbers of personnel and the movement of personnel within the suite during surgery is kept to a minimum. The organisms most frequently associated with surgical wound infection are *S. epidermidis* and *S. aureus*, organisms that are found on skin. The higher the number of personnel in the operating room, the higher the number of these microorganisms (Merrill et al., 1975, p. 149). As personnel shed these microorganisms they settle on dust particles. The greater the amount of movement, the greater the amount of airborne contamination that can be expected (Garner & Schultz, 1987, p. 226).
152. Certain areas and items are designated as clean or sterile and are separated from items and areas designated as contaminated, soiled, or dirty. Movement of clean and sterile items and supplies should be separated by time; space and traffic patterns; and from contaminated, soiled, or dirty items and supplies.
153. Items that are considered contaminated, soiled, or dirty should not be transported through the same corridors as clean and sterile items. In those facilities where design does not permit this, contaminated, soiled, or dirty items should be transported at times other than when clean or sterile items are transported through the same area.
154. Items delivered to the operating room from sources outside the health care facility should be removed from packing and external shipping cartons before being permitted into the operating room. Outside shipping cartons may harbor insects and dirt collected during transport.
155. Items and supplies prepared or selected for surgical cases that are delivered to the operating room from departments within the health care facility should be transported in closed or covered carts to reduce the potential for contamination.

Operating Room Sanitation

156. Operating room sanitation practices play a significant role in creating a surgical environment for patient and personnel that is clean and contains a minimum of microorganisms. Adherence to specified cleaning practices is essential to control and minimize the numbers of pathogens present in the suite.
157. Although cleaning and housekeeping protocols may vary among health care institutions, cleaning procedures are generally carried out prior to the beginning of the day's schedule, during the procedure, between procedures, at the end of the daily schedule, and periodically, e.g., weekly or monthly.
158. Persons responsible for cleaning and who, in the course of their work, have the potential to contact contaminated items or blood or body fluids must practice universal precautions by wearing personal protective attire that is appropriate to the task to be performed. Such attire includes gloves, masks, eye wear, and gowns.
159. Prior to the first procedure of the day, furniture, equipment, and surgical lights should be damp dusted with a detergent germicide using a lint-free cloth. Particular attention should be paid to horizontal surfaces because dust and lint that transport microorganisms settle on these surfaces. Equipment from other areas, such as x-ray machines and tourniquet devices that are necessary for the procedure, are damp dusted before they are brought into the room.
160. Throughout the procedure, an effort is made to confine and contain contamination to as small an area around the patient and sterile field as possible. During the procedure, spills or splashes of blood and body fluids may occur in the immediate vicinity of the sterile field. These should be promptly absorbed with a cloth and

cleaned with a germicide. Spills or splatters of other organic debris, such as patient tissue, should also be promptly cleaned.

161. Disposable items that become contaminated should be discarded into leakproof and tear-resistant containers to prevent contact with the environment and with personnel who are responsible for handling operating-room waste. Sponges are deposited into a plastic-lined bucket. They are counted as soon as possible and sealed in an impervious receptacle. They are not left to hang over the sides of the bucket where they can drip onto the floor. Blood, body secretions, and other fluids from the sterile field are collected in leakproof containers.
162. Specimens should be placed in clean leakproof containers. Upon receipt from the sterile field they are sealed and wiped with a germicide. Care is taken to prevent contamination of supporting specimen documents and other records.
163. Contaminated reusable items that fall or are removed from the sterile field should be wiped with a germicide and placed in an impervious container. Gloves must be worn by persons who handle contaminated items.
164. All items that come in contact with the patient or the sterile field are considered contaminated and should be discarded according to local, state, and national waste regulations, which specify what constitutes infectious waste. Disposable items contaminated with infectious waste are deposited in color-coded hazardous-waste bags displaying the biohazard symbol. Examples of such waste are gowns, gloves, sponges, and suture threads.
165. Infectious waste fluids may be poured down a drain connected to a sanitary sewer if regulations permit, or the collection container must be sealed and placed in a hazardous-waste bag.
166. Hazardous-waste bags are sealed prior to removal from the room.
167. Disposal and treatment of infectious waste is significantly more costly than disposal and treatment for noninfectious waste. For this reason noninfectious waste should not be placed into hazardous-waste bags. This is also the reason it is important to know the definition of infectious waste in the area in which one practices, and to deposit only those items that meet the definition of *infectious* into the hazardous-waste bag.
168. Noninfectious disposable items are deposited into leakproof bags that are sealed and removed from the room.
169. Sharp items, such as needles, staples, and scalpel blades, are deposited in a designated leakproof, puncture-resistant sharps container. Sharps containers are sealed and exchanged by designated personnel when they become full.
170. Reusable linen is deposited in specifically designated linen receptacles and sealed before removal from the room.
171. All instruments opened for a procedure, *whether or not they were actually used*, are considered contaminated and must be appropriately cleaned and processed. They should be placed in designated closed carts and transported to instrument cleaning areas. Where designated carts are not available, the instruments should be covered and transported.
172. Furniture, including operating lights, linen hamper frames, suction canisters, and other equipment used during the procedure, is wiped with a detergent germicide. Kick buckets are cleaned and relined. The operating room table, including the mattress, is cleaned with a detergent germicide and the bed is remade. Patient transport vehicles are wiped with detergent germicide.
173. A 3- to 4-foot area of the floor around the operating room table should be cleaned with a detergent germicide. The preferred method of cleaning is a wet-vacuum system. If a wet-vacuum system is not available, a clean mop and fresh detergent germicide solution may be used. A fresh mop head and fresh solution is used for every patient. Individual institutional policies for cleaning the floor may vary and floor cleaning may not be necessary for all procedures.
174. Walls, doors, push plates, handles, cabinets, and other areas that have come in contact with patient blood or body fluids are cleaned.
175. At the conclusion of the day's schedule, operating rooms, scrub-utility areas, corridors, furnishings, and equipment should be terminally cleaned (AORN, 1995, p. 251).
176. Areas that should be cleaned with a detergent germicide at the conclusion of the day include but are not limited to
    - surgical lights and tracks
    - ceiling-mounted equipment
    - scrub sinks
    - faucet heads
    - horizontal surfaces
    - furniture
    - drawer, door, and cabinet handles
    - push plates

- vent face plates
- furniture castors and wheels
- cabinet and operating room doors
- kick buckets and other trash receptacles
- utility carts
- refillable soap dispensers
- floors in the operating room, scrub sink area, and corridor

177. Reusable cleaning equipment is disassembled, cleaned, and dried prior to storage.
178. Many items and areas within the operating room are cleaned periodically. Cleaning may be weekly, monthly, or as otherwise indicated in the policies of the institution. Each facility should have written policies that address cleaning schedules, techniques, and persons responsible for the following:
    - lounges, locker areas, offices
    - holding areas
    - cabinet shelves
    - walls
    - ceilings
    - air conditioning vents, grills, filters
179. Every facility should also have a cleaning schedule for the cleaning of anesthesia equipment. The anesthesia department is generally responsible for cleaning and caring for its own equipment. The Association of Operating Room Nurses has written guidelines for cleaning and processing anesthesia equipment.

Additional Considerations—Cleaning and Scheduling

180. Under the concept of universal precautions, all recipients of health care, i.e., all surgical patients, are considered infectious and the potential for cross infection exists for all procedures. Therefore, no special cleaning technique is required after procedures on patients known to be infected with HIV or other infectious microorganisms. Routine cleaning, however, must be adequate and thorough.
181. At one time it was believed that patients known to be infected with HIV, hepatitis, or other infectious diseases should be scheduled as the last patient of the day to prevent possible cross contamination with other patients who would subsequently be brought into the room where surgery had been performed on the known infected patient. Because every surgical patient is considered infectious, because universal precautions is practiced, and because cleaning practices should be consistent across patients and procedures, there is no need to schedule known infected patients as the last procedure for the day.
182. The exception to this is for patients with airborne transmitted infectious diseases. These patients should be scheduled when personnel and patient traffic is minimal and exposure is therefore reduced. Scheduling as the last case of the day is appropriate for these patients.

Section Questions

Q32. Air flow in the operating room (Ref. 140, 141, 142):

a. flows from ceiling to floor
b. is directed into the room under positive pressure
c. to be effective requires that operating room doors be closed
d. is filtered before it enters the room
e. must have a minimum of 10 air exchanges an hour

Q33. Scrubs are required in the semirestricted area of the operating room. (Ref. 148)

True False

Q34. Explain why supplies are removed from their external shipping cartons before being permitted entry into the operating room. (Ref. 154)

____

____

Q35. When a specimen is received from the sterile field and placed in a specimen container, the container should be sealed and sterilized before it is transported to the laboratory. (Ref. 163)

True False

Q36. Under no circumstances should infectious waste fluids be poured down a drain. (Ref. 165)

True False

Q37. Infectious waste is deposited in specially marked color-coded bags. Explain why it is prudent to include only infectious waste in these bags and to exclude noninfectious waste. (Ref. 167)

____

____

Q38. Instruments that were opened for a procedure, but not used, should be transported to the instrument cleaning area in a closed or covered cart. (Ref. 171)

True False

Q39. Universal precautions necessitates that patients known to be infected with HIV must be scheduled as the last patient of the day in order to protect all other patients. (Ref. 181)

True False

NOTES

Association of Operating Room Nurses (AORN). (1995). *Standards and recommended practices.* Denver, CO: AORN.

Association of Operating Room Nurses (AORN). (1996). Proposed recommended practices for establishing and maintaining a sterile field. *AORN Journal*, *63*(1), 211–216.

Association for Practitioners in Infection Control (APIC). In Mathias, J. (1995). APIC guideline recommends shortened surgical scrub. *OR Manager*, *11*(11), 13.

Bartley, J.M. (1993, Oct.). Environmental control: Operating room air quality. *Today's O.R. Nurse*, *15*(5), 13.

Baumgardner, C., Maragos, C., Walz, J., & Larson, E. (1993, July). Effects of nail polish on microbial growth of fingernails. *AORN Journal*, *58*(1), 84–89.

Belkin, N. (1992). Barrier materials: Their influence on surgical wound infection. *AORN Journal*, *55*(6), 1522.

Cardo, M., Falk, P., & Mayhall, C. (1993, April). Validation of surgical wound surveillance. *Infection Control and Hospital Epidemiology*, 211–215.

Cruise, P., & Foord, R. (1980, Feb.). The epidemiology of wound infection: A 10 year prospective study of 62,939 wounds. *Surgical Clinics of North America*, *60*, 27–40.

Ellis, H. (1990, Dec.). The hazards of surgical glove dusting powders. *Surgery, Gynecology & Obstetrics*, *171*, 521–527. In Fay, M. (1992, June). Surgical gloves: Measuring cost and effectiveness. *AORN Journal*, 1500–1519.

Garner, J.S., & Schultz, J.K. (1987). Absence of infection in perioperative patient care: The nursing perspective (2nd. ed.). In J. Kneedler and G. Dodge, (Eds.) Boston: Blackwell Scientific Publications, Inc. In: Association of Operating Room Nurses (AORN). (1995). *Standards and recommended practices.* Denver, CO: AORN.

Groah, L. (1990). *Operating room nursing: Perioperative practice* (2nd ed.). San Mateo, CA: Appleton & Lange.

Johnson & Johnson Medical, Inc. (1992). *Bloodborne infections: A practical guide to OSHA compliance.* Arlington, TX: Johnson & Johnson Medical Inc.

Meeker, M.H., & Rothrock, J.C. (1995). *Alexander's care of the patient in surgery.* St. Louis: Mosby Year Book.

Merrill, A., et al. (1975, September). The operating room environment as affected by people and the surgical face mask. *Clinical Orthopedics*, *3*, 149.

Olsen, M., MacCallum, J., & McQuarrie, D.G. (1986, Feb.). Preoperative hair removal with clippers does not increase infection rate in clean surgical wounds. *Surgery, Gynecology and Obstetrics*, *162*, 182.

Pittet, D., & Ducel, G. (1994, July). Infectious risk factors related to operating rooms. *Infection Control and Hospital Epidemiology*, *15*(5), 459.

Pottinger, J., Burns, S., & Manske, C. (1989, Dec.). Bacterial carriage by artificial versus natural nails. *American Journal of Infection Control*, 340–341.

ADDITIONAL READING

Beck, W.C. (1989). The hole in the surgical glove: A change in attitude. *Bulletin of the American College of Surgeons*, *74*, 15.

Everett, W.D., & Kipp, H. (1991). Epidemiologic observations of operating room infections resulting from variations in ventilation and temperature. *American Journal of Infection Control*, *19*(6), 277–282.

Grinbaum, R., Mendonca, J., and Cardo, D. (1995). An outbreak of handscrubbing-related surgical site infections in vascular surgical procedures. *Infection Control and Hospital Epidemiology*, *16*(4), 198–201.

O'Neale, M. (1994). Floor cleaning. *AORN Journal*, *59*(5), 1086.

Smith, C. (1995). Cover gowns, surgical hand scrubs. *AORN Journal*, *61*(4), 671.

Wynd, C.A., Samstag, D., and Lapp, A.M. (1994). Bacterial carriage on the fingernails of OR nurses. *AORN Journal*, *60*(5), 796–805.

Appendix 5–A

Chapter 5 Post Test

1. Surgical wound infection is one of the most common nosocomial infections. (Ref. 1, 5, 6)

   True False

2. Aseptic technique (Ref. 7, 8, 9):
   a. eliminates all the microorganisms in the surgical suite
   b. is an important measure to protect the patient from developing a surgical wound infection
   c. includes nursing practices that prevent contamination
   d. includes the surgical scrub
   e. is the responsibility of all team members

3. The patient who sustains a surgical wound infection cannot be the source of that infection. (Ref. 11)

   True False

4. The premature infant is at increased risk for surgical wound infection. (Ref. 14)

   True False

5. Explain why the patient who has sustained severe burns is at increased risk of infection. (Ref. 18)

   ____

6. Proper hand washing is a component of universal precautions. (Ref. 32)

   True False

7. Explain why an ordinary pair of glasses is not sufficient protective eye wear to be in compliance with universal precautions. (Ref. 33)

   ____

   ____

8. Under no circumstances should an item be used in surgery if it appears that the wrapper may possibly have been subject to strike-through. (Ref. 38c)

   True False

9. A wrapped heavy item, such as a surgical drill, may be tossed onto the sterile field by the unscrubbed person so long as the portion of the unscrubbed person's hand that extends over the sterile field is covered by a sterile wrapper. (Ref. 38d)

   True False

10. The sterile field (Ref. 38e):
    a. should be set up as close to the time of surgery as possible
    b. should be covered if surgery is delayed
    c. should be monitored at all times
    d. could include an x-ray cassette if it were covered with a sterile drape

11. If a scrub person is asked during surgery to move to the other side of the table the scrub person should (Ref. 38f):
    a. move to the other side all the while facing the sterile field
    b. pivot away from the sterile field, keep back to the sterile field, and move to the other side
    c. pass other scrubbed persons at the sterile field in a back-to-back manner

12. With regard to infection prevention (Ref. 40, 41, 43, 44):
    a. a dry shave of the operative site is preferable
    b. a wet shave of the operative site is preferable
    c. no shave is preferred unless hair interferes with the intended procedure

13. One quality that the antiseptic agent used to prep the patient's skin should have is that it is nonirritating to the skin. List two additional desirable properties. (Ref. 51)

    ____

    ____

14. When alcohol is used as a prep agent it should be allowed to evaporate before electrosurgery is begun. Explain why. (Ref. 57)

    ____

15. In restricted areas in the presence of open sterile supplies the following attire should be worn by nonscrubbed personnel (Ref. 60, 61, 62, 65):
    a. hat
    b. scrub clothes
    c. mask
    d. shoe covers

16. Wearing of warm-up jackets is advisable for unscrubbed personnel in restricted areas. (Ref. 63)

    True False

17. One mask may be worn for consecutive cases provided it is not permitted to dangle from the neck between cases. (Ref. 68)

    True False

18. Both mechanical washing and chemical antisepsis are necessary to achieve the objectives of a surgical hand scrub. (Ref. 76)

    True False

19. A person with a cut on the hand (Ref. 78):
    a. should not function in the scrub role
    b. may scrub if two pairs of gloves are worn
    c. may scrub if the cut is appropriately bandaged

20. A scrub that lasts less than 5 minutes cannot be effective. (Ref. 88)

    True False

21. During the scrub the water should (Ref. 90):
    a. run from the elbows down the arms and flow off the fingertips
    b. run from the fingertips down the arm and flow off the elbows

22. The scrub person's sterile gown should be opened on the same table as the sterile instruments. (Ref. 91)

    True False

23. Closed gloving by the scrub person is a preferred technique to prevent contamination; however, the open-glove technique should be used in the event that the scrub person's glove becomes contaminated and the scrub person must reglove. (Ref. 110, 117, 119)

    True False

24. If the surgeon's glove becomes contaminated during surgery (Ref. 117):
    a. the scrub person should remove the contaminated glove and reglove the surgeon
    b. the unscrubbed person should remove the surgeon's glove and the scrub person should reglove the surgeon.

25. If the gown of a sterile team member becomes contaminated and a new gown is donned (Ref. 118):
    a. the team member should first remove gloves, then gown, and then regown and reglove
    b. the team member should first remove gown, then gloves, and then regown and reglove
    c. the team member should keep gloves on, remove gown, and then regown as there is no need to change gloves since only the gown was contaminated

26. Following surgery it is necessary to wash hands after glove removal. (Ref. 122)

    True False

27. Reusable drapes should (Ref. 130, 136):
    a. be tracked for number of times used because laundering will reduce barrier effectiveness over time
    b. be inspected after each use
    c. have defects repaired with a vulcanized heat seal patch

28. Explain why it is so important to limit access to the operating room and to limit the number of personnel in the operating room during surgery. (Ref. 145, 151)

    ____

    ____

29. Contaminated items should not share the same passageways as sterile or clean items; however, in the event the physical plant does not permit separate corridors, soiled items should be covered before transport. (Ref. 153)

    True False

30. All horizontal surfaces should be damp dusted with a detergent germicide prior to the first case of the day. (Ref. 159)

    True False

31. Spills of blood that occur in the vicinity of the sterile field during surgery should (Ref. 160):
    a. be left untouched until the end of surgery when the floor can be cleaned
    b. vigorously wiped with a detergent germicide
    c. absorbed with a cloth then cleaned with a germicide

32. All items that were opened for a procedure, whether or not they were actually used during the procedure, are considered contaminated. When disposable items are opened for a procedure, whether or not they are used during the procedure, they should be deposited in color-coded biohazard-waste bags designated for infectious waste. (Ref. 164)

    True False

Appendix 5–B
Competency Checklist: Asepsis

Under observer's initials enter initials upon successful achievement of competency. Enter N/A if competency is not appropriate for institution.

NAME ____

	OBSERVER'S INITIALS	DATE
Universal Precautions		
1. Blood and body fluids of all patients are considered infectious. Universal precautions are practiced as follows:	________	________
a. gloves worn when direct contact with blood and body fluids is expected to occur	________	________
b. masks and protective eye wear worn when aerosolation or splattering of blood and body fluids is anticipated	________	________
c. gowns worn that provide a barrier appropriate to the procedure	________	________
d. needles not recapped	________	________
e. sharps deposited in sharps containers	________	________
f. infectious waste deposited in designated container	________	________
g. contaminated laundry deposited in designated laundry bags	________	________
Aseptic Technique		
1. Gloved hands are kept in sight at or above the level of the sterile field.	________	________
2. (Circulating role) Items are checked for sterility prior to being dispensed to the sterile field (package integrity, chemical indicator, evidence of strike-through, expiration date if applicable).	________	________
3. (Scrub role) Sterility of items is checked prior to accepting for delivery to sterile field (packaging, chemical indicator, expiration date).	________	________
4. Items of questionable sterility and unsterile items are not entered into the sterile field.	________	________
5. Items that fall below the level of the sterile field are not brought back into the sterile field.	________	________
6. Items are dispensed to the sterile field without contamination.	________	________
7. Ungloved hands and arms are not extended over the sterile field.	________	________
8. Fluids		
a. are dispensed to receptacle placed at the edge of the sterile field	________	________
b. are poured carefully to prevent splashing	________	________

NAME ____________________________________

	OBSERVER'S INITIALS	DATE
9. Sterile field:		
a. is set up as close to time of surgery as possible	________	________
b. is not left unattended	________	________
c. is not covered	________	________
10. Scrubbed nurse touches only sterile items.	________	________
11. Scrubbed nurse remains close to sterile field.	________	________
12. Movement around sterile field is back to back and front (sterile) to front (sterile).	________	________
13. Circulating nurse maintains safe distance from sterile field.	________	________
14. Circulating nurse approaches sterile field by facing sterile field.	________	________
Skin Prep		
1. Skin condition and sensitivities are assessed and assessment is documented.	________	________
2. Prep is implemented as follows:		
a. awake patient is informed	________	________
b. unnecessary exposure is avoided	________	________
c. prep begins at incision site and continues outward to periphery	________	________
d. prep progresses from clean to dirty and never in reverse	________	________
e. prep solutions are not permitted to pool	________	________
f. dirtiest areas are prepped last	________	________
3. Prep is documented for:		
a. solution used	________	________
b. person performing prep	________	________
c. patient response to prep	________	________
Attire		
1. Hat/hood is worn so that all head and facial hair is covered.	________	________
2. Surgical attire that becomes visibly soiled is removed and fresh attire donned.	________	________
3. Masks		
a. cover nose and mouth and do not permit venting	________	________
b. are not left to dangle around the neck	________	________
4. Appropriate attire is worn in restricted and semirestricted areas.	________	________

NAME ____________________________

	OBSERVER'S INITIALS	DATE
Surgical Scrub		
1. Jewelry is removed.	______	______
2. Scrub includes all surfaces of nails, subungual areas, hands, and arms to 2 inches above the elbow.	______	______
3. Timed or anatomical scrub adheres to institutional policy.	______	______
Gowning and Gloving		
1. Hands are dried without contamination of towel.	______	______
2. Gown is donned without contamination.	______	______
3. Open gloving is performed without contamination.	______	______
4. Closed gloving is performed without contamination.	______	______
5. Assistance in gowning and gloving other team members is performed without contamination.	______	______
6. At end of procedure gown is removed before gloves.	______	______
7. Gloves are removed in manner that bare skin does not contact contaminated glove.	______	______
8. Hands are washed after gown and glove removal.	______	______
Draping		
1. Equipment is draped without contamination:		
a. back table	______	______
b. Mayo stand	______	______
c. ring stand	______	______
2. Patient is draped without contamination:		
a. abdomen	______	______
b. perineum (lithotomy)	______	______
c. extremity	______	______
3. Patient is draped from the operative site to the periphery.	______	______
4. A cuff is formed from drape to protect gloved hand.	______	______
5. Drapes are not repositioned once placed.	______	______

NAME ______________________________

	OBSERVER'S INITIALS	DATE
Sanitation		
1. Spills or splashes of blood and body fluids that occur in the immediate vicinity of the sterile field are absorbed and cleaned with a germicide.	________	________
2. Soiled sponges are deposited into a plastic-lined bucket, counted, and sealed in an impervious receptacle.	________	________

OBSERVER'S SIGNATURE INITIALS

______________________________ ________

ORIENTEE'S SIGNATURE

____

CHAPTER 6

Prevention of Injury—Positioning the Patient

Learner Objectives

At the end of Prevention of Injury—Positioning the Patient, the learner will

- list the desired patient outcomes relative to positioning
- identify six criteria for evaluating achievement of desired patient outcome relative to positioning of the patient in surgery
- discuss the responsibilities of the perioperative nurse in patient positioning
- describe the impact of surgical position upon the respiratory, circulatory, musculoskeletal, and integumentary systems
- identify body structures at risk in supine, prone, lateral, lithotomy, Trendelenburg, and sitting positions
- describe nursing interventions to prevent patient injury in supine, prone, lateral, lithotomy, Trendelenburg, and sitting positions

Lesson Outline

I. **NURSING DIAGNOSES**

II. **DESIRED PATIENT OUTCOMES—AORN OUTCOME STANDARDS/CRITERIA**

III. **IMPACT OF SURGICAL POSITIONING—OVERVIEW OF INJURIES**
- A. Respiratory and Circulatory System Compromise
- B. Musculoskeletal System Injury
- C. Nervous System Injury
  1. Facial Nerves
  2. Brachial Plexus
  3. Lower Extremity Nerves
- D. Integumentary System Injury

IV. **RESPONSIBILITIES OF THE PERIOPERATIVE NURSE**
- A. Patient Advocate
- B. Nursing Considerations
  1. Patient Assessment
  2. Planning Care

V. **ADDITIONAL CONSIDERATIONS FOR POSITIONING**
- A. Surgical Procedure
- B. Anesthesia
- C. Patient Dignity

VI. **POSITIONING DEVICES**

VII. **IMPLEMENTATION OF PATIENT CARE**
- A. Transportation and Transfer
- B. Initial Position Techniques

VIII. **BASIC SURGICAL POSITIONS**
- A. Supine (Dorsal Recumbent)
- B. Trendelenburg
- C. Reverse Trendelenburg
- D. Lithotomy
- E. Sitting (Modified Fowler's)
- F. Semisitting
- G. Prone
- H. Jackknife (Kraske's)
- I. Lateral

IX. **EVALUATING IMPLEMENTATION OF POSITIONING**

X. **POSTOPERATIVE TRANSFER**

XI. **DOCUMENTATION OF NURSING ACTIONS**

CHAPTER 6

Prevention of Injury—Positioning the Patient

NURSING DIAGNOSES

1. Nursing diagnoses derived from assessment data are patient specific; however, the nursing diagnosis of high risk for injury related to positioning is appropriate for most patients. The degree of risk for injury is relative to whether or not the patient receives general or regional anesthesia, the type and length of the procedure, the required position, and the patient's overall condition at the time of surgery. Specific nursing diagnoses that may be applicable include high risk for impaired skin integrity, high risk for ineffective breathing pattern, high risk for altered tissue perfusion, and high risk for musculoskeletal injury.
2. Positioning the patient for surgery is a critical component of perioperative nursing practice. Improper positioning can result in severe and permanent patient injury and can hinder the surgeon's ability to perform surgery.

DESIRED PATIENT OUTCOMES—ASSOCIATION OF OPERATING ROOM NURSES (AORN) OUTCOME STANDARDS/CRITERIA

3. Desired patient outcomes related to positioning are stated in the following AORN Outcome Standards: "The patient is free from injury related to positioning. . ." and "The patient's skin integrity is maintained" (AORN, 1995, pp. 125, 126).
4. Although desired outcomes are patient specific, there are desired patient outcomes relative to positioning that are applicable to all patients. At the completion of surgery the patient should have sustained no injury as a result of positioning.
5. Criteria for measuring achievement of the desired outcomes (Perry, 1994, pp. 265–266) include:
   a. Skin integrity is maintained—no signs and symptoms of
      - physical injury reported by the patient
      - impaired skin integrity or breakdown
   b. Breathing pattern is unaltered—no signs and symptoms of
      - ineffective breathing
      - abnormal blood gas values due to ineffective respirations
   c. Tissue perfusion is unaltered—no signs and symptoms of
      - edema
      - cold or discolored extremities
      - diminished arterial pulsations
      - altered blood pressure in extremities
   d. There is no injury to musculoskeletal or nervous system—no signs and symptoms of
      - postoperative cramping or pain in joints or muscles (excluding the surgical site)
      - inability to resume preoperative range of motion without pain or discomfort
      - weakness in extremities
      - tingling, numbness
      - uncompensated sensory deficit (touch or kinesthesia)
6. To achieve these outcomes, the perioperative nurse must have the knowledge of
   - principles of anatomy and physiology
   - anatomical and physiological changes related to anesthesia and surgical position
   - the surgical procedure to be performed
   - proper positioning technique
   - appropriate positioning equipment
   - proper use of equipment
7. In addition to absence of injury, maintenance of dignity and comfort are also desired outcomes.

IMPACT OF SURGICAL POSITIONING—OVERVIEW OF INJURIES

8. Some of the complications that can arise from improper positioning are postoperative musculoskeletal pain, joint dislocation, peripheral nerve damage, skin breakdown including necrosis, and cardiovascular and respiratory compromise.
9. The anesthetized patient is at increased risk of positioning injury. General anesthetic and regional blocks prevent the body's normal defense of pain from warning of exaggerated stretching, twisting, and compression of body parts. Subsequent damage to nerves and vascular structures and compromise to respiratory and circulatory functions occur without patient awareness.

Respiratory and Circulatory System Compromise

10. Extreme or unnatural positions such as Trendelenburg, where the head and upper body are lower than the feet and lower body, affect circulation and oxygen–carbon dioxide exchange. Pulmonary capillary blood volume, and therefore the amount of blood available for oxygenation, is altered by gravity. When the lung becomes engorged with blood, the amount of space for alveolar expansion is decreased and therefore the amount of oxygenated blood is reduced. In addition, the air inspired in the lungs is redistributed and affects the amount of air that is available to oxygenate the blood.
11. Unfavorable positions can also decrease compliance or stretchability of the lung and the ability of the thoracic cage to expand. The amount of air that may be taken in for gas exchange can be reduced and hypoventilation can result. In positions that compromise respiratory mechanics, muscles become fatigued as the patient attempts to compensate and hypoventilation may occur. Even where respiratory function is supported through mechanical assistance, hypoxia and hypercarbia can still occur.
12. Lung expansion may be decreased by mechanical restriction of the ribs or sternum. Lung expansion may also be decreased by the diaphragm's reduced ability to push down against abdominal contents or retractors that are used during surgery.
13. General and regional anesthetics disrupt normal vasodilatation and constriction and frequently cause dilation of peripheral blood vessels and result in a drop in blood pressure. Dilated vessels allow venous blood to pool in areas that are dependent. This reduces the amount of blood returned to the heart and lungs for oxygenation and redistribution. In some operations, certain body parts may be placed in a dependent position for an extended period of time, causing a significant amount of pooling to occur.
14. Cardiac contractibility is impacted by certain positions and anesthetic agents. The result is a relaxation of skeletal muscles that normally support vein walls and help to propel blood, interference with the venous sucking action of unhampered breathing, and compromise of vasopressor mechanisms (Guendemann & Fernsebner, 1995, p. 391).
15. Positions or pressure that obstructs the flow of blood in the legs also has the potential to result in phlebothrombosis. Venous thrombosis can result when superficial veins are occluded by pressure, straps, or other positioning devices. Safety straps should be tight enough to secure the patient but not so tight as to impair superficial venous return.

Musculoskeletal System Injury

16. In the awake patient, normal pain and pressure receptors of muscle groups warn against unnatural stretching and twisting of tendons, ligaments, and muscles. Opposing muscle groups also prevent strain on muscle fibers. The anesthetized patient, subjected to an exaggerated range of motion, is unable to indicate pain. Anesthetic agents and muscle relaxants further exacerbate the potential for injury by inducing loss of muscle tone and exaggerated muscle relaxation, which interferes with normal defense mechanisms against unnatural or excessive range of motion.
17. Evidence of hyperextension injury can range from mild postoperative joint pain to dislocation.
18. Musculoskeletal injury is minimized with adequate support of the extremities while being positioned and adequate padding at final positioning. Extremities should not be allowed to hang unsupported over the edge of an armboard or the operating table. Lower extremities should be moved slowly and in unison to prevent sacroiliac joint dislocation.
19. Crushing and pressure injuries to fingers, toes, ears, and nose are possible whenever the operating table, instrument table, or Mayo stands are adjusted. Team members are cautioned to visualize these parts when positioning and repositioning. Equipment must not be allowed to rest or exert pressure contact against the patient. Surgical team members must not lean on the patient.

Nervous System Injury

Facial Nerves

20. Injury to the facial nerve (buccal branch), resulting in motor injury to the mouth, can occur if the nerve is compressed from an improperly fitting face mask.
21. Injury to the suborbital nerve, resulting in numbness of the forehead, can occur from pressure on the nerve by endotracheal tube connectors.
22. Prolonged stretching or compression of nerves may result in postoperative numbness, tingling, or pain. Severe injury can result in permanent loss of sensation and paralysis in the affected area.

Brachial Plexus

23. Because of its superficial position and close proximity to bony structures, brachial plexus nerve injury is one of the more common positioning injuries.
24. Brachial plexus injury may result from improper positioning of the arm and/or armboard. The supine position, with one or both arms extended on armboards, is

the most common surgical position. Brachial plexus nerve injury can occur in this position if the armboard is positioned to cause hyperextension of the arm. Unintentional movement of an armboard, causing the arm to be hyperabducted, may not be noticed because the arm is hidden by surgical drapes.

25. When the arm is positioned on an armboard, pronated, and extended more than 90 degrees, damage to the plexus can occur. To minimize pressure on the brachial plexus, the patient's head may be turned toward the extended arm and the palm supinated.
26. Injury to the brachial plexus may occur when shoulder braces are improperly applied. In Trendelenburg position, shoulder braces, used to prevent the patient from slipping from the table, can cause compression of the brachial plexus. If the brace is placed too far laterally and the arm is abducted, the head of the humerus can be pushed into the axilla, causing compression of the plexus. If the brace is positioned too far medially and the arm is abducted, the plexus can be compressed between the clavicle and the first rib.
27. Motor and sensory loss to the arm and shoulder may be evidenced postoperatively if damage has occurred to the brachial plexus.
28. The radial or ulnar nerve may be injured if the elbow slips off the mattress onto the metal edge of the operating table and the nerve is compressed between the table and the medial epicondyle. Such an injury can occur when the surgical team leans against the table and is unaware that the patient's arm has slipped and is being compressed against the table.
29. The possibility of damage to the radial or ulnar nerve caused by compression against the table can be minimized by securing the arm with a draw sheet. The draw sheet begins from under the patient and is brought up over the arm and then tucked back under the patient.
30. Ulnar nerve injury can also occur during anesthesia if the upper extremity of a supine patient is allowed to rest on a flexed elbow with the forearm pronated across the ventral trunk. Supination of the arm on an armboard is preferable because this shifts the elbow pressure away from the cubital tunnel onto the olecranon process of the ulnar and relieves compression from the ulnar nerve. Padding around the elbow can also help to protect the nerve (Martin, 1991, p. 70).
31. A malfunctioning automatic blood pressure cuff that recycles without allowing sufficient time between compressions can also cause ulnar nerve damage (Martin, 1991, p. 70).
32. Symptoms of ulnar nerve injury include tingling, pain, and numbness in the fourth and fifth fingers. Severe injury can result in a weak grip or contractures leading to a "claw hand."
33. Radial nerve damage may be evidenced by wrist drop.

Lower Extremity Nerves

34. Improper placement in stirrups, or improper movement of the legs, can result in extension, flexion, compression, or stretching that can cause injury to lower extremity nerves.
35. The peroneal, posterior tibial, femoral obturator nerves, and sciatic nerves are at risk for injury in lithotomy position.
36. Injury to the peroneal nerve on the lateral aspect of the knee can occur if the nerve is compressed between the fibula and a laterally positioned stirrup bar. This injury can result in footdrop.
37. Injury to the posterior tibial nerve, resulting in numbness of the foot, can occur if the nerve is compressed. Popliteal knee supports should be padded to prevent compression injury of the tibial and femoral obturator nerves.
38. Injury to the femoral obturator nerve, resulting in paralysis and numbness of the calf muscles, can occur if the nerve is compressed between a metal popliteal knee support stirrup and the medial tibial condyle.
39. Padding at these potential compression sites can prevent injury.
40. Injury to the sciatic nerve, resulting in footdrop, can occur if the nerve is compressed or stretched. Compression and stretching can occur if the legs are fully extended in high lithotomy position and the thighs are flexed more than 90 degrees on the trunk.

Integumentary System Injury

41. Integumentary injuries are cause by friction, shearing, and pressure. Friction injuries occur when the skin moves across coarse surfaces such as bed linen or blankets. Friction injury can also be caused from excessive rubbing. Friction injuries are usually superficial and result in an abrasion or blister. These, however, can contribute to the more serious injury of a pressure ulcer.
42. Shearing injuries occur when the skin remains stationary and the tissue beneath is shifted. This can occur when linen or blankets underneath the patient are pulled or when the patient is pulled rather than lifted. Shearing injuries result in the stretching or tearing of subcutaneous capillaries and can lead to ischemia and contribute to the development of a pressure ulcer.
43. Lesions caused by unrelieved pressure are referred to as pressure ulcers. These occur most commonly over bony

prominences where tissue tends to be thin. Injury is caused by tissue hypoxia that leads to eventual necrosis. The duration of unrelieved pressure impacts the extent of the injury. Any patient on the operating table for more than 2 hours is at risk for developing a pressure ulcer (Stewart & Magnano, 1988, p. 36). Surgeries lasting longer than 8 hours put the patient at increased risk of pressure ulcers leading to necrosis (Hoyman & Gruber, 1992, p. 15).

44. A pressure ulcer can develop during surgery and go unnoticed for some time because actual skin breakdown is not immediately visible postoperatively. Operating room–acquired pressure ulcers typically appear as a bruise and rapidly progress to a pressure ulcer. The damage originates from deep within the tissue and progresses to subcutaneous tissue damage and eventual skin rupture.
45. Areas most at risk for pressure ulcer formation are heels, elbows, scapula, sacrum, and coccyx. Prevention of pressure ulcer formation is achieved through adequate padding and relief of pressure after 2 hours (see Figures 6–1, 6–2, 6–3, and 6–4).

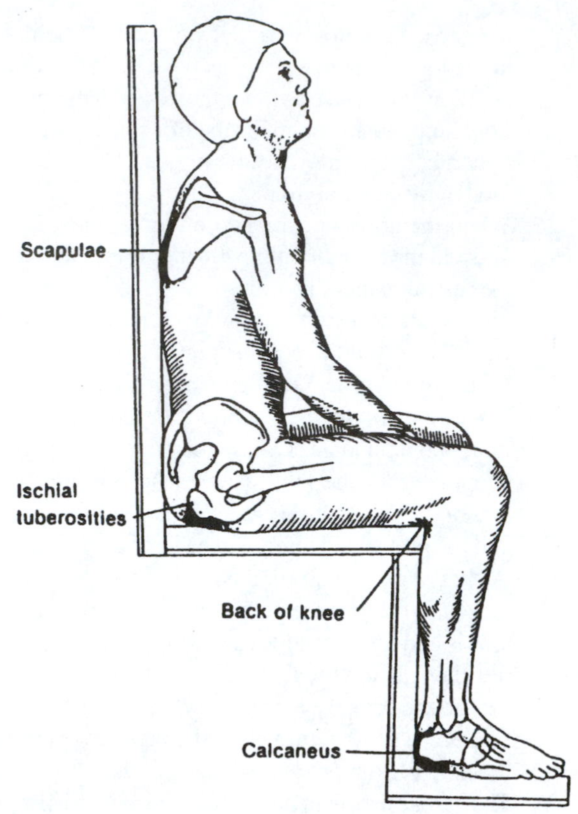

Figure 6–2 Potential Pressure Points in Sitting Position. *Source:* Reprinted from *Operating Room Nursing: The Perioperative Role,* by L.K. Groah, p. 268, Reston Publishing Company, Inc., © 1983. Reprinted with permission of Appleton & Lange.

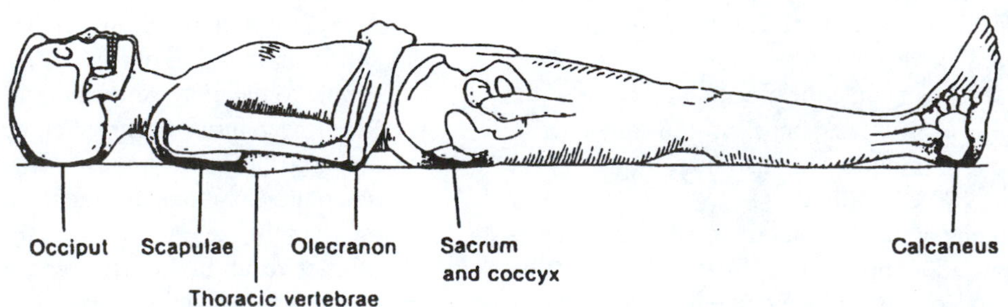

Figure 6–1 Potential Pressure Points in Supine Position. *Source:* Reprinted from *Operating Room Nursing: The Perioperative Role*, by L.K. Groah, p. 265, Reston Publishing Company, Inc., © 1983. Reprinted with permission of Appleton & Lange.

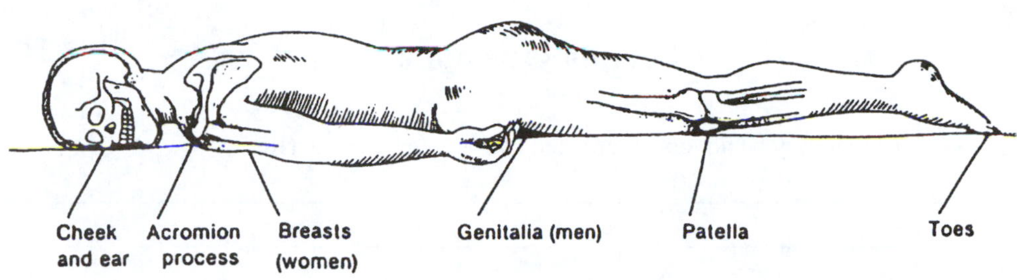

Figure 6–3 Potential Pressure Points in Prone Position. *Source:* Reprinted from *Operating Room Nursing: The Perioperative Role*, by L.K. Groah, p. 271, Reston Publishing Company, Inc., © 1983. Reprinted with permission of Appleton & Lange.

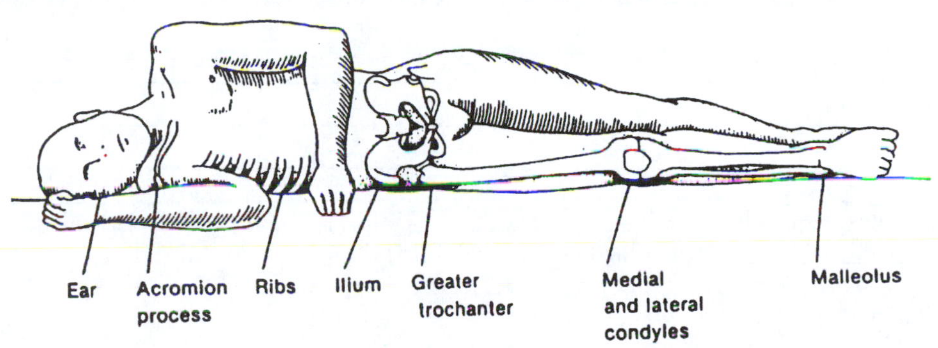

Figure 6–4 Potential Pressure Position. *Source:* Reprinted from *Operating Room Nursing: The Perioperative Role*, by L.K. Groah, p. 273, Reston Publishing Company, Inc., © 1983. Reprinted with permission of Appleton & Lange.

Section Questions

Q1. List four body systems that may be adversely affected by poor positioning. (Ref. 5, 8)

____

____

____

____

Q2. List four criteria that may be used to evaluate whether the patient has sustained injury to the musculoskeletal or nervous system. No postoperative evidence of (Ref. 5):

____

____

____

____

Q3. List three respiratory system changes that occur with extreme or unnatural positions such as Trendelenburg. (Ref. 10, 11, 12)

____

____

____

Q4. General anesthetics frequently cause ____________________ of peripheral blood vessels and also a(n) ________________ in blood pressure. (Ref. 13)
a. dilation/drop
b. constriction/increase

Q5. An improperly positioned safety strap can result in venous thrombosis. (Ref. 15)

True False

Q6. What severe musculoskeletal injury may result from hyperextension? (Ref. 17)

____

Q7. An improperly fitting face mask can result in injury to the (Ref. 20):
a. suborbital nerve
b. buccal branch of the facial nerve
c. hypoglossal nerve

Q8. Why is brachial plexus injury one of the more common positioning injuries? (Ref. 23)

____

____

Q9. Hyperabduction of the arms on armboards is a common cause of brachial plexus injury. (Ref. 24)

True False

Q10. To minimize pressure on the brachial plexus, the patient's head may be turned _____ the extended arm and the palm_________ . (Ref. 25)
a. toward/pronated
b. away from/supinated
c. toward/supinated
d. away from/pronated

Q11. List two causes of ulnar nerve injury. (Ref. 28, 29, 31)

____

____

Q12. Ulnar nerve injury is evidenced by tingling, pain, and numbness in the fourth and fifth fingers. (Ref. 32)

True False

Q13. The following nerves may be injured by improper positioning with stirrups (Ref. 35):
a. peroneal
b. posterior tibial
c. radial
d. saphenous

Q14. Footdrop may occur as a result of peroneal nerve damage caused by pressure on the nerve from a laterally positioned stirrup bar. (Ref. 36)

True False

Q15. An anesthetized surgical patient who remains on the table for an hour is at high risk for development of a pressure ulcer. (Ref. 43)

True False

Q16. A pressure ulcer that develops during surgery will be immediately noticeable following surgery. (Ref. 44)

True False

RESPONSIBILITIES OF THE PERIOPERATIVE NURSE

Patient Advocate

46. The patient undergoing surgery is vulnerable to positioning injury particularly when the procedure is performed under general anesthesia. Musculoskeletal, integumentary, and physiologic systems can be severely compromised at a time when the patient is unable to indicate that there is a problem.
47. Although it is most frequently the perioperative nurse who positions the patient, the surgeon, surgical assistants, anesthesia personnel, and other members of the nursing team may all participate in patient positioning.
48. Every team member must serve as a patient advocate. The perioperative nurse is a crucial patient advocate and at no time should the responsibility to ensure proper positioning be assumed to belong to another team member. The unconscious surgical patient is unable to self-advocate, and the responsibility for advocacy becomes a perioperative nursing responsibility for which the nurse is accountable.

Nursing Considerations

Patient Assessment

49. Planning for positioning begins with a nursing assessment of the patient. Assessment relative to positioning should include surgical procedure, age, height, weight,

activity level, muscle tone, nutritional status, skin condition, and respiratory and cardiac status.

50. The surgical procedure will determine the position in which the patient will be placed. Lengthy procedures under general anesthesia require extended periods of immobility and increase the risk for injury. Surgeries performed on areas where access is difficult may result in unnatural positions that increase the risk for injury.
51. Any physical limitations, injuries, or previous operations should also be noted.
52. Elderly patients have decreased muscle tone, poor skin turgor, and less subcutaneous fat and muscle to cushion bony prominences. These factors place the elderly patient at increased risk for impaired skin integrity.
53. Height and weight data are useful to determine appropriate positioning aids. Activity level and muscle tone data provide information about how well the patient moves and the degree to which the patient may participate in transfer to and from the operating room bed. Drugs and anesthetic agents can alter the patient's ability to move. Baseline data provide information that is useful for evaluating the impact of drugs and anesthesia on movement and muscle tone.
54. Patients with poor nutritional status are at increased risk for tissue injury. Malnourished patients lack protein reserves necessary to maintain healthy skin cells and are at increased risk for skin impairment. Obese patients may trap moisture and fluids from skin prep solutions in tissue folds, which may lead to skin breakdown. Adipose tissue is not well perfused, and the pressure resulting from positioning can cause a decrease in circulation to peripheral body areas. Excess body weight increases the strain on joints and ligaments. Respiratory function is compromised in obese patients because of increased weight on the chest. Anesthetic agents and positioning for surgery place additional strain on respiratory function. Obesity places an increased workload on the heart and circulatory system. Positioning that increases venous blood return to the heart can further compromise circulation.
55. Underweight patients experience greater than normal pressure on bony prominences and are therefore at greater risk for impaired skin integrity.
56. Patients with existing integumentary damage are at increased risk for further skin impairment. Diminished body fat provides little protection for peripheral nerves, and the underweight patient is at high risk for nerve damage.
57. Certain preexisting injuries or conditions and certain surgical procedures may require additional planning to prevent injury.
58. Preexisting conditions requiring additional considerations include
    - demineralized bone conditions such as osteoporosis and malignant metastasis—increased risk of fracture
    - diabetes, anemia, and paralysis—increased risk for skin breakdown
    - arthritis and joint prosthesis—limited joint movement
    - edema, infection, obstructive pulmonary disease, and other conditions that reduce respiratory and cardiac reserves
    - immunocompromised—increased risk of skin breakdown
59. Surgical procedures requiring additional considerations include:
    - surgeries lasting 2 hours or longer—increased risk for skin breakdown
    - vascular surgery compromises blood perfusion to tissues—increased risk for skin breakdown
    - surgeries where prolonged traction or sustained pressure is required—increased risk for skin breakdown and nerve damage

Planning Care

60. The perioperative nurse should communicate with surgical and anesthesia personnel to determine any specific needs. This information, the procedure, assessment data, and nursing diagnoses serve as the basis for planning the care necessary to correctly position the patient. Appropriate positioning equipment is selected, and decisions are made regarding the number of persons needed to implement positioning and whether aspects of positioning can be assigned to ancillary personnel.

ADDITIONAL CONSIDERATIONS FOR POSITIONING

Surgical Procedure

61. The procedure being performed determines the necessary position. The surgical site should be readily accessible by the surgeon and assistants. Surgeon preference may also be a factor in positioning.

Anesthesia

62. Patients who are awake or lightly sedated are able to state objection to a particular position or a sensation of pain. Patients under general anesthesia are totally dependent on the surgical team to prevent injury from incorrect positioning. Patients who receive regional anesthesia will not feel or report pain and are at risk for

injury to anesthetized regions that are improperly positioned.

63. Anesthesia personnel (anesthesiologist or nurse anesthetist) are concerned with airway access, respiratory and circulatory functions, and monitoring lines. Anesthesia has a profound effect on cardiac and respiratory function.
64. The anesthesiologist or nurse anesthetist will perform a patient assessment prior to delivering anesthesia. The assessment data coupled with the specialized body of knowledge of anesthesia will determine the limitations to positioning with regard to anesthesia.

Patient Dignity

65. Patient dignity should be a major consideration during positioning. The patient should not be exposed unnecessarily and, once positioning is complete, a final check should be made to ensure that the patient is appropriately covered. The patient should be made to feel that even when he or she is anesthetized dignity will be maintained with adequate covers.
66. For some patients the response to entering the operating room is to turn all control over to the personnel providing care. Even an awake patient who feels a loss of dignity while being exposed during positioning may not feel the confidence to cover an area inadvertently left exposed. The perioperative nurse, as patient advocate, must preserve the patient's dignity whether the patient is awake or asleep.

POSITIONING DEVICES

67. Each operating room facility will have its own routine supplies and devices to be used for positioning. These should be clean, in good repair, and used only by staff who are knowledgeable in the mechanics of the equipment.
68. Every operating room must have some type of operating bed or table. A table may be designed for general, urologic, ophthalmic, dental, neurological, orthopedic, or minor surgery. Tables have multiple parts and specific functions. Persons who operate tables and utilize attachments should have demonstrated competency to do so.
69. Table attachments include the following:
    - head rest
    - anesthesia screen
    - padded armboards
    - shoulder braces
    - kidney brace
    - table strap
    - leg stirrups
    - table extensions
    - table attachment holders
70. In addition to attachments for the table, there are a number of positioning accessories that are needed to achieve certain positions and to provide patient safety and comfort.
    - Blankets and sheets are for patient warmth. They are also used to form rolls and bolsters. A draw sheet under the patient's body can serve as a lift sheet. A draw sheet may be used to secure the patient's arms at the sides.
    - A donut that is made of foam, contoured gel silicone, or fashioned from towels is used as a head rest and to protect the ears and nerves of the head and face. If sized properly, donuts can be used to protect knees and heels.
    - Pillows are used to support and elevate body parts.
    - Sandbags are used for immobilization.
    - Padding made of sheepskin, foam, felt, cotton, or contoured silicone gel can be used to protect bony prominences and pressure areas such as elbows, knees, and heels. Disposable foam and reusable contoured gel silicone pads are available in a variety of sizes and shapes.
    - Tape is sometimes used to secure the patient or an extremity in a flexed position. A patient assessment for tape allergy should precede the use of tape as a positioning aid.
    - A laminectomy frame, or body rolls made from sheets that extend from the acromioclavicular joint to the iliac crest, are used to support the body off the chest while in a prone position.
    - Eye pads may be used to protect the eyes and maintain them in a closed position.
    - Pneumatic sequential compression devices, elastic bandages, or antiembolectomy stockings are all appropriate for reducing venous pooling in certain positions and for certain conditions. A pneumatic sequential compression device consists of a sleeve that is wrapped around the leg and is automatically inflated and deflated in sequential progression along the extremity.

IMPLEMENTATION OF PATIENT CARE

Transportation and Transfer

71. Verification of the patient's identity and of the surgical procedure is completed before the patient is transported to the operating room.

72. The patient's condition, the presence of invasive lines, the planned procedure, and institutional policy determine whether the patient may ambulate to the operating room or whether a wheelchair or stretcher is used.
73. Stretchers used for transportation should have side rails, a safety strap, a locking mechanism, and the capability to alter the patient's position. Pediatric transport cribs should have side rails on all four sides, bumper pads, and a canopy that prevents escape.
74. During transport, stretcher side rails are up and the safety strap is secured. The patient is covered to maintain body temperature and to preserve dignity.
75. The patient's condition, as determined from the nursing assessment, will aid in determining whether special equipment is necessary for transport to the operating room and whether additional personnel are required. (For example, patients on ventilators are transported to the operating room in a bed rather than on a stretcher, and additional personnel are required to wheel the bed and maintain the patient's respirations during transport.) Institutional policy may require the presence of nursing and/or medical personnel during transport of critically ill or ventilator-dependent patients.
76. Verification of patient identity and the incision site is made before the patient is transferred to the operating table. Patient transfer from the stretcher to the operating table begins only when sufficient personnel are in attendance. Before transfer, the stretcher is brought adjacent to the operating table and the side rail that is proximal to the table is lowered. Both the stretcher and the table are locked in place and raised or lowered to equal height. All patient intravenous lines and catheters need to be visible and free from entanglement. All team members must be ready for patient transfer.
77. During transfer to the operating table, one team member stands at the far side of the table to receive the patient. Another team member stands at the near side of the stretcher to assist the patient to transfer and to ensure that the stretcher does not move away from the table should the lock fail. Operating room personnel must use good body mechanics to prevent injury to themselves.
78. If the patient is unable to move unaided, he or she is lifted or may be transferred with the assistance of a roller. The patient is not pushed or pulled. Pushing and pulling create a shearing effect that stretches blood vessels and obstructs blood flow, thus promoting the potential for a pressure ulcer.
79. Intravenous lines, monitoring devices, and endotracheal tubes are supported during transfer. The anesthesiologist supports the head and indicates readiness for any move.

Initial Position Techniques

80. Prior to being anesthetized, the patient is positioned supine with careful attention to proper body alignment. Legs are secured with the table strap applied 2 inches above the knees. The arms may be initially secured at the patient's side with a draw sheet drawn over the arm and tucked under the patient.
81. The patient is never left unattended while on the operating table.
82. If the patient is awake, all actions should be explained. The patient should be asked if he or she is comfortable, and if not, appropriate adjustments are made.
83. Because the temperature in the operating room is generally cool, a warm blanket may be applied to the patient. This can prevent hypothermia. Many patients are uncomfortable lying flat on their back, and when possible, a pillow is placed under the patient's head until anesthesia preparations necessitate removal.
84. To reduce the potential for compression injury and/or electrical burn, no part of the patient is allowed to contact a metal surface.
85. Extremities do not extend beyond the table. All body parts are supported and not allowed to hang free where they may be compressed or stretched and thus injured.
86. To prevent compression and trauma to blood vessels, skin, and the tibial nerve, legs must not be crossed at the ankles.

Section Questions

Q17. The perioperative nurse is accountable for providing safety during positioning. (Ref. 48)

True False

Q18. In preparation to position a patient scheduled for a thoracotomy the perioperative nurse should assess (Ref. 49, 50, 70):

a. bowel habits
b. nutritional status
c. height
d. cardiac status
e. respiratory status
f. skin condition
g. anticipated length of surgery
h. tape allergy

Q19. The patient who is underweight or anemic is at increased risk for ____________________ injury. (Ref. 55, 58)

a. musculoskeletal
b. integumentary
c. respiratory
d. circulatory

Q20. What type of positioning device may be used to protect the patient's ears and nerves of the face? (Ref. 70)

____

Q21. All patients should be transported to the operating room in either a wheelchair or a stretcher and should not be allowed to ambulate. (Ref. 72)

True False

Q22. If the patient is unable to move, the safest way to transfer the patient is to use a draw sheet to pull the patient. (Ref. 78)

True False

Q23. It is appropriate to secure the patient's arm at the side with a draw sheet drawn over the arm and tucked under the patient. (Ref. 29, 70)

True False

BASIC SURGICAL POSITIONS

Supine (Dorsal Recumbent)

87. The supine position is the most common surgical position (see Figure 6–5). Procedures in this position include abdominal surgeries and those that require an anterior approach. Head, neck, and most extremity surgery is performed in the supine position.
88. In the supine position, the patient is positioned flat on the back with the head and spine in a horizontal line. Hips are parallel to each other and the legs are positioned in a straight line, uncrossed, and not touching each other.
89. The head may be supported by a small donut, headrest, or pillow to prevent stretching of neck muscles that support the head.

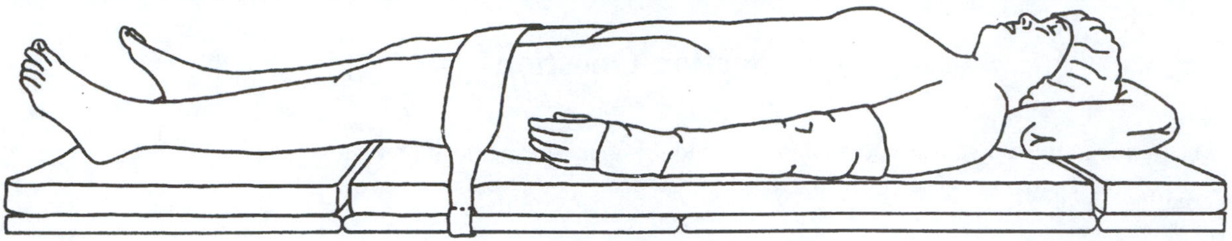

Figure 6–5 Supine Position. *Source:* Courtesy of Reichert Consulting, Olmsted Falls, Ohio.

90. Arms may be placed on padded armboards or at the patient's side. If the arm is extended on an armboard, it must be positioned at less than a 90 degree angle from the body and palms are supinated (palms up) to prevent ulnar nerve compression (Martin, 1991, p. 70). If the arm is positioned next to the body, the elbows must not be flexed or extend beyond the mattress. The arm is secured with a draw sheet.
91. A small pillow may be placed under the lumbar curvature to prevent back strain that occurs when paraspinal muscles are relaxed from anesthetic and muscle relaxant agents. An anesthetized patient lying on the back for hours will likely experience temporary lumbar pain without a small pillow for support.
92. The table strap is applied loosely over the waist or mid thighs. The strap should be at least 2 inches above the knees to prevent hyperextension of the knees. It should be secure but not constricting and should not be applied over a bony prominence.
93. If surgery is anticipated to extend beyond 2 hours or if the patient's condition indicates an increased risk of skin injury, protective padding is placed at pressure points. To prevent plantar flexion and crushing injuries to the toes, the foot board must extend beyond the toes.
94. Pressure points at risk for skin injury in the supine position include skin over bony prominences, occiput, spinous processes, scapulae, styloid process of the ulnar and radius, olecranon process, sacrum, and calcaneus. Skin breakdown from pressure is most common on the styloid process of the ulnar and radius (elbows), the sacrum, and the calcaneus (heels).
95. Nerves or nerve groups at risk include the brachial plexus, radial, ulnar, median, common peroneal, and tibial nerves.
96. Vital capacity can be reduced because of restriction of posterior chest expansion.

Trendelenburg

97. Trendelenburg is a supine position with the table tilted head down so that the head is lower than the feet (see Figure 6–6). This position is used for surgery on the lower abdomen and pelvis. It is also indicated for patients who develop hypovolemic shock.
98. The patient is positioned supine with knees over the lower break in the table. All safety measures are applied before the table is tilted. To help maintain this position, the lower part of the table may be adjusted so that the patient's legs are parallel with the floor.
99. Padded shoulder braces may be positioned against the acromion and spinous process of the scapula. Care is taken to ensure that they are not placed incorrectly over soft tissue of the shoulder where they can cause brachial plexus injury. Because of the high risk of injury, shoulder braces should not be used unless absolutely necessary.
100. The position of the arm and hand is checked to make certain that the elbow does not extend beyond the table and that the fingers are not at the lower break in the table where they can be crushed when the table is adjusted.
101. Before the patient is placed in Trendelenburg position, Mayo stands, tables, and other equipment are adjusted. When the position is attained, the toes are checked to ensure that the Mayo stand or other equipment is not pressing on them.
102. All movements are done slowly to allow the body enough time to adjust to the change in blood volume, respiratory exchange, and displacement of abdominal contents.
103. Respiratory and circulatory changes occur as a result of redistribution of body mass that limits diaphragm expansion and decreases ventilation-perfusion ratio.

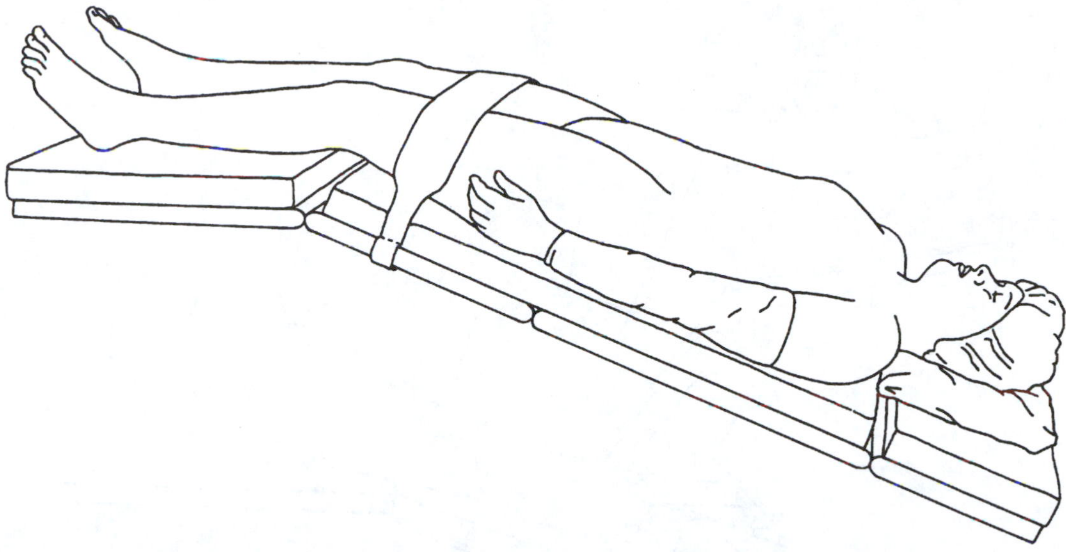

Figure 6–6 Trendelenburg. *Source:* Courtesy of Reichert Consulting, Olmsted Falls, Ohio.

Trendelenburg position increases intrathoracic and intracranial pressure. Because of these changes, the patient should remain in Trendelenburg position for as short a time as possible.

Reverse Trendelenburg

104. Reverse Trendelenburg is a variation of the supine position in which the table is tilted feet down (see Figure 6–7). This position is used for head and neck procedures.
105. A padded foot board may be used to support the patient's body.
106. A pneumatic compression device, elastic bandages, or antiembolectomy stockings are used to prevent pooling of blood in the legs.
107. Movement in and out of reverse Trendelenburg is performed slowly to allow sufficient time for the heart to adjust to change in blood volume.

Lithotomy

108. The lithotomy position is an extreme modification of the supine position in which the legs are elevated, abducted, and supported in stirrups (see Figure 6–8). This position is used for procedures involving the perineum region, pelvic organs, and genitalia.

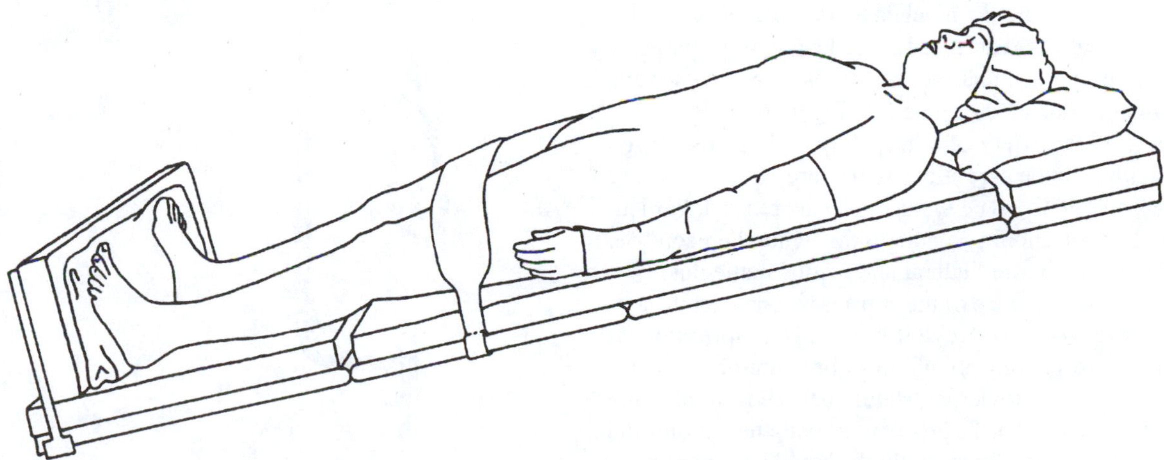

Figure 6–7 Reverse Trendelenburg. *Source:* Courtesy of Reichert Consulting, Olmsted Falls, Ohio.

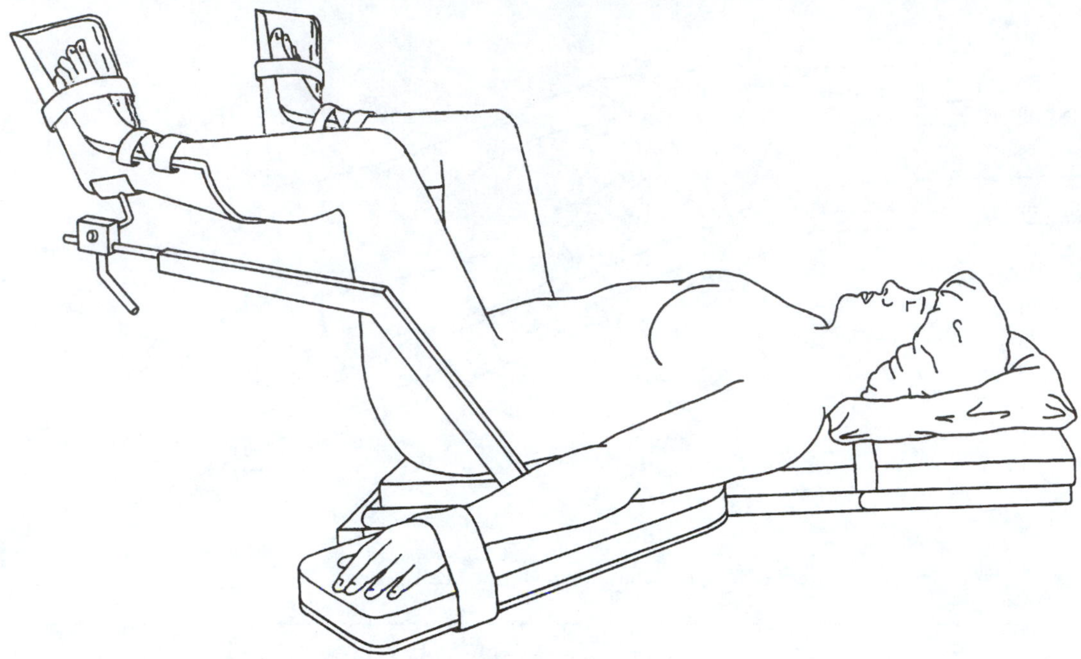

Figure 6–8 Lithotomy. *Source:* Courtesy of Reichert Consulting, Olmsted Falls, Ohio.

109. The patient is positioned supine with buttocks even with the lower break in the table. For lengthy procedures antiembolectomy stockings or elastic bandages are applied to decrease pooling of blood in the lower legs.
110. Arms are secured on padded armboards to prevent injury to fingers and hands that can be compressed in the mechanism of the table when the bottom section of the table is lowered or raised.
111. Stirrups are securely attached to the table, positioned at equal height, and adjusted to the length of the patient's legs. This adjustment prevents pressure at the knee and lumbar region of the spine (see Figure 6–9).
112. There are a variety of stirrups available and selection should be made carefully. At-risk pressure points vary according to the type of stirrups that are used. Particular attention should be paid to the femoral epicondyle, tibial condyles, and lateral and medial malleolus.
113. Padding on portions of the stirrups that contact the legs is appropriate to prevent external compression of nerves. To prevent injury from pressure on the peroneal nerve, the lower leg should be free from pressure against the stirrup. To prevent injury to the femoral and obturator nerve, the inner thigh should be free of pressure from the stirrup.
114. Although rare, compartment syndrome—characterized by pain, muscle weakness, and loss of sensation—can result if calf muscles remain in prolonged contact with leg supports (Walsh, 1993, p. 56).

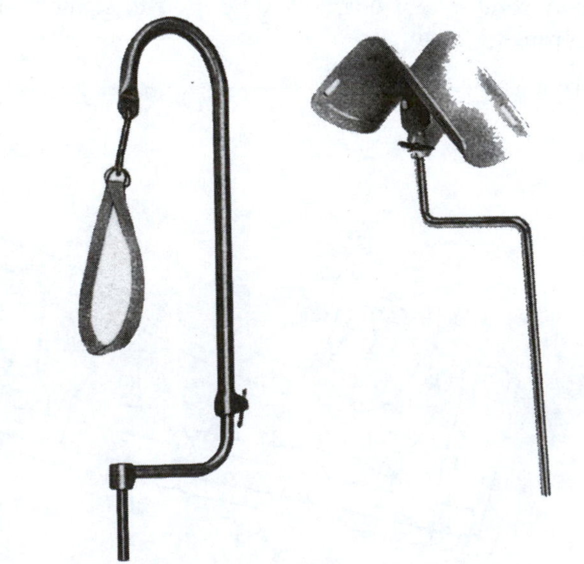

Figure 6–9 Stirrups

115. To prevent hip dislocation or muscle strain from an exaggerated range of motion, the legs are raised or lowered simultaneously by two members of the surgical team. During leg elevation, the foot is held in one hand and the lower leg in the other. The legs are flexed slowly, and the padded foot is secured in the stirrup.
116. After the legs are safely secured, the bottom section of the table is lowered or removed.
117. Padding is placed under the sacrum to prevent lumbosacral strain.
118. Following the procedure, the lower section of the table is raised to align with the rest of the table, the legs are removed from the stirrups, extended fully to prevent abduction of the hips, and lowered slowly onto the table. The table strap is then applied.
119. When the legs are lowered, 500 to 800 mL of blood is diverted from the visceral area to the extremities, which can result in hypotension. To prevent severe sudden hypotension, the legs must be lowered very slowly.
120. Lithotomy position reduces respiratory efficiency because pressure from the thighs on the abdomen and pressure from the diaphragm on the abdominal viscera restrict thoracic expansion. Lung tissue becomes engorged with blood, and vital capacity and tidal volume are decreased.
121. If nursing assessment suggests a limited range of hip motion because of contractures, arthritis, prosthesis, or another condition, the patient may be placed in lithotomy position while awake to permit vocalization of pain or discomfort so that appropriate modifications can be made.

Sitting (Modified Fowler's)

122. The sitting position is generally used for cranial procedures.
123. The patient is initially positioned supine. The foot of the table is slowly lowered, flexing the knees and thighs. The upper portion of the table is then raised to become the back rest and the torso is in an upright position. The head is supported in a cranial head rest. The feet are supported on a padded foot rest.
124. The torso and shoulders should be supported with a loose body strap. The arms should be flexed at the elbows and the arms rest on a pillow on the patient's lap or on an adjustable pillow in front of the patient.
125. Pressure points at increased risk for skin impairment include the scalp, scapulae, olecranon process, back of the knees, sacrum, ischial tuberosities, and calcaneus.
126. Padding at these pressure points is essential. Ischial tuberosities and the sacral nerve are especially at risk because most of the patient's body weight rests here. For this reason it is critical that the operating table be well padded.
127. Antiembolism stockings or elastic bandages are used to prevent postural hypotension and pooling of blood in lower extremities (see Figure 6–10).

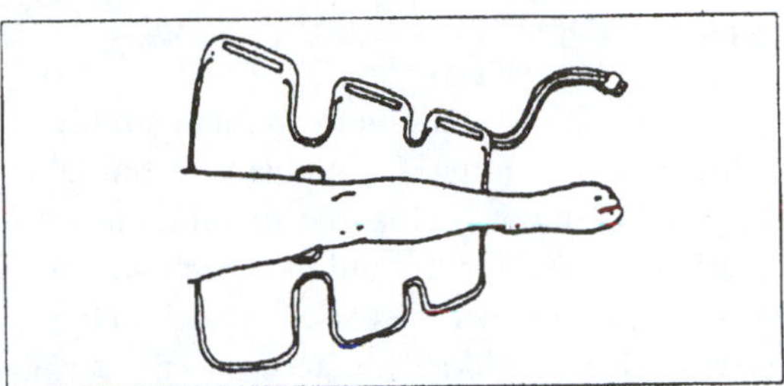

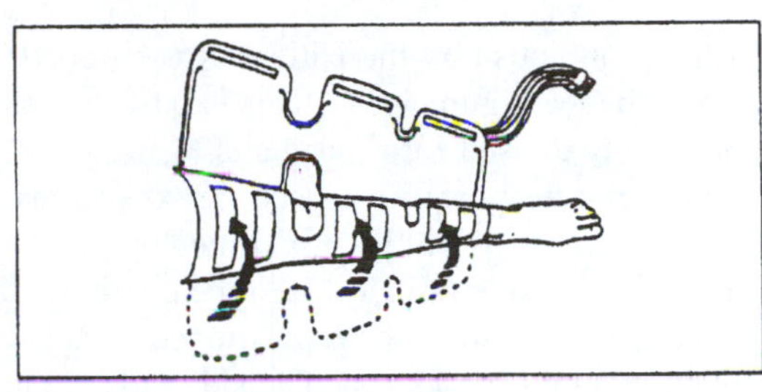

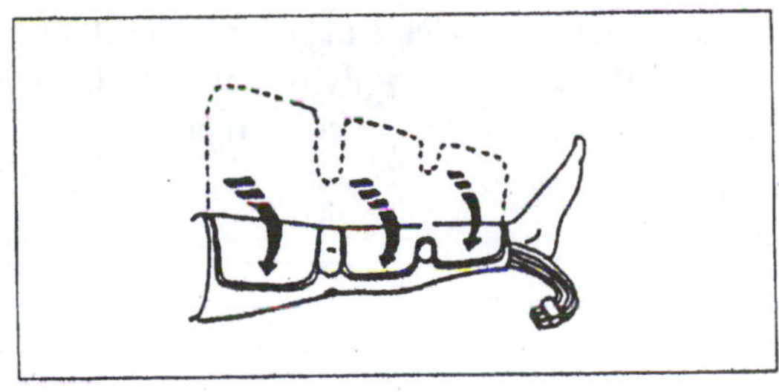

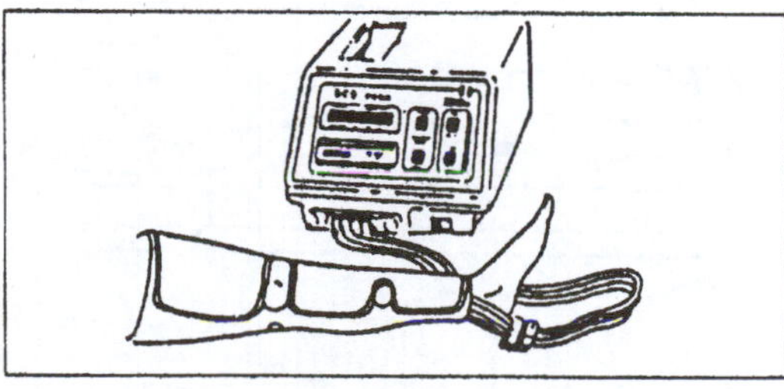

Figure 6–10 Application of Sequential Compression Device. *Source:* Courtesy of Kendall Healthcare Products, Mansfield, Massachusetts.

128. Because the sitting position causes negative venous pressure in the head and neck, the patient is at risk for air embolism. A central venous line with a Doppler ultrasound flowmeter is used to monitor the patient in this position. The Doppler is used to detect an air embolism and the central venous pressure line is used to extract the air.

Semisitting

129. In the semisitting position the patient's body is flexed at the pelvis and knees. The back of the table is not upright and the patient is in a reclining position. This position is used for thyroid and neck surgery. A roll may be placed under the patient's neck to hyperextend the neck and provide better access to the surgical site.

Prone

130. In the prone position the patient is positioned on the abdomen (see Figure 6–11). This exposure of the posterior body is used for procedures of the spine, back, rectum, and the posterior aspects of extremities.
131. The patient is initially positioned supine on the stretcher. The side rail closest to the operating table is lowered and the stretcher is positioned adjacent to the operating table and locked. The side rails are lowered and anesthesia is administered prior to placing the patient in a prone position. Following induction, the anesthesiologist will secure the endotracheal tube to prevent dislocation, and apply ointment to the eyes and tape them shut to prevent corneal abrasion. The anesthesiologist will indicate readiness of any movement of the patient.
132. A minimum of four persons is necessary to safely turn the patient from supine position on the stretcher to prone position on the operating table; one person supports and moves the head, one supports and moves the torso, one supports and moves the lower body, and one controls the body as it is rolled onto the operating table. All necessary equipment must be available. This includes padded armboards, a donut, body rolls or laminectomy frame, pillows, and padding.
133. All movement of the patient is done slowly and gently to allow the body time to adjust to the change in position. The anesthesiologist supports the head and neck and protects the patient's airway. A second person turns the patient from the stretcher onto the operating table into the waiting arms of a third person who supports the patient's chest and lower abdomen. A fourth person supports and turns the patient's legs. During turning, the patient's arms and hands are placed at the sides. The body is maintained in alignment and all team members work in concert to turn the patient in a single motion.
134. After the patient is turned, the arms are brought down and forward in a normal range of motion and then placed on armboards positioned next to the head. The arms are flexed at the elbows with the hands pronated. When the arms are in place, the person receiving the patient may then remove the patient's arms from under the patient. Elbows should be padded.
135. The patient's head is turned to one side and supported on a small pillow or donut, and the airway is secured.

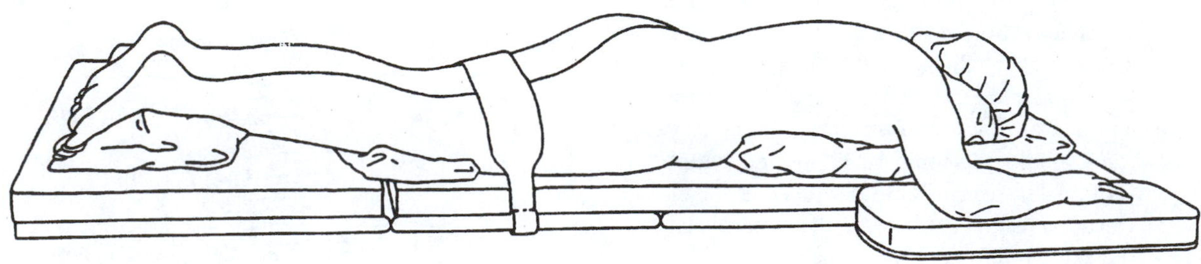

Figure 6–11 Prone. *Source:* Courtesy of Reichert Consulting, Olmsted Falls, Ohio.

The eyes are checked to ensure that they are closed in order to prevent corneal abrasion and free them from pressure, which can cause permanent eye injury. The ears are checked to ensure that they are not folded unnaturally. Neck and spine must be in good alignment.

136. The chest is supported by rolls or a laminectomy frame, such as the Wilson frame, which is positioned lengthwise from the acromioclavicular joint to the iliac crest. This facilitates respiratory expansion because the chest is lifted off the operating table and the weight of the abdomen is removed from the diaphragm. This is important because female breasts and male genitalia must be free of crushing pressure.
137. A pillow is placed under the ankles to prevent stretching of the anterior tibial nerve and to prevent pressure on the toes and feet that can cause plantar flexion and footdrop.
138. In the prone position, the table strap is placed over the mid thighs, which are covered with a sheet and/or a blanket. The strap should be at least 2 inches above the knees so as not to impede superficial venous return.
139. A small donut under the knees prevents pressure on the patellas.
140. If the patient has a stoma, precautions must be taken prevent ischemic compression of the stoma against the frame or body rolls. Such pressure can lead to tissue necrosis and sloughing.

Jackknife (Kraske's)

141. In the jackknife position the patient is positioned prone with the table flexed at the center break in the table. This position is often used for proctological procedures (see Figure 6–12).
142. Venous pooling in the chest and feet can cause a decrease in mean arterial blood pressure. Restriction of diaphragm movement, combined with increased blood volume in the lungs, can cause a decrease in ventilation and cardiac output. Because of its adverse effect on the respiratory and circulatory systems, the jackknife position is considered one of the most precarious surgical positions.
143. In the jackknife position the patient is positioned as for prone with the hips placed over the center table joint. Arms are positioned on padded angled armboards placed next to the head. Elbows are flexed and palms are pronated. Chest rolls are placed to raise the patient's chest, and the head is turned to one side. (Chest rolls are not necessary if the patient is awake.) A pillow is placed under the ankles and the table strap is applied to the thighs. The table is then flexed to a 90 degree angle, causing the hips to be raised and the head and legs to be lowered.
144. All precautions that are taken with the prone position are also taken with the jackknife position.

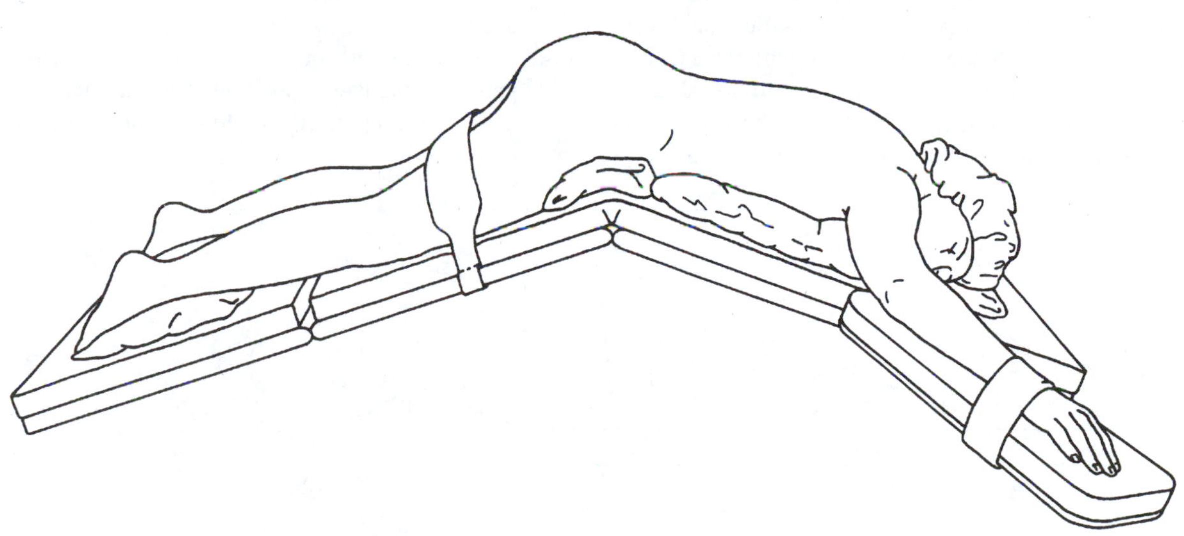

Figure 6–12 Kraske. *Source:* Courtesy of Reichert Consulting, Olmsted Falls, Ohio.

Lateral

145. In the lateral position the patient lies on one side (see Figure 6–13). In the right lateral position the patient is placed on the right side for surgeries on structures on the left side of the body. The reverse is true for the left lateral position.
146. The lateral position is used for access to the thorax, kidney, retroperitoneal space, and hip.
147. The patient is initially positioned supine on the operating table and anesthetized. A team of four persons will then lift and turn the patient onto the nonoperative side. The anesthesiologist's responsibility is to support the head and neck, guard the airway, and initiate any movement. A second person will lift and support the chest and shoulders, while a third will lift and support the hips. A fourth person is needed to support and turn the legs.
148. The patient is lifted in supine position to the edge of the operative side of the table and then turned on the side toward the center of the table. For kidney procedures, it is important that the patient's flank be positioned over the kidney rest with the iliac crest just below the table break. The patient's head is supported with a pillow or donut, and the body is checked for proper alignment. The head must be placed in cervical alignment with the spine. The bottom leg is flexed. The lateral aspect of the lower knee is well padded to prevent peroneal nerve damage, resulting in footdrop that is caused by pressure from the fibula on the nerve. A pillow is placed between the legs, and the upper leg is extended out straight. Feet and ankles are padded and supported to prevent footdrop and pressure injuries of the malleolus. The patient is secured with the table strap or with wide tape applied across the upper hip and fastened to the table.
149. A small roll or padding is placed under the patient's lower axilla to relieve pressure on the chest and axilla, to allow sufficient chest expansion, and to prevent compression of the brachial plexus by the humeral head. The lower arm is slightly flexed and placed on a padded armboard. The upper arm may rest on a padded elevated armboard or other padded support. Care must be taken not to abduct the arm more than 90 degrees, which can cause brachial plexus injury.
150. For kidney procedures the patient is supported on the operating table with well-padded braces, rolls, or sandbags. Extra padding is applied to bony prominence areas of the ankles, knees, greater trochanter, iliac crest, shoulders, elbows, and wrists.
151. The table is flexed at the center break in the table. The kidney elevator (kidney rest) portion of the table is raised to provide greater exposure of the area from the twelfth rib to the iliac crest. Kidney braces that fit over the kidney elevator may be used to support and maintain the patient in this position. Kidney braces must always be well padded.
152. Respiratory efficiency is affected by pressure from the weight of the body on the lower chest. The lower lung receives more blood from the right side of the heart, so has increased perfusion but has less residual air because of mediastinal compression and weight from abdominal contents.
153. Circulation is compromised by pressure on abdominal vessels and pooling of blood in the lower extremities. In the right lateral position, compression on the vena cava impairs venous return. If the kidney elevator is raised, additional pressure on abdominal vessels can further compromise circulation (Atkinson, 1992, p. 350).
154. Injury of the eye or ear is a special concern with the patient in the lateral position. The ear must be laid flat against the operating table and the eyelid must be closed.

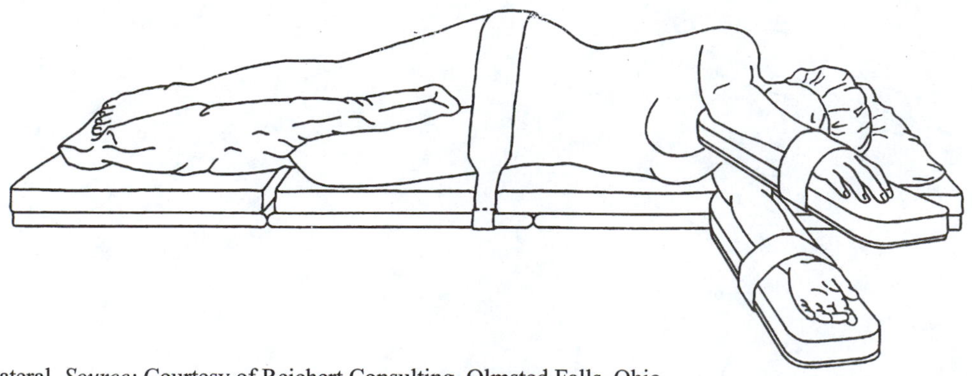

Figure 6–13 Lateral. *Source:* Courtesy of Reichert Consulting, Olmsted Falls, Ohio.

Section Questions

Q24. In the supine position the arms may be positioned at the patient's side, flexed, and secured with a draw sheet. (Ref. 90)

True False

Q25. In the supine position what intervention may be taken to prevent back strain and lumbar pain? (Ref. 91)

____

____

Q26. List five bony prominence areas that are susceptible to pressure injury in the supine position. (Ref. 94)

____

____

____

____

Q27. Explain why all movement of the patient into Trendelenburg position should be done slowly. (Ref. 102)

____

____

____

Q28. In lithotomy position the patient's buttocks are positioned even with the lower break in the table. (Ref. 109)

True False

Q29. One person is sufficient to place an anesthetized patient in stirrups provided the legs are raised slowly. (Ref. 115)

True False

Q30. Explain why sudden hypotension can occur when a patient's legs are lowered from stirrups. (Ref. 119)

____

____

____

Q31. Explain why lithotomy position reduces respiratory efficiency. (Ref. 120)

____

____

Q32. Explain why a central venous pressure line with a Doppler ultrasound is used to monitor a patient in a sitting position. (Ref. 128)

____

____

____

Q33. Which member of the team initiates readiness to move the patient from supine to prone position? (Ref. 131)
a. perioperative nurse
b. anesthesiologist
c. surgeon
d. scrub person

Q34. In the prone position the patient's arms will be brought down and forward, placed on armboards with the elbows flexed, and the hands pronated. (Ref. 134)

True False

Q35. When the prone position is used in surgery, the perioperative nurse facilitates diaphragmatic expansion by (Ref. 136):
a. repositioning the patient several times during surgery
b. pressing down on the OR table mattress periodically throughout the procedure
c. placing supporting rolls from the acromioclavicular joint to the iliac crest under the patient
d. placing the patient's head on a neck roll

Q36. Describe an intervention for the patient in the prone position to prevent stretching of the anterior tibial nerve and pressure on the toes that can cause plantar flexion and footdrop. (Ref. 137)

____

____

Q37. A patient who is having a hemorrhoidectomy will be placed in which position for surgery? (Ref. 141)
a. right lateral
b. jackknife
c. prone

Q38. A team of four persons is necessary to safely position the patient in the lateral position. (Ref. 147)

True False

Q39. In the lateral position the patient's lower leg is positioned straight and the upper leg is flexed with a pillow between them. (Ref. 148)

True False

Q40. In the lateral position it is appropriate to place a small roll under the patient's upper axilla to relieve pressure on the chest and promote chest expansion. (Ref. 149)

True False

EVALUATING IMPLEMENTATION OF POSITIONING

155. The anesthetized patient cannot report discomfort or pain related to positioning, and the effects of improper positioning are not generally known until the patient recovers form anesthesia and is able to report pain and injury. The patient relies on the surgical team to ensure that positioning injuries do not occur.
156. Once the patient is in position for the surgery, the perioperative nurse should do a thorough, once-over check to ensure that the patient's body is in alignment, extremities are not extended beyond their natural range of motion, bony prominences are padded, pressure is removed from nerves where injury can occur, respiratory and circulatory efforts are restricted as little as possible, and positioning devices are appropriately positioned and padded and hold securely without excessive restriction on body structures. Intermittent revaluation of the patient's position throughout the procedure is important. If the patient is repositioned during the procedure a thorough reevaluation is critical, with adjustments made as necessary.

POSTOPERATIVE TRANSFER

157. When surgery is completed and the anesthesiologist indicates that the patient is stable and can be moved, the postoperative bed or stretcher is brought adjacent to the operating table. It is raised or lowered to the level of the operating table and locked into place.
158. Four staff should be available to transfer the anesthetized patient in a slow and smooth manner to the bed or stretcher. The airway and proper body alignment must be maintained. Lines and catheters must be transferred intact and free from entanglement.
159. The patient is lifted or rolled onto the bed or stretcher. Pushing and pulling is avoided. Side rails are raised and locked for safe patient transfer and recovery.

DOCUMENTATION OF NURSING ACTIONS

160. Nursing documentation related to positioning should include but not be limited to the following:
    - assessment, considerations for positioning
    - overall skin condition on arrival and discharge from the perioperative suite
    - position
    - placement of extremities
    - placement of positioning devices such as rolls, padding, and restraints
    - precautions to protect eyes
    - any changes made in positioning during the procedure
    - presence and position of safety strap

Section Questions

Q41. Once the patient is in final position the perioperative nurse should do an overall check to ensure that positioning will not cause injury. Describe what the perioperative nurse should assess. (Identify at least four implementations to check for.) (Ref. 156)

____

____

____

____

Q42. Assessment of the patient's position should be performed (Ref. 156):

a. just prior to surgery
b. intermittently throughout the procedure
c. whenever the patient is repositioned
d. following the procedure

Q43. Information that should be included in nursing documentation relative to positioning should include at least five items. (Ref. 160)

____

____

____

____

____

NOTES

Association of Operating Room Nurses (AORN). (1995). *Standards and recommended practices.* Denver, CO: AORN

Atkinson, L. (1992). Positions. *Operating room technique* (7th ed.). St. Louis: Mosby Year Book.

Gruendemann, B., & Fernsebner, B. (1995). *Comprehensive perioperative nursing.* (Vol. 1, Principles). Boston: Jones and Bartlett Publishers.

Hoyman, K., & Gruber, N. (1992). A case study of interdepartmental cooperation: Operating room acquired pressure ulcers. *Journal of Nursing Care Quality, Special Report, 15*, 12–17.

Martin, J. (1991). Updating the concepts of patient positioning during anesthesia and surgery. *Current Reviews for Nurse Anesthetists, 14*, 67–76.

Perry, S. (1994). Positioning the patient. In M. Phippen, & M. Wells (Eds.), *Perioperative nursing practice* (pp. 264–278). Philadelphia: W.B. Saunders.

Stewart, T.P., & Magnano, S.J. (1988). Burns or pressure ulcers in the surgical patient. *Decubitus, 1*(1), 36–40.

Walsh, J. (1993, Feb.). Postop effects of OR positioning. *RN*, 50–57.

ADDITIONAL READING

Foster, C., Mukai, G., et al. (1979). Effects of surgical positioning. *AORN Journal, 30*, 219–232.

Groah, L. (1996). *Perioperative nursing* (3rd ed., pp. 251–271). Stamford, CT: Appleton & Lange.

Appendix 6–A

Chapter 6 Post Test

1. The patient undergoing surgery for a thoracotomy is at high risk for (Ref. 1)
   a. impaired skin integrity
   b. ineffective breathing pattern
   c. altered tissue perfusion
   d. musculoskeletal injury

2. A sign of possible altered tissue perfusion is altered blood pressure in the extremities. (Ref. 5)

   True False

3. List four things necessary for the perioperative nurse to know for safe positioning of the patient. (Ref. 6)

   ____

   ____

   ____

   ____

4. Maintenance of patient dignity is a desired patient outcome relative to positioning. (Ref. 7, 65, 66)

   True False

5. Complications that can occur as a result of improper positioning include (Ref. 8):
   a. pain
   b. joint dislocation
   c. fracture
   d. cardiovascular compromise
   e. paralysis and paresis
   f. necrosis

6. Trendelenburg position can result in hypoventilation. (Ref. 10, 11)

   True False

7. Muscle relaxants decrease risk of hyperextension injury. (Ref. 16)

   True False

8. When the Mayo stand or operating room table is repositioned during surgery, what should the perioperative nurse check for to prevent injury to the patient? (Ref. 19)

   ____

   ____

9. Select the correct statement(s) concerning brachial plexus nerve injury. (Ref. 25, 26, 27, 90)
   a. The arm is positioned on an armboard at a greater than 90 degree angle and the palm pronated.
   b. The arm is positioned on an armboard at a less than 90 degree angle to the body and the palm supinated.
   c. Injury can occur if a shoulder brace is positioned too far medially with the arm abducted.
   d. Motor and sensory loss to the arm and shoulder may occur as a result of brachial plexus injury.

10. Ulnar nerve injury (Ref. 31, 32):
    a. may occur as a result of a malfunctioning blood pressure cuff
    b. may result in symptoms of numbness in the fourth and fifth fingers
    c. may result in a weak grip

11. The position most likely to lead to injury of the peroneal nerve is (Ref. 35, 36):
    a. prone
    b. supine
    c. lithotomy
    d. jackknife

12. Shearing injury can contribute to the development of a pressure ulcer. (Ref. 41, 42)

    True False

13. An anesthetized patient is at risk for pressure ulcer after (Ref. 43):
    a. 30 minutes
    b. 1 hour
    c. 2 hours

14. The elderly are at greater risk for skin breakdown during surgery because (Ref. 52):
    a. surgery on the elderly generally lasts longer than on young people
    b. they have less subcutaneous fat and muscle tissue
    c. they are usually malnourished

15. Immunocompromised patients are at increased risk of (Ref. 58):
    a. joint dislocation
    b. skin breakdown
    c. circulatory insufficiency

16. List three safety features that should be present in a pediatric transport crib. (Ref. 73)

    ____

    ____

    ____

17. Explain why two persons should be present when a patient transfers from a stretcher to the operating room bed. (Ref. 77)

    ____

    ____

18. The longer that pressure is applied, the more severe is the tissue damage. (Ref. 43, 59, 93)

    True False

19. Concerning positioning (Ref. 18, 19, 82, 84, 86):
    a. All actions are explained to the awake patient.
    b. The safety strap is applied 2 inches below the knee.
    c. No part of the patient is touching metal.
    d. No extremity is allowed to hang free.
    e. Legs are not crossed at the ankles.

20. Match the position to the pressure areas. (Ref. 94, 135, 136, 148, 150)
    a. Supine _____ occiput, scapulae, spinous processes, medial epicondyle of the humerus, sacrum, olecranon process, calcaneus
    b. Prone _____ ear, patella, breasts, genitalia, cornea, toes
    c. Lateral _____ malleolus, greater trochanter, iliac crest, lateral aspect of the knee

21. In which position are the ischial tuberosities and sacral nerve are at high risk of injury? (Ref. 125, 126)
    a. supine
    b. lateral
    c. lithotomy
    d. sitting

22. Another name for the dorsal recumbent position is ______________________. (Ref. 87)

23. Although rare, compartment syndrome injury can occur when calf muscles remain in prolonged contact with leg stirrups. (Ref. 114)

    True False

24. Explain why in the lithotomy position it is safer to position the patient's arms on armboards than next to the body. (Ref. 110)

    ____

    ____

25. Modified Fowler's position is used most often for (Ref. 122):
    a. perineal procedures
    b. cranial surgeries
    c. neck surgery
    d. gastrointestinal surgery

26. Describe the position of the patient in reverse Trendelenburg. (Ref. 104)

    ____

    ____

27. What intervention may be undertaken to prevent pooling of blood in lower extremities during a procedure? (Ref. 109, 127)

    ____

    ____

28. List three positioning devices that are necessary when positioning the patient in prone position. (Ref. 135, 136)

____

____

____

29. Explain the purpose of placing a pillow under the feet and ankles in the prone position. (Ref. 137)

____

____

30. In which position is the female at greatest risk for injury to breasts? (Ref. 136)

____

____

31. Because of its adverse effects on the respiratory and circulatory systems, the jackknife position is considered one of the most dangerous positions. (Ref. 142)

    True False

32. Venous thrombosis can result from an improperly placed safety strap. (Ref. 138)

    True False

33. When positioning a patient in the lateral position (Ref. 148)
    a. a team of three people is needed for positioning
    b. a pillow is placed between the patient's legs
    c. the lateral aspect of the lower knee is well padded
    d. the lower leg is flexed and the upper leg is straight
    e. feet and ankles are supported and padded

34. For surgery on the left side the patient is positioned in the ______________ lateral position. (Ref. 145)
    a. right
    b. left

35. In the right lateral position circulation is compromised from pressure on the vena cava. (Ref. 153)

    True False

36. Which statement(s) concerning patient transfer from the operating room table are correct? (Ref. 158, 159)
    a. Four persons should be available to transfer.
    b. The surgeon initiates transfer of the patient.
    c. The stretcher is positioned lower than the operating table.
    d. The patient may be lifted or rolled onto the stretcher.

37. List five items of information that should be included in nursing documentation relative to positioning. (Ref. 160)

____

____

____

____

____

Appendix 6–B

Competency Checklist: Positioning the Patient for Surgery

Under observer's initials enter initials upon successful achievement of competency. Enter N/A if competency is not appropriate for institution.

NAME ______________________________

	OBSERVER'S INITIALS	DATE
1. Patient Transfer		
a. side rails up and secure	________	________
b. patient covered	________	________
c. stretcher adjacent to table with proximal side rail lowered	________	________
d. stretcher and table locked	________	________
e. stretcher and table are equal height	________	________
f. two team members present during transfer	________	________
g. patient lifted or rolled, not pulled	________	________
2. Supine		
a. patient is flat on back with head and spine in a straight, horizontal line	________	________
b. hips are parallel and legs are in a straight line and uncrossed	________	________
c. safety strap is placed at least 2 inches above the knees (secure but nonconstricting)		
d. small pillow is placed beneath the patient's head	________	________
e. arms extended on armboards are at less than a 90 degree angle from the body and supinated	________	________
f. arms at patient's side are not flexed and do not extend beyond the mattress; arms are secured with a draw sheet	________	________
g. protective padding is placed at pressure points	________	________
3. Trendelenburg		
a. patient is positioned supine	________	________
b. knees are over lower break of the table	________	________
c. table is tilted head down	________	________
d. following table tilt patient's toes are checked	________	________
4. Reverse Trendelenburg		
a. patient is positioned supine	________	________
b. table is tilted feet down	________	________

NAME ______________________________

	OBSERVER'S INITIALS	DATE
5. Lithotomy		
a. equipment assembled		
• appropriate stirrups	________	________
• OR table stirrup holders	________	________
• padding	________	________
b. patient is initially positioned supine	________	________
c. buttocks are positioned directly above the break in the table	________	________
d. both legs are simultaneously and slowly raised and positioned in stirrups by two people	________	________
e. both stirrups are at even height	________	________
f. metal stirrups are not placed in close proximity to the fibular head	________	________
g. stirrups are not exerting pressure against the upper inner aspect of the calf	________	________
h. padded stirrups do not compress vascular structures in the popliteal space	________	________
i. padding is placed beneath the sacrum	________	________
j. both legs are slowly and simultaneously lowered to the bed by two people	________	________
6. Sitting		
a. patient is initially positioned supine	________	________
b. foot of table is slowly lowered	________	________
c. upper portion of table is raised	________	________
d. feet are supported on a padded foot rest	________	________
e. torso and shoulders are secured with table strap	________	________
f. arms are flexed and positioned on a pillow on the patient's lap	________	________
g. pressure points are padded	________	________
7. Prone		
a. equipment assembled		
• chest roll or laminectomy frame	________	________
• donut	________	________
• pillows and padding	________	________
b. patient is logrolled from the stretcher to the OR table onto chest rolls or laminectomy frame by four people	________	________
c. arms are rotated through their normal range of motion and positioned on padded armboards next to the patient's head	________	________
d. arms are not abducted beyond 90 degrees	________	________
e. elbows are padded	________	________
f. patient's head is positioned to one side and supported on a donut	________	________
g. eyes and ears are checked for pressure points	________	________
h. male genitalia are checked for pressure points	________	________

NAME ______________________________

	OBSERVER'S INITIALS	DATE
i. female breasts are checked for pressure points	______	______
j. knees to toes are padded	______	______
8. Jackknife (Kraske's)		
a. patient is positioned prone	______	______
b. hips are placed over the center table break	______	______
c. arms are positioned on padded armboards next to the patient's head	______	______
d. elbows are flexed; palms are pronated	______	______
e. pillow is placed beneath the ankles	______	______
f. table strap is placed across thighs	______	______
g. table is flexed to a 90 degree angle	______	______
9. Lateral		
a. equipment assembled		
• tape	______	______
• pillows	______	______
• axillary roll	______	______
b. patient is initially positioned supine	______	______
c. patient is turned to the nonoperative side by four people	______	______
d. patient's head is in cervical alignment with the spine	______	______
e. bottom leg is flexed	______	______
f. lateral aspect of lower knee is padded	______	______
g. upper leg is extended	______	______
h. pillow is placed between the legs	______	______
i. patient is secured with table strap and tape across hips	______	______
j. axillary roll is placed at the lower axilla	______	______
k. lower arm is flexed on a padded armboard	______	______
l. upper arm is supported on a padded elevated armboard	______	______
m. arms are not abducted more than 90 degrees	______	______
n. lower ear is flat and eyes are closed	______	______

OBSERVER'S SIGNATURE INITIALS

______________________________ __________

ORIENTEE'S SIGNATURE

____

CHAPTER 7

Prevention of Injury—Counts in Surgery

Learner Objectives

At the end of Prevention of Injury—Counts in Surgery, the learner will

- identify the desired patient outcome relative to counts in surgery
- list three criteria for evaluating achievement of desired patient outcome relative to counts in surgery
- discuss nursing responsibilities related to counts in surgery
- describe the procedure for sponge, sharp, and instrument counts

Lesson Outline

I. **DESCRIPTION**
II. **NURSING DIAGNOSIS**
III. **DESIRED PATIENT OUTCOMES/CRITERIA**
IV. **OVERVIEW**
V. **NURSING RESPONSIBILITIES—COUNT PROCEDURE**
   A. Sponge Counts
   B. Sharp Counts
   C. Instrument Counts

CHAPTER 7

Prevention of Injury—Counts in Surgery

DESCRIPTION

1. Surgical counts refers to the counting of sponges, sharps such as blades and needles, and instruments that are opened and delivered to the field for use during surgery.

NURSING DIAGNOSIS

2. The nursing diagnosis of high risk for injury related to a retained foreign body is appropriate for a patient undergoing an invasive surgical procedure.

DESIRED PATIENT OUTCOMES/CRITERIA

3. A desired outcome at the end of surgery is that the patient is free from injury related to extraneous objects (Association of Operating Room Nurses [AORN], 1995, p. 126). Extraneous objects such as sponges, sharps, or instruments if unintentionally retained inside the patient constitute serious patient injury. Unnecessary pain, possible readmission to the hospital or an extended hospital stay, additional surgery, and delayed healing result when a foreign body is unintentionally retained.
4. The desired patient outcome relative to surgical counts is that the patient is free of an unintended foreign body at the end of surgery.
5. The criteria for measuring achievement of the desired outcome includes no signs and symptoms of
   - retained foreign body upon x-ray
   - cramping, fever, pain, or cavity abscess of unknown origin

   Cramping, fever, pain, or cavity abscess are often not identified until some time after surgery and may not be recognized until well after the patient has returned home.

OVERVIEW

6. In addition to the harm incurred by the patient, malpractice litigation frequently results when foreign objects are retained. Because a retained foreign body in a patient is almost always indefensible, such cases usually do not come before a jury. Any or all members of the surgical team may be held liable.
7. One mechanism to reduce the potential for a retained foreign body is surgical counts.
8. Counts are usually performed by the scrub person and the circulating nurse. However, the entire surgical team has a responsibility to protect the patient from foreign body injury.
9. The Association of Operating Room Nurses recommends counting all sponges, sharps, and instruments on all procedures and that counts be documented (AORN, 1995, pp. 261–263).
10. Many health care facilities have established count policies that reflect the AORN recommended practice; however, there are many facilities where count policies differ from the recommended practice. With the advent of minimally invasive surgery, the opportunity for a retained foreign body has been reduced and count policies have often been developed that do not mandate instrument counts unless an open procedure is performed. All

policies, however, should specify when counts are to be taken, by whom, and what is counted.

11. Policies determining what is counted are often based on the nature of the procedure and the probability of a retained item, the anticipated size of the incision, and the supplies required for the procedure. Some institutions have policies that identify specific procedures for which a count may be eliminated. Presently more than 60% of hospitals and ambulatory surgery centers are not performing initial instrument counts on all procedures (*Healthcare Purchasing News*, 1995, p. S26).
12. Some institutions use a count record to record count results. Others employ a wall board where counts are recorded during the procedure and the only the final results are recorded on the patient's record.

NURSING RESPONSIBILITIES

13. Counts in surgery provide a mechanism to provide patient safety during surgery. As patient advocates, perioperative nurses have a responsibility to ensure that count procedures are carried out according to institutional policy.
14. Surgical counts are not a guarantee that items will not be retained in a patient. Existence of a documented correct count usually accompanies a lawsuit for a retained item. The item was not intentionally retained nor does the documentation intentionally misrepresent the count. An error in the count process accounts for this phenomenon. All counts must be performed carefully, and the responsibility must be shared equally by the scrub person and the circulating nurse. Counts must be done together, concurrently, and aloud. Items being counted must be visible to both persons.
15. When an incorrect count occurs, it is the responsibility of the nurse to inform the surgeon and for all team members to assist in locating the missing item.
16. In an extreme emergency situation, a count may not be possible. In such an instance, the omission and the rationale should be documented, and institutional policy for this occurrence should be followed.
17. As a general procedure, counts are performed and documented prior to the beginning of the surgery, during surgery when items are added to the field, before closure of a body cavity or deep incision, before closure of a cavity within a cavity (cesarean section), and at skin closure. Additional counts may be performed as needed to verify accuracy.
18. All counted items should be removed from the room at the end of surgery. Items left in the room may cause an incorrect count in a following procedure.
19. When either the scrub person or the circulating nurse is relieved by a new team member, counts should be verified.
20. The results of all counts and the persons who performed the counts should be documented for all patients.

Section Questions

Q1. List three categories of items that surgical counts refer to. (Ref. 1)

____

____

____

Q2. The nursing diagnosis of high risk for injury related to retained foreign body is appropriate for the patient who undergoes an invasive procedure such as a total joint replacement. (Ref. 2)

True False

Q3. The Association of Operating Room Nurses recommends counting all sponges, sharps, and instruments on all surgical procedures, which may differ from hospital or health care facility policy. (Ref. 9, 10, 11)

True False

Q4. Perioperative nurses have a responsibility to ensure that count procedures are carried out according to (Ref. 13):
a. institutional policy
b. the Association of Operating Room Nurses' recommendations
c. the surgeon's recommendation

Q5. Counts are performed (Ref. 17, 19):
a. prior to the procedure
b. when items are added to the sterile field
c. following all x-rays
d. when either scrub person or circulator is relieved
e. as needed

Sponge Counts

21. The word *sponges* refers to materials designed to absorb blood and fluids. All sponges placed on the sterile field should incorporate a radiopaque strip or thread that makes them x-ray detectable. An x-ray–detectable strip facilitates location of sponges presumed to be retained in the patient should a count discrepancy occur. Sponges include
    - Lap pads (also referred to as tapes and lap packs)—square or rectangular gauze pads with an x-ray–detectable tape sewn in the corner of the pad. These are used where a moderate to large amount of blood or fluids is encountered.
    - Gauze sponges (also referred to as raytec and swabs). These are used where a small amount of blood or fluid is anticipated. They may be folded and clamped to forceps to be used for swabbing an area.
    - Peanuts—very small sponges approximately the size of a peanut. They are clamped to forceps and used for dissection or to absorb a small amount of fluid or blood on delicate tissue.
    - Kitner dissectors—a small roll of heavy cotton tape that is clamped to forceps and used for dissection or absorption.
    - Tonsil sponges—cotton-filled gauze in the shape of a ball. They have a long tape attached to them and are used in tonsil surgery, where they are inserted into the mouth to absorb blood and stop bleeding. The tape extends outside the mouth and is used for retrieval.
    - Cottonoid patties (also referred to as neuro sponges)—small sponges made of compressed cotton and supplied in a variety of sizes. They are used for surgeries on delicate structures such as the brain and spinal cord. Small patties include a long radiopaque thread. When these patties become saturated with blood they are difficult to see. The thread facilitates location.
    - Pledgets—small pieces of felt used as a support under sutures in friable tissues.

22. Before surgery begins, the scrub person and the circulating nurse count all sponges on the field and document the count. The count is performed aloud and together. Sponges must be handled so that both persons can visually verify the count.
23. Sponges are generally supplied from the manufacturer in packs of five and ten and are held together with a paper strip. It must never be assumed that the amount indicated on the package label is accurate. The paper strip must be removed and all sponges must be separated and individually counted.
24. If additional sponges are needed during the procedure, they are delivered to the sterile field, counted together and aloud, and the addition is documented.
25. During surgery the scrub person discards used sponges into a plastic-lined kick bucket provided for this purpose.
26. When a unit of five or ten sponges accumulates, the circulating nurse counts them aloud together with the scrub person and places them in an impervious bag. At the end of the procedure the bags containing sponges are deposited in a regulated waste bag. Soiled sponges are handled with an instrument or with gloved hands and never with bare hands.
27. Bagging units of sponges in impervious containers is an appropriate infection-control technique and reduces the risk of transmission of bloodborne diseases (Centers for Disease Control [CDC], 1987, p. 378).
28. As wound closure begins, the scrub person and the circulating nurse count aloud and together all sponges on the sterile field and any in the bucket. This number is added to the number of bagged sponges. The total should equal the number supplied for the surgery.
29. The surgical team is informed of the results of the count. If the count is accurate, closure will continue. As skin closure begins, a final count of sponges is conducted in the same manner. The results are reported to the surgical team and are documented.
30. If a count is found to be incorrect at the time of wound closure, the surgical team is notified and a thorough search, beginning within the wound and including the operative field, the room, and the trash, is initiated for any missing sponge.
31. Common institutional policy is that if the count remains incorrect after skin closure, an incident report is filed and an x-ray taken before the patient leaves the operating room. If an x-ray reveals a retained sponge, appropriate measures are taken to retrieve it and complete the surgery.
32. The names and/or signatures of the scrub person and circulating nurse should appear on the count record or operative record according to institutional policy.
33. Steps to minimize the possibility of an incorrect sponge count include keeping to a minimum the amount, size, and types of sponges opened for a procedure, and containing all sponges in the room by not removing any linen, trash, or supplies from the operating room until after the patient leaves the room.

Section Questions

Q6. Only sponges that contain a(n) ______________________ strip should be used on the surgical field. (Ref. 21)

Q7. List four types of sponges that should be counted. (Ref. 21)

____

____

____

____

Q8. Sponge counts should be (Ref. 22):
- a. performed silently
- b. performed by the scrub person and the circulating nurse
- c. visually verified

Q9. Sponges are generally supplied by the manufacturer in packs of five and ten and are held together by a strip. It is acceptable practice to accept the amount on the package label as accurate. (Ref. 23)

True False

Q10. As sponges are discarded during surgery they should be counted in units of five and ten and placed on a sheet until wound closure, when they are placed in an impervious bag. (Ref. 26)

True False

Q11. Steps to minimize the possibility of an incorrect sponge count include (Ref. 33):
- a. keeping the type of sponges used for a procedure to a minimum
- b. containing all sponges in the room until the patient leaves the room
- c. counting together each time a sponge is discarded from the sterile field during the procedure

Sharp Counts

34. Sharps include but are not limited to scalpel blades, suture needles, hypodermic needles, cautery blades and needles, and safety pins.
35. The procedure for counting sharps is essentially the same as for counting sponges. Counting must be done concurrently, visibly, and aloud by the scrub person and the circulating nurse. Sharp counts are documented.
36. When counting atraumatic sutures it is acceptable practice to count needles according to the number indicated on the label of each suture packet. However, once the scrub person opens a suture package, the number of needles inside must be verified (Fogg, 1994, p. 848).
37. Occasionally a needle or blade will break during a surgical procedure. When this occurs the sharp(s) in question must be accounted for in their entirety. On occasion, the risk of injury to a patient may be greater if a needle or piece of a needle is retrieved than if it is left to encapsulate in tissue. The decision not to retrieve a needle rests with the surgeon. Individual institutional policy dictates documentation of such an occurrence.
38. If a sharp is removed from the sterile field for any reason during a procedure, the circulating nurse should isolate it and keep it a designated place in the operating room until the final count is performed and the procedure is complete.
39. During some surgical procedures a large number of suture needles are used. During these cases frequent needle counts can help reduce the risk of an incorrect count.

40. Sharps should be contained on a magnetic needle mat or other device designed for this purpose. Sharps pose a risk of inflicting injury and permitting transmission of infectious disease to patients and personnel. Loose sharps should never be permitted on the sterile field.
41. Following the procedure, sharps must be disposed of in containers that are leakproof, puncture resistant, and color coded, or labeled as biohazardous waste.

Instrument Counts

42. Although the risk of a retained instrument is small, there are documented cases where it has occurred. Instrument counts are a means to reduce this risk. Instrument counts should be mandated for procedures where a body cavity is entered or where an incision is large enough to permit an instrument to be accidentally retained (Bruning, 1995, p. 150).
43. In addition to being a means of providing safe patient care, instrument counts are a means of inventory control and cost containment. Instruments are less likely to be lost if they must be accounted for.
44. The procedure for counting instruments is essentially the same as for counting sponges and sharps; however, instruments are generally counted two times: once just prior to the procedure and again at wound closure. Instrument counts must be done concurrently, visibly, and aloud by the scrub person and the circulating nurse. Instrument counts are documented.
45. Instruments that are removed from the sterile field should be retained in the operating room until the final count is performed and the patient leaves the room. Removal of an instrument from the room increases the potential for an incorrect count.
46. Reducing the numbers and types of instruments on a set and standardization of instrument sets are mechanisms that facilitate counting practices (see Exhibits 7–1 and 7–2).

Exhibit 7–1 Instrument/Sponges/Needle Count Record

ST. VINCENT'S MEDICAL CENTER OF RICHMOND
INSTRUMENT/SPONGES/NEEDLE COUNT RECORD

OPERATION	DATE

SECTION A	COUNT BEFORE SURGERY	ADDED DURING SURGERY	COUNT BEFORE PERITONEUM	FINAL COUNT (BEFORE SKIN CLOSE)
Raytec Sponges (4x4)				
Laparotomy Sponges				
Cottonoid				
Peanuts				
Tonsil Sponges				
Umbilical Tapes				
Vessel Loops				
Scalpel Blades				
Reel Ties				
Retention Sutures				
Free Needles				
Atraumatic Needles				

SECTION B	BEFORE SURGERY	ADDED	BEFORE PERITONEUM	FINAL COUNT INSTS. AFTER PERITONEUM	SECTION B CONTINUED	BEFORE SURGERY	ADDED	BEFORE PERITONEUM	FINAL COUNT INSTS. AFTER PERITONEUM
Mosquitos (curv)					Richardson Retractors				
Criles					Deaver Retractors				
Kelly (med)					Ribbon Retractors				
Allis					Balfour, Blade, Screw				
Babcock					Self-Retaining				
Kelly (lg)					McBurney Retractors				
Allis (lg)					Vein Retractors				
Babcock (lg)					Allen (anastomosis)				
Kochers					Bowel (rt) Angle				
Adson					DeMartel Applier				
Mixters					DeMartel Clamps				
Metzenbaum Scissors					Mayo Robson Clamps				
Mayo Scissors (curv)					Payr Pylorus Clamps				
Mayo Scissors (str)					Bakes (dilators)				
Metzenbaum (lg)					Randall Stone				
Mayo (lg str)					Trocar				
Potts Scissors					Heaney				
Needle Holders					Kochers (curv)				
Sponge Sticks					Phaneuf				
Adson Forceps (plain)					Tenaculum				
Adson Forceps (mt)					Uterine Packing				
Forceps (plain)					Pedicle				
Forceps (mt)					Bronchus				
Forceps (plain/long)					Lung Clamps				
Forceps (mt/long)					Bulldog Clamps				
Arterial Forceps					Vascular Clamps				
Rings					Baby Mosquitos				
Suction					Baby Rt. Angles				
Towel Clips					Skin Hooks				
Scalpel Handle #3					Lahey				
Scalpel Handle #7					Hemoclip appliers				
Scalpel Handle #3L					Other				
Rakes									
Army/Navy									
Parker Retractors					COUNTS ARE:				

SCRUB NURSE	RELIEF-SCRUB NURSE	CIRC. NURSE	RELIEF CIRC. NURSE

FORM 998 (9/86) MADISON BUSINESS FORMS

Source: Courtesy of St. Vincent's Medical Center of Richmond, Staten Island, New York.

Exhibit 7–2 Instrument/Sponge/Needle Count Record

GENERAL INSTRUCTIONS:

1. Instruments will be counted on all procedures which include invasion of peritoneum and an anticipated incision of more than three inches.
2. Instruments will be counted on all other procedures which do not invade the peritoneum but where incision is anticipated to be greater than three inches.
3. Sponges and needles will be counted on all procedures.
4. Incorrectly numbered packaged sponges must be isolated and not used during the procedure.
5. Instruments, counted sponges, and needles should never be taken from the O.R. for any reason during a procedure.
6. Instruments or needles broken or disassembled during a procedure must be accounted for in their entirety.
7. Used needles should be kept on a needle pad to insure their containment on the table.

PROCEDURE:

1. Before surgery begins, the scrub nurse and circulating nurse count instruments, sponges, and needles together and out loud as each item is separated in the counting procedure.
2. This original count is recorded immediately after being taken by the circulating nurse, on the Instrument/Sponge/Needle count Record Form #998A.
3. All instruments/sponges and needles added to the operative field during surgery are counted together and out loud by the scrub and circulating nurses and recorded immediately by the circulating nurse on Form #998A in the column marked "Added".
4. During the operative procedure, the circulating nurse:

   a) counts all sponges that are discarded from the operative field together and out loud with the scrub nurse.
   b) separates sponges into units.
   c) place counted sponges by units into plastic bags.
5. Before closure of peritoneum begins, the scrub nurse and the circulating nurse count together and out loud:

   a) all instruments/sponges/needles contained within the operative field which were counted before surgery and which were added during surgery.
   b) all instruments/sponges/needles which have been discarded from the operative field which were counted before surgery and which were added during surgery.
   c) the circulating nurse records the tally in the column marked "Before Peritoneum Closure".
   d) the circulating nurse reports to the surgeon, out loud, the results of this count.
6. Before skin closure begins the scrub and circulating nurses count out loud and together all instruments which were used after the peritoneum closure and all items included in Section A of the Instrument/Sponge/Needle Count Record Form #998A.

   a) This final count is recorded by the circulating nurse in the column marked "Final Count" on Form #998A.
   b) Result of this count e.g. correct or incorrect is recorded on Form #998A in the appropriate space.
   c) The scrub nurse and circulating nurse write their name and status in the appropriate space on Form #998A.

Source: Courtesy of F. Zarnick, Director of Nursing Services, St. Vincent's Medical Center of Richmond, Staten Island, New York.

Section Questions

Q12. If a sharp is removed from the sterile field for any reason during the surgical procedure, the circulating nurse should immediately dispose of it in a proper sharps container. (Ref. 38, 41)

True False

Q13. Instrument counts (Ref. 43, 44):
   a. do not require documentation
   b. are a means of inventory control
   c. reduce risk of patient injury

Q14. Contaminated instruments removed from the sterile field should be retained in the operating room until the patient leaves the room. (Ref. 45)

True False

NOTES

Association of Operating Room Nurses (AORN). (1995). *Standards and recommended practices.* Denver, CO: AORN.

Bruning, L. (1995). Environmental safety in the surgical suite. In R. Roth (Ed.), *Perioperative nursing core curriculum* (pp. 143–181). Philadelphia: W.B. Saunders.

Centers for Disease Control (CDC). (1987, Aug.). Recommendations for prevention of HIV transmission in healthcare settings. *Morbidity and Mortality Weekly Report*, *36*, 2S.

Fogg, M. (1994, Nov.). Clinical issues: Counting multipack suture. *AORN Journal*, *60*(5), 848–850.

Healthcare Purchasing News. (1995, May 15), S26.

Appendix 7–A

Chapter 7 Post Test

1. Surgical counts guarantee that unintended items will not be retained in the patient. (Ref. 7, 8)

   True False

2. The consequences for a patient who experiences an unintended retained foreign body include (indicate three consequences; Ref. 3):

   ____

   ____

   ____

3. A correct count at the end of a procedure is a guarantee that no unintended foreign body has been retained. (Ref. 4)

   True False

4. What information regarding counts should be documented? (Ref. 10)

   ____

   ____

5. Soiled sponges may be handled with gloved hands or with an instrument. (Ref. 26)

   True False

6. If a count is found to be incorrect during the procedure the ____________________ is notified immediately so that a search may be initiated. (Ref. 30)
   a. surgeon
   b. surgical team
   c. O.R. director

7. List three items besides scalpel blades that are considered to be sharps and should be counted. (Ref. 34)

   ____

   ____

   ____

8. Suture needles (Ref. 36, 37):
   a. should be accounted for in their entirety
   b. should always be retrieved in their entirety
   c. should be counted according to the amount indicated on the label but confirmed when they are opened
   d. should be stored in a medicine cup to keep them together

9. Instruments removed from the sterile field during a surgical procedure requiring an instrument count should be immediately sent to the instrument processing room for decontamination. (Ref. 45)

   True False

10. Surgical counts (Ref. 45):
    a. are a means to reduce the patient's risk of injury
    b. are a shared responsibility
    c. should be documented
    d. should be performed according to institutional policy
    e. that are incorrect may incur liability for any or all members of the surgical team

Appendix 7–B

Competency Checklist: Counts in Surgery

Under observer's initials enter initials upon successful achievement of competency. Enter N/A if competency is not appropriate for institution.

NAME ____________________________________

	OBSERVER'S INITIALS	DATE
1. Counts are performed and documented:		
a. prior to procedure	________	________
b. during procedure when items are added	________	________
c. before closure of a body cavity	________	________
d. prior to skin closure	________	________
e. at time of relief	________	________
2. Count is performed together, concurrently, and aloud by scrub person and circulating nurse.	________	________
3. Items being counted are visible to scrub person and circulating nurse.	________	________
a. sponges are separated for visibility		
4. Sharps are maintained on a needle mat (or other device designed for this purpose).	________	________
5. Contents of multipack sutures are verified by scrub person when opened.	________	________
6. Names of all persons who performed counts during procedure are documented.	________	________

OBSERVER'S SIGNATURE INITIALS

____________________________________ ________

ORIENTEE'S SIGNATURE

____

CHAPTER 8

Prevention of Injury—Hemostasis, Tourniquet, and Electrosurgical Equipment

Learner Objectives

At the end of Prevention of Injury—Hemostasis, Tourniquet, and Electrosurgical Equipment, the learner will

- identify three potential patient injuries related to use of tourniquet
- list two criteria for evaluating achievement of desired patient outcome relative to use of tourniquet
- describe nursing interventions to prevent patient injury when tourniquet is used
- identify three potential patient injuries related to the use of electrosurgical equipment
- identify and define general electrosurgical terms
- define capacitive coupling and describe related injury
- identify the desired patient outcome relative to use of electrosurgical equipment
- list four criteria for evaluating achievement of desired patient outcome relative to electrosurgical equipment
- describe nursing interventions to prevent patient injury when electrosurgical equipment is used

Lesson Outline

I. **HEMOSTASIS**
   A. Natural Methods of Hemostasis
   B. Artificial Methods of Hemostasis
      1. Chemical Hemostasis
         a. Thrombin
         b. Gelatin Sponge
         c. Oxidized Cellulose
         d. Microfibrillar Collagen
         e. Styptic
      2. Mechanical Hemostasis
         a. Instruments, Ties, Suture Ligatures, Ligating Clips
         b. Bonewax
         c. Pressure

II. **TOURNIQUET**
   A. Overview
   B. Potential Injury—Desired Patient Outcome/Criteria
   C. Nursing Interventions

III. **ELECTRICAL HEMOSTASIS—ELECTROSURGERY**
   A. Overview
   B. Electrosurgical Components
      1. The Generator
      2. The Active Electrode
      3. The Dispersive Electrode
   C. Application
   D. Potential for Patient Injury
   E. Desired Patient Outcome/Criteria
   F. Nursing Interventions

CHAPTER 8

Prevention of Injury—Hemostasis, Tourniquet, and Electrosurgical Equipment

HEMOSTASIS

1. Hemostasis is the arrest of bleeding. Historically, attempts to achieve hemostasis have included applications of egg yolk, dust, cobwebs, tree bark, boiling oil, turpentine, and various combinations thereof (Atkinson, 1992, pp. 368–369). Until the advent of modern hemostatic methods, blood loss made surgery difficult and was a serious surgical complication.
2. Modern hemostatic methods, including electrosurgery and tourniquet application, have greatly enhanced the surgeon's ability to perform slow, deliberate surgery and to operate in a field where control of bleeding permits excellent visualization of anatomical structures.
3. Hemostasis may be achieved by natural or artificial methods.

Natural Methods of Hemostasis

4. When an injury occurs to a blood vessel, a roughened surface is created. Platelets are attracted to and adhere to this surface. Several layers accumulate and a platelet plug is formed. A platelet plug is often sufficient to seal small injuries. As the platelets break down, they release thromboplastin into the blood. Thromboplastin is necessary for coagulation to occur.
5. Platelet plug formation is not the same as coagulation. In coagulation a fibrin clot is formed. Coagulation is a complex mechanism involving multiple clotting factors and a series of reactions. During coagulation, prothrombin, which is present in blood, reacts with thromboplastin, which is released when tissues are injured and platelets break down. Prothrombin, thromboplastin, and calcium ions in the blood form thrombin. In the final step, thrombin unites with fibrinogen, a blood plasma, to form fibrin. Fibrin is the basic structure of the clot and reinforces the platelet plug. Initially this fibrin is white. As platelets, white cells, and red cells become entangled in the fibrin, the clot becomes red, taking on the appearance of a blood clot. The process of coagulation is regulated so that, as blood loss is controlled, coagulation ceases.
6. In spite of the complexity of the coagulation process, it is rapid and sufficient to prevent blood loss from most small wounds.

Artificial Methods of Hemostasis

7. Natural hemostasis is not sufficient to control bleeding during surgery. Gross bleeding and oozing occur during surgery and both are controlled through artificial hemostatic methods. Chemical, mechanical, or thermal methods may be used and can include the use of thrombin, gelatin sponge, oxidized cellulose, microfibrillar collagen, collagen pads, styptics, pressure, instruments, ties, suture ligatures, ligating clips, bonewax, tourniquet, and electrosurgery. Tourniquet and electrosurgery have significant patient safety implications and are addressed in depth in this chapter.

Chemical Hemostasis

Thrombin.

8. Thrombin is an enzyme made from dried beef blood. It combines with fibrinogen and accelerates the coagulation process. Thrombin is useful in controlling capillary

bleeding, and it is supplied as a dry white powder that may be sprinkled on an oozing site. More often, it is mixed with water or saline to form a solution and is used in conjunction with a gelatin sponge. Thrombin is for topical use only and must never be injected.

Gelatin Sponge.

9. Gelatin sponge is made from a purified gelatin solution. It is available as a powder, a film (Gelfilm), or a pad (Gelfoam). Gelfoam, which resembles Styrofoam, is the form used most often. It absorbs 45 times its weight in blood. Gelfoam is available in a variety of sizes and may be used by itself, but is frequently dipped in a thrombin solution. When placed on an area of capillary bleeding, fibrin will be deposited in the interstices of the pad, the pad will swell, and clot formation will progress. Gelfoam may be cut to the desired size. It is not soluble; however, when left in the body it will be absorbed in 20 to 40 days. Gelfoam may also be soaked in epinephrine before application.

Oxidized Cellulose.

10. Oxidized cellulose (Oxycel, Surgicel, and Surgicel Nu-Knit) is a specially treated gauze or cotton applied directly to an oozing surface to control bleeding. It absorbs seven to eight times its own weight. When oxidized cellulose contacts whole blood it increases its size, forms a gel, and causes clot formation. The pressure of the swollen cellulose also encourages hemostasis. Oxidized cellulose is used to control bleeding in areas that are difficult to control by other means of hemostasis. It may be left on an oozing surface and will be absorbed by the body in 7 to 14 days. It must, however, be removed when used around the optic nerve or spinal cord, where swelling of the cellulose can exert harmful pressure on these structures.

Microfibrillar Collagen.

11. Microfibrillar collagen (Avitene) is a fluffy, white, absorbable material made from purified bovine dermis. It is applied directly over the source of bleeding. Its form allows it to be placed in crevices and areas of irregular contour. Hemostasis is achieved when platelets and fibrin adhere to the collagen and clot formation progresses. Microfibrillar collagen is useful where tissue is friable. Collagen pads (Helistat), sponges (Superstat and Collastat), and felt (Lyostypt) are also available and are applied directly to a bleeding surface.

Styptic.

12. Styptics are agents that cause blood vessel constriction. Epinephrine is a frequently used styptic. It is often added to a local anesthetic, such as lidocaine, to decrease bleeding at the site of the surgery.
13. Silver nitrate in the form of a stick or pencil with a silver nitrate crystal head is another form of styptic. It is applied topically to small vessels.
14. Tannic acid and Monsel's solution, a ferric subsulfate salt, are two less frequently used topical agents.

Mechanical Hemostasis

Instruments, Ties, Suture Ligatures, Ligating Clips.

15. A hemostatic clamp may be used to occlude the end of a bleeding vessel. As long as the clamp is in place, bleeding will not occur. Clamping is a temporary means of hemostasis and is followed by the application of a tie, a suture ligature, a ligating clip, or electrosurgery. A tie is a strand of material tied around the vessel to occlude the lumen. A suture ligature is a tie with an attached needle that is used to anchor the tie through the vessel. A ligating clip (hemoclip) is a stainless steel, tantalum, or titanium clip used to permanently clamp a vessel. Except for polymeric clips, which are absorbable, clips remain permanently within the patient.

Bonewax.

16. Bonewax is made from beeswax and is used to stop bleeding from bone. It is used most often in neurosurgery and orthopedic surgery. A small amount rubbed over a cut bone surface will control bleeding.

Pressure.

17. Pressure is applied when sponges are used to blot areas of bleeding. When a sponge is removed it is possible to identify the area of bleeding and to employ additional methods of hemostasis. Manual pressure applied directly to small vessels may delay bleeding long enough for clot formation to begin.

Section Questions

Q1. Coagulation (Ref. 5, 6):
a. is a natural process
b. is the same as a platelet plug formation
c. is a complex process that involves multiple clotting factors
d. is a slow deliberate process
e. ceases as blood loss is controlled
f. is a process that is sufficient to prevent blood loss from most small wounds

Q2. Artificial means of hemostasis include (Ref. 7):
a. gelatin sponge
b. suture ligatures
c. blood transfusion
d. ligating clips
e. electrosurgery

Q3. Match the word in column A with the description in column B. (Ref. 8–15)

A	*B*
a. gelatin sponge	_____ lidocaine
b. thrombin	_____ stainless steel clip used to clamp a vessel
c. oxidized cellulose	_____ specially treated gauze or cotton used to control oozing
d. styptic	_____ enzyme made from dried beef blood used to control capillary bleeding
e. hemoclip	_____ resembles Styrofoam, used to control capillary bleeding, may be dipped in thrombin

Q4. ________is used in orthopedic surgery to control bleeding from bone. (Ref. 16)

TOURNIQUET

Overview

18. Application of a tourniquet prior to surgery provides a bloodless surgical field. A pneumatic tourniquet is frequently used for surgery on an extremity. The resultant bloodless field greatly increases the surgeon's ability to complete the surgery and prevents blood loss for the patient.
19. Once the tourniquet is released the severed vessels will bleed and cauterization or ligation will be necessary to stop bleeding.
20. Tourniquets of various types are available. The simplest tourniquet is a piece of rubber tubing, such as a Penrose drain, that is used around an extremity in preparation for a venipuncture. An Esmarch bandage is a long piece of rolled latex that is wrapped tightly around an extremity from the distal end toward the proximal end. The extremity is raised to permit gravity to drain blood from the extremity and the Esmarch applied. The Esmarch compresses superficial blood vessels and further forces the blood from the extremity. The Esmarch is removed and a pneumatic tourniquet is then applied.

21. Pneumatic tourniquets are inflated and maintained at a specified pressure required for the surgery and requested by the surgeon. Pneumatic tourniquets contain an internal bladder housed in a pressure cuff. The bladder is inflated with either ambient air or compressed gas from a cartridge, tank, or compressed-air line.

Potential Injury—Desired Patient Outcome/Criteria

22. The nursing diagnosis of high risk for injury related to use of tourniquet is appropriate for the patient on whom a tourniquet is used. Tourniquet injury can include skin injury, such as chemical burn from prep solutions; bruise or blister formation; and nerve injury, including paralysis.
23. The Association of Operating Room Nurses (AORN) outcome standard states, "The patient is free from injury related to positioning, extraneous objects, or chemical, physical, and electrical hazards" (AORN, 1995, p. 126). The patient should experience no injury as a result of tourniquet use.
24. Successful achievement of the desired outcome is indicated if at the completion of surgery there is no evidence of
    - skin blisters, abrasions, necrosis, swelling
    - chemical burn
    - paralysis or other sign of nerve injury (Phippen & Wells, 1994, p. 184)

Nursing Interventions

25. Nursing interventions to prevent injury from tourniquet application require knowledge of equipment use and appropriate safety precautions. Institutional policy and practice may dictate who has responsibility for tourniquet application. Regardless of who actually applies the tourniquet, patient safety with regard to its use is a shared responsibility. The perioperative nurse must be able to select a tourniquet that is in working condition and that is the appropriate size, and the nurse must be knowledgeable regarding the principles of application.
26. Prior to tourniquet application the patient's skin should be assessed for integrity and turgor, and the extremity size should be evaluated in order to select an appropriate size tourniquet cuff.
27. The pneumatic tourniquet should be tested and inspected prior to use. Testing should be performed according to the manufacturer's written instructions and health care facility policy. Most policies for tourniquet testing require periodic testing to ensure that the pressures are accurate and that the tourniquet functions properly.
28. Inspection should include the cuff, console, tubing, connections, and electrical cords. When nitrogen gas is used to inflate the cuff, the level of gas in the tank should be checked before each use to ensure that there is an adequate amount for the duration of the intended surgery. Close inspection of the cuff for cleanliness is important. Velcro fasteners are areas where microorganisms and other debris can collect. Water left in a tourniquet cuff port can cause microbial growth with the potential for entry of microorganisms into the tourniquet-regulating mechanism when the cuff is deflated (AORN, 1995, pp. 227–228).
29. The selection of a tourniquet cuff should take into consideration the size of the patient's extremity. As wide a cuff as possible should be selected because a wider cuff occludes blood flow at a lower pressure. The length of the cuff should permit an overlap that is adequate to provide even pressure on the circumference of the extremity. Overlap should be approximately 3 to 6 inches. Too much overlap can cause increased pressure in the area of the overlap (AORN, 1995, p. 228).
30. Except where the manufacturer specifies in writing that padding is not required, the tourniquet should not be applied to unprotected skin. A Webril or stockinette material should be wrapped around the extremity where the tourniquet will be applied. Care must be taken to prevent bunching or wrinkling the material, which can result in uneven pressure against the skin and create the potential for the impairment of skin integrity.
31. The tourniquet should be placed on the limb at the most proximal point of maximum circumference, according to the manufacturer's written instructions for use. This area provides the greatest amount of soft tissue and therefore protection of underlying nerves and blood vessels (AORN, 1995, p. 229).
32. The area of tourniquet application should be protected from any potential or actual pooling or collection of fluids, which can irritate the skin. Prepping agents, if allowed to pool under the cuff, have the potential to cause a chemical burn to the skin. The nurse should remove excess liquid resulting from the prep, and should protect the area from subsequent pooling of fluids during surgery by applying a protective fluid barrier. Such a barrier may be included as part of the extremity drape and will be applied during the draping procedure.
33. Exact tourniquet inflation pressures have not been determined. The lowest pressure needed to create a bloodless field should be used. Patient age, extremity size, systolic blood pressure, and tourniquet cuff size are factors that determine inflation pressures.

34. The exact length of time for tourniquet inflation has not been determined; however, inflation times should be kept to a minimum. Excessive inflation times can damage underlying tissue and cause injury as severe as permanent paralysis. For an adult, an hour for an arm and an hour and a half for a leg are usual inflation times. A lower pressure is used for children and for patients where blood supply to the extremity is diminished. Insufficient pressure and subsequent prolonged venous congestion can also result in nerve injury.
35. During the surgery the nurse should periodically report to the surgeon the length of time that the tourniquet has been inflated. Intervals for reporting inflation times should be agreed upon between the surgeon and the nurse. Anesthesia personnel may also monitor inflation times. All team members must work in concert to ensure adequate and appropriate communication.
36. Throughout the surgery the nurse should refer to the tourniquet gauge to determine fluctuations in pressure that may indicate a tourniquet failure.
37. In the case of inadvertent loss of pressure, the tourniquet should be totally deflated, and an elastic bandage or the action of gravity should be used to force the blood out of the extremity before the tourniquet is reinflated. The tourniquet should not be reinflated over an area already engorged with blood. To do so creates a risk for intravascular thrombosis (AORN, 1995, p. 229).
38. The tourniquet should be deflated upon instructions from the surgeon.
39. AORN recommended practices for use of the pneumatic tourniquet state that the perioperative nurse document

    - the assessment of skin and tissue integrity under the cuff before and after tourniquet use
    - the location of cuff
    - the cuff pressure
    - the time of inflation and deflation
    - the identification/serial number and model of the equipment used
    - the identification of the person who applied the cuff (AORN, 1995, p. 230)

40. Documentation should also include an evaluation of the achievement of desired outcome.

Section Questions

Q5. What is the purpose of an Esmarch bandage? (Ref. 20)

Q6. The patient on whom a tourniquet is used is at high risk for injury. List three potential injuries that can result from pneumatic tourniquet use. (Ref. 22)

Q7. Prior to the application of a tourniquet the patient's extremity should be assessed for (Ref. 26):
a. size
b. skin turgor
c. skin integrity
d. capillary fill

Q8. Explain why a cuff as wide as possible should be selected for use with a pneumatic tourniquet. (Ref. 29)

Q9. Tourniquet pressure is determined by (Ref. 33):
a. patient age
b. size of extremity
c. make of tourniquet
d. tourniquet cuff size

Q10. Monitoring of inflation time and pressure is not the responsibility of the perioperative nurse. (Ref. 35)

True False

Q11. Documentation regarding tourniquet application and use should include (Ref. 39, 40):
a. skin assessment before and after cuff application
b. location of cuff
c. tourniquet cuff pressure
d. inflation time
e. evaluation of achievement of desired patient outcome

ELECTRICAL HEMOSTASIS—ELECTROSURGERY

Overview

41. Electrosurgery is used routinely in most surgical procedures. Radio frequency electrical current is passed through the patient's body for the purpose of cutting tissue or coagulating bleeding points.
42. As the current passes through the tissue, heat is generated in sufficient amounts to produce cutting and/or coagulation.

Electrosurgical Components

43. Three components are required to perform electrosurgery: (1) an electrosurgical unit (ESU) or generator, (2) an active electrode, and (3) a dispersive electrode.

The Generator

44. The unit that supplies the current is referred to as an electrosurgical unit or generator (see Figure 8–1).
45. In the 1920s Dr. William Bovie was instrumental in the development of the first spark-gap vacuum tube generator that produced cutting with hemostasis. This was the basis of electrosurgical units until the 1970s when solid state electrosurgical units were introduced. Solid state units with small printed circuit boards and transistors have replaced the vacuum tube. However, many persons still refer to the solid state electrosurgical units as "Bovie" machines.
46. Current is provided by the generator to the active electrode accessory and is used to introduce current into the patient. The dispersive electrode is an accessory that is in contact with the patient and returns the current from the patient to the electrosurgical generator.
47. Early electrosurgical units presented significant risk for a burn or shock injury. Generators manufactured today are both solid state and isolated systems and have dramatically reduced the risk of injury.
48. Early generators were the ground-referenced type. In a ground-referenced system the generator acts as a ground to earth. If the circuit whereby the current returns to the machine is broken, the current may seek an alternate pathway and cause a burn at the site of contact. Alternate sites might include electrocardiogram electrodes and sites where the patient is touching a grounded metal item. If there is not proper contact between the patient and the dispersive electrode, there will be an interruption in the current. Although isolated-system generators are most commonly used, ground-referenced generators may still be found in some operating rooms.

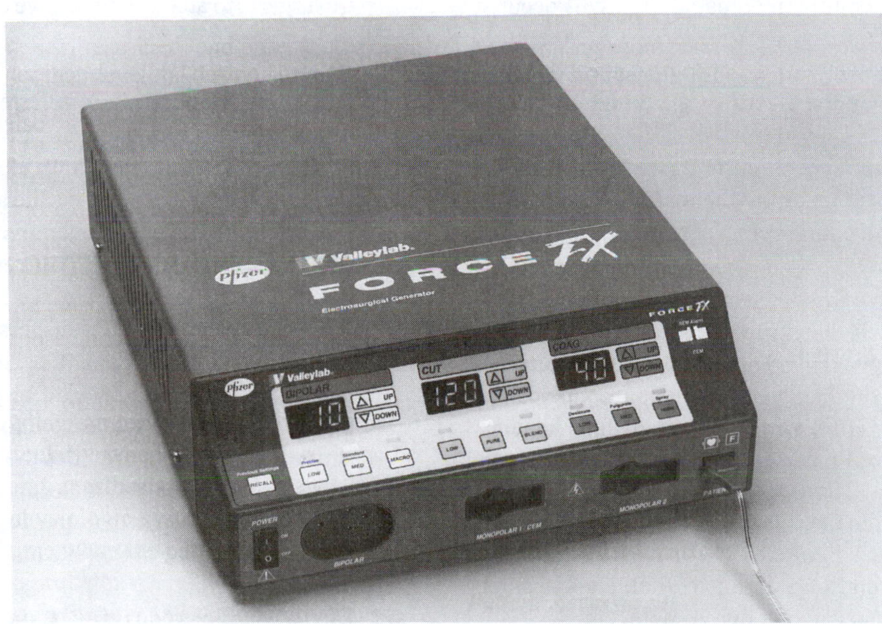

Figure 8–1 Electrosurgery Unit. *Source:* Courtesy of Valley Lab, Inc., Pfizer Hospital Products Group, Boulder, Colorado.

49. Isolated systems are a significant improvement over ground-referenced systems. In an isolated system there is a transformer within the generator that isolates the current from the ground. Current is restricted to pathways to and from the generator. In addition to isolated currents, newer systems include a patient return electrode-monitoring system. The current that enters the patient is measured and compared with current returning to the dispersive electrode. If the currents are not sufficiently balanced the unit will alarm and deactivate. These systems have virtually eliminated burns under the dispersive electrode.
50. Electrosurgical units are designed to deliver current that will cut, coagulate, or combine the two. The type of waveform that is selected determines whether cutting, coagulation, or a combination of the two will occur.
51. A continuous-frequency waveform will cause cutting to occur. In the cutting mode, tissue is severed as intense heat is delivered from the active electrode and focused at the intended site. The active electrode is held slightly above the tissue.
52. An interrupted-frequency waveform will cause coagulation to occur. In the coagulation mode, when the active electrode is in direct contact with the tissue, the ends of small to moderate size vessels are seared and bleeding is controlled. When the active electrode is slightly above the tissue, a spark is produced and tissue is charred.
53. When a combination of the cut and coagulation waveform is selected, cutting and coagulation will occur simultaneously.
54. The amount of power and the type of current are regulated by controls on the electrosurgical unit and the accessories.
55. The selection of the type of current (waveform) and the amount of power is made by the surgeon and is determined by the procedure being performed and by surgeon preference.

The Active Electrode

56. The active electrode delivers current from the generator to the operative site. Active electrodes may be disposable or reusable. Most active electrodes are handheld devices with a cord that attaches to the electrosurgical generator. Active electrodes may be shaped as a blade, ball, loop, or needle that fits into a pencil-shaped handle or other device (see Figure 8–2). Active electrodes may also be a combination suction catheter and cautery where the tip of the catheter delivers current.
57. Active electrodes are activated by either a foot control or a control on the handpiece.
58. Active electrodes may be bipolar or monopolar. A monopolar electrode has one active pole or tip. This tip carries the current to the operative site. The current is then dissipated through the tissue, dispersed through the dispersive electrode, and returned to the generator.
59. Bipolar electrodes are shaped as forceps with two poles or tips. One tip acts as the active electrode, the other tip acts as the return or dispersive electrode. Current flows from the generator down one tine of the forceps, through the tissue between the forceps, and is returned to the generator through the other tine of the forceps. The current flows only between the tips of the forceps and only low wattage is necessary. Precise hemostasis is provided and current does not disperse throughout the patient. Because one tip of the forceps acts as a dispersive electrode, it is not necessary, as it is in monopolar electrosurgery, to attach a dispersive electrode to the patient.

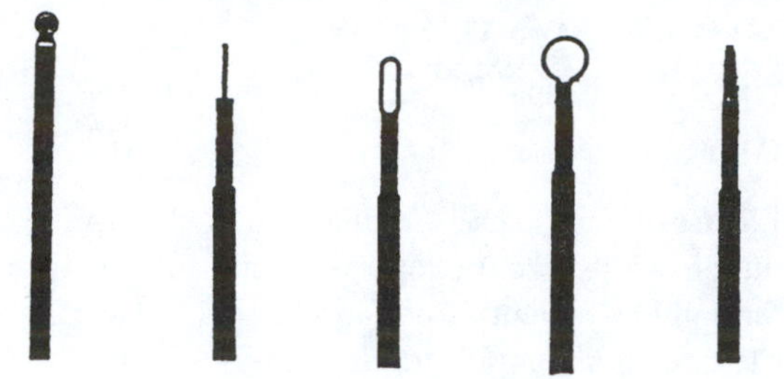

Figure 8–2 Examples of Active Electrode Tips

The Dispersive Electrode

60. Dispersive electrodes are referred to by many names. These include grounding pad, inactive electrode, patient plate, "Bovie" pad, and return electrode.
61. Current enters the patient via the active electrode, where it is concentrated at the operative site and where tissue destruction is achieved. Current is then dissipated through the patient and returned to the generator via the dispersive electrode. The dispersive electrode is in direct contact with the patient's skin. It has a cord that attaches to the generator. The dispersive electrode disperses the current released into the patient from the active electrode and provides the return path to the generator (see Figure 8–3). Because the dispersive electrode is much larger than the active electrode, the current density is low at this site and therefore burns do not normally occur.
62. Dispersive electrodes may be disposable or reusable.
63. Reusable dispersive electrodes are metal plates made of stainless steel that are positioned under the patient. Conductive gel is used to enhance the conductivity of the patient's skin and to fill in gaps between the plate and

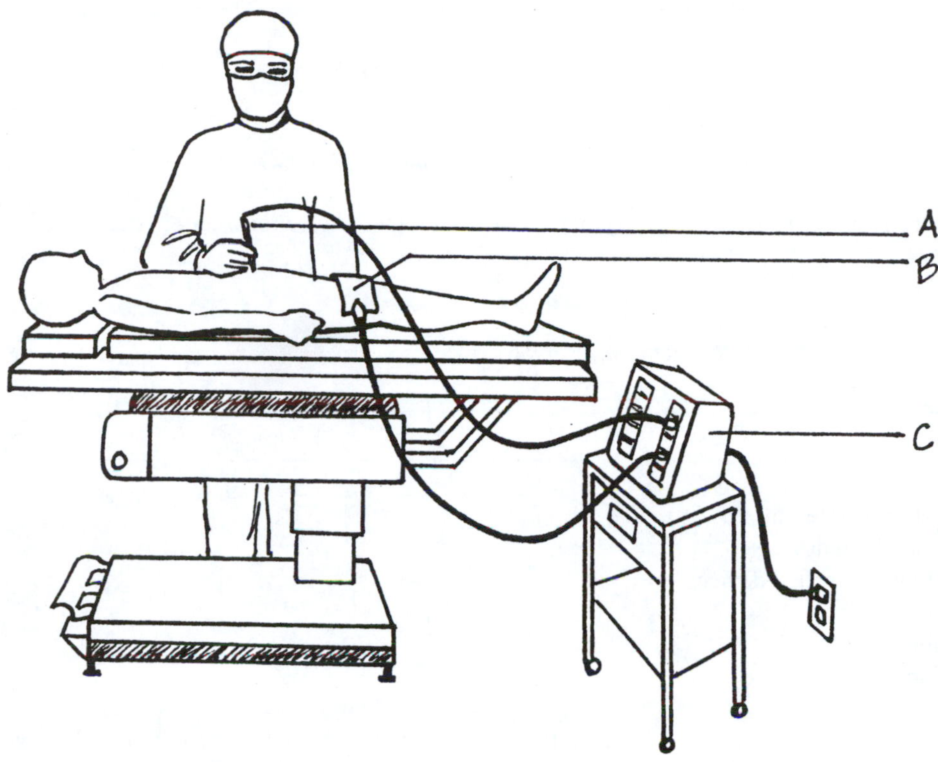

Figure 8–3 Electrosurgery. A. Active electrode. B. Dispersive electrode. C. Generator. *Source:* Courtesy of Jeanne Spry.

the patient's skin. Metal plates do not conform to the patient's body contour and are not adhesive. Disposable, adhesive dispersive electrodes have been available since the 1970s and have almost entirely replaced metal plates.

64. The most commonly used dispersive electrode is a disposable adhesive foil pad covered with a foam and impregnated with electrolyte gel. The pad easily conforms to the patient's body contour and provides uniform contact with the patient. The adhesive promotes good conductivity. Newer electrosurgical systems employ a dispersive electrode that works with the generator to identify potential current concentration sufficient to cause a burn. When this occurs the machine will alarm and deactivate.

Application

65. Many surgeons prefer electrosurgery to other methods of hemostasis that involve cutting and tying tissue. Use of electrosurgery permits rapid achievement of cutting and coagulation and may reduce surgical time. However, coagulated tissue produces a foreign-body reaction and must be absorbed during the healing process. If there is an excessive amount of coagulated tissue in the wound, sloughing may occur and healing by first intention may not occur.
66. Electrosurgery is used in many types of surgery. A single power setting is not appropriate for all surgery. Differences in generator performance, surgical technique, and active electrode size determine power settings. Generally, low power is used in neurosurgery, dermatology procedures, and oral and plastic surgery.
67. Fulguration and desiccation are two types of coagulation. Fulguration is the use of sparking to coagulate large bleeders and to char tissue. In fulguration the active electrode does not actually contact the tissue. As sparks contact tissue, superficial coagulation results initially. As the sparking continues, this superficial coagulation is followed by deep necrosis. Fulguration is frequently used by urologists in transurethral resections where the intent is to cause necrosis and destroy tissue.
68. Coagulation in which the active electrode contacts the tissue is referred to as desiccation and is the type of coagulation used in most surgeries. Desiccation results in hemostasis but does not always result in necrosis.

Section Questions

Q12. Electrosurgery may be used to __________ or __________ tissue. (Ref. 42)

Q13. An isolated electrosurgery system is _____ than a ground-referenced electrosurgery system. (Ref. 49)
a. safer
b. less safe

Q14. Explain the function of the active electrode. (Ref. 56)

____

____

Q15. The active electrode (Ref. 56, 57, 58):
a. may be a handheld device
b. may be a foot-controlled device
c. disperses current
d. may be monopolar
e. may be bipolar

Q16. The dispersive electrode provides a return path for electrical current from the patient to the electrosurgical generator. (Ref. 61)

True False

Q17. Coagulated tissue causes a foreign-body reaction. Describe a complication of healing that can occur if there is an excessive amount of coagulated tissue in the wound. (Ref. 65)

____

____

Q18. Desiccation and fulguration are forms of coagulation. (Ref. 67)

True False

Q19. Explain the difference between desiccation and fulguration. (Ref. 67, 68)

____

____

Potential for Patient Injury

69. The nursing diagnosis of high risk for injury related to use of electrosurgery is appropriate for the patient on whom electrosurgery is used. Although improvements in electrosurgical equipment have minimized the risk of patient burn at an alternate ground site, the risk of patient injury remains. All operating rooms are not equipped with the most modern equipment and even modern machines do not eliminate the potential for injury. Older dispersive electrode pads can permit concentration of current and subsequent burn if there is poor contact, i.e., poor electrical connection between the patient and the dispersive electrode. Poor contact can be caused by the incorrect placement of the pad.
70. A patient burn can occur from inadvertent contact with the patient at an unintended site if the generator is accidentally activated and the active electrode is not housed in a protective receptacle.
71. The advent of minimally invasive laparoscopic surgery has brought with it an increased risk of burn injury from electrosurgery. One study indicated a reported incidence of injury in 331 laparoscopic procedures during a 1-year period, 75% of which were not recognized at the time of surgery (Tucker & Randle, 1995, p. 63)
72. In laparoscopic surgery the active electrode is introduced into the patient through the abdominal wall via a cannula. The internal view is limited and the shaft of the laparoscope and the cannula are not visualized. Unintended transfer of energy along the laparoscope or cannula shaft, or along the active electrode shaft, can result in an internal burn that may go unnoticed. Inadvertent activation of the active electrode outside the visible field can also cause an internal burn. The result may be an undiagnosed burn that perforates the bowel and results in postoperative peritonitis, which is then life threatening because of the time lapse between when a patient is discharged and when the infection is diagnosed.
73. Electrosurgical complications in laparoscopic surgery are caused by three mechanisms: (1) insulation failure in the active electrode, (2) direct coupling between the active electrode and other metal instruments or with tissue, and (3) capacitive coupling (Tucker & Randle, 1995, p. 58)
74. Insulation failure occurs when the insulation of an active electrode is not intact and causes current to flow to an unintended area where it may contact tissue and result in a burn injury to the abdominal viscera. Insulation failures occur in laparoscopic instruments such as a suction cautery where the tip of the suction cannula acts as an active electrode. The shaft of the instrument is insulated to prevent current from exiting other than at the active electrode end, but if the insulation is not intact, current can flow unimpeded to tissue where it can burn through abdominal viscera and cause life-threatening injury. A less serious injury will occur if the current is directed to the cannula in which the electrode is housed. In this instance the patient will experience a burn to the abdominal wall or skin where there is contact with the cannula.
75. Insulation defects may be so small as to go unnoticed during routine instrument examination.
76. In direct coupling the tip of the active electrode touches another metal instrument. The current is transferred to that instrument, which in turn acts as an active electrode, causing a burn at the contact site.
77. This type of injury is within the surgeon's view, and repair can be attempted before the completion of surgery.
78. Capacitive coupling is the transfer of electrical current from the active electrode through the coupling of stray current into other conductive surgical equipment (Tucker, Voyles, & Silvis, 1992, p. 304). When radio frequency currents flow through an electrode, the flow induces stray currents onto other nearby conductors. Currents are induced onto the nearby conductors even though the insulation on the active electrode is intact (Tucker & Randle, 1995, p. 61). The current may be passed on to a metal cannula or working channel of a laparoscope or other metal instrument through which the electrode is passed. This creates the potential for a burn most probably at the abdominal wall or on external skin.
79. Recent advances in laparoscopic instrumentation include laparoscopic bipolar active electrodes and shielded monopolar active electrodes with monitors designed to detect insulation failure. Bipolar electrodes localize current. Shielded monopolar monitoring systems detect insulation failure and will automatically deactivate in such an event. Both systems offer safety advantages.
80. The risk for capacitive coupling injury increases when high voltage and fulguration are used.
81. Two other risks associated with the use of electrosurgery are fire and plume inhalation.
82. The current from an active electrode is sufficient to initiate a fire. An active electrode that has been engaged and is in contact with a flammable item, such as linen or drapes, has the potential to start a fire. The operating room is an oxygen-enriched environment that quickly helps to spread fire, which can become intense in just a few minutes.

83. Fire in the operating from electrosurgical equipment is not unknown. Patient injury and death have been reported.
84. Plume or surgical smoke resulting from electrosurgical application is a concern. The National Institute for Occupational Safety and Health (NIOSH) has detected chemicals in surgical smoke that may be harmful and has identified electrosurgical smoke as a potential health hazard. A Japanese study has shown that electrosurgical smoke is mutagenic (Patterson, 1993, pp. 6–7). NIOSH, the American National Standards Institute, and the Association of Operating Room Nurses recommend smoke evacuation when there is electrosurgical smoke. In the absence of a dedicated smoke evacuator a suction should be used.

Desired Patient Outcome/Criteria

85. The desired patient outcome is that the patient will experience no injury as a result of the use of electrosurgery.
86. The criteria to evaluate successful achievement of the desired outcome are no evidence of
    - impaired skin integrity (burn) at dispersive electrode site or alternate current path such as electrocardiograph monitoring leads
    - burn at an unintended site
    - burn at the entrance site of laparoscopic instrumentation
    - fever or abdominal pain associated with peritonitis

Nursing Interventions

87. Although electrosurgery is performed by the surgeon and/or assistants, perioperative nursing interventions are critical to a safe patient outcome.
88. Prior to surgery the patient's skin should be assessed overall for the placement of dispersive electrode. The presence of scar tissue, excessive adipose tissue, metal prosthetic implant, pacemaker, or automatic implantable cardioverter defibrillator (AICD) should be noted. This information is necessary for selecting a site for dispersive electrode placement.
89. Implementation of the following guidelines and safety measures will minimize the risk of electrosurgical burn. Some of the measures will be implemented by the scrub person, others by the circulating nurse.
    - Inspect the generator for frayed cords, loose connections, and an intact and activated alarm system.
    - Test the alarm and set it loud enough to be heard during surgery.
    - Place the generator close enough to the patient to prevent cords from being pulled taut and thus creating tension at the connection sites.
    - Orally confirm the power settings with the surgeon. Power settings should be kept as low as possible. If a request is made for an unusually high setting because the present setting is no longer adequate, check for loose connections and malfunction. In older equipment this may signal that the current is seeking an alternate path. Replace the generator if a malfunction is discovered or suspected.
    - Do not place liquids on the generator as these may spill, leak into the generator, and cause the equipment to malfunction. Foot pedals must also be kept dry. Placing the foot pedal into a plastic bag will keep it dry.
    - Do not use electrosurgery in the presence of flammable agents. Prep solutions containing flammable agents should be permitted to dry before electrosurgical application.
    - Position the active electrode on the sterile field, close to the operative site, and in a protective container or holster so that accidental activation will not cause incidental burn or ignite drapes. When two active electrodes are in use and both are attached to the same generator, it is especially important to avoid incidental contact of both electrodes with the patient. In older generators, both active electrodes will be energized whenever either one is activated. For a few seconds after deactivation, the active electrode can retain heat sufficient to melt some plastics (ECRI, 1992, p. 1). When the active electrode is not in use it should be placed in the holster.
    - Keep the active electrode clean during surgery by removing charred tissue from the electrodes.
    - Prior to surgery, inspect the active electrodes for insulation defects. If a defect is noted, the electrode must not be used. If the defect is noted during the surgery or after the procedure, inform the surgeon that the patient may have sustained an inadvertent internal burn.
    - Do not use single-use electrodes that have been reprocessed. The insulation may not be designed to withstand reprocessing.
    - When available, request active electrode monitoring equipment for use during laparoscopic surgery.
    - Select a dispersive electrode appropriate to the patient's size and in accordance with the manufacturer's guidelines. Do not cut the dispersive electrode to modify its size or shape.
    - Check the dispersive electrode to ensure that there is adequate adhesive and gel, and that cord connections

are secure. If the dispersive electrode is designed to accept an application of gel, an even, smooth application is made to ensure uniform conductivity.

- Place the dispersive electrode on the patient over clean dry skin that covers a large muscle mass and as close to the operative site as possible. Such placement will help ensure good contact with the patient's skin, will ensure sufficient current dispersal, and will minimize current through the patient's body. Because bony prominences and scar tissue can concentrate current, these areas should not be selected as placement sites for the dispersive electrode. Areas of excessive hair and areas where fluids can accumulate and compromise the adhesive should be avoided. Areas of excess adipose tissue should also be avoided. Fatty undervascularized tissue can impede conductivity of electrical current and dissipation of heat. Muscular areas generally have adequate blood circulation and promote conductivity of the electrical current. Suitable areas of placement include the anterior and posterior thigh, the calf, the upper arm, the buttock, the midback, and the abdomen. Areas close to electrocardiographic electrodes are avoided because current may be attracted to these electrodes and cause a patient burn at these sites.
- Position the patient free from contact with metal surfaces, such as the operating room table.
- Do not include metal implants in the circuit path from the active electrode to the dispersive electrode. Metal implants can carry a fraction of the electrosurgical energy (AORN, 1995, p. 158).
- During lengthy procedures, or when the patient is repositioned during surgery, verify patient contact with the dispersive electrode.
- Suction electrosurgical smoke from the field.
- In the event of the failure of any of the electrosurgical components, retain the defective items for follow-up with biomedical personnel and for reporting of medical instrumentation failure as required.
- Do not use reusable active electrodes beyond their intended life. Refer to manufacturer's guidelines for the permitted number of uses.

90. The patient who has an AICD will need to have the device deactivated prior to surgery and reactivated after surgery. The presence of an AICD should be noted, and procedures designed to implement deactivation and reactivation should be followed. Regardless of who has the responsibility for activation and deactivation, the perioperative nurse must ensure that the AICD has been noted and appropriate action has been taken.
91. The use of electrosurgery in patients with a pacemaker represents a potential electrical hazard. Electrosurgery can interfere with the operation of some pacemakers. The tip of the active electrode should be as far from the pacemaker as possible. The dispersive electrode should not be placed near the pacemaker. Safety guidelines for patients with a pacemaker should be prepared in advance of surgery according to manufacturer's instructions.
92. Patients with a pacemaker or AICD should have continuous electrocardiogram monitoring during procedures where electrosurgery is used, and a defibrillator should be readily available.
93. Following surgery, the dispersive electrode should be removed slowly and carefully to prevent denuding the skin. The placement area should be inspected for injury. The patient should be checked for incidental burns with particular attention given to electrocardiogram electrode sites and temperature probe entry sites (AORN, 1995, p. 158).
94. Documentation of electrosurgical use should include the following:
    - assessment of the skin preoperatively
    - identification of electrosurgical equipment and setting
    - site of dispersive electrode placement and person who applied electrode
    - assessment of skin postoperatively

Section Questions

Q20. The patient undergoing laparoscopic surgery in which electrosurgery is used is at risk of (Ref. 72):
   a. internal burn from unintended transfer of energy along the laparoscope cannula
   b. internal burn from inadvertent activation of the active electrode outside the field of vision
   c. excessive tissue desiccation

Q21. When nonintact insulation on an active electrode results in patient injury during electrosurgery application, the injury can be life threatening. (Ref. 74)

True False

Q22. If insulation is intact on an active electrode used in laparoscopic surgery there is no risk of injury from capacitive coupling. (Ref. 78)

True False

Q23. In addition to patient burn, hazards associated with electrosurgery include (Ref. 83, 84):
   a. cardiac arrest
   b. fire
   c. plume

Q24. List four criteria used to evaluate successful achievement of the desired patient outcome of no injury as a result of electrosurgery. (Ref. 86)

____

____

____

____

Q25. Suitable areas for placement of the dispersive electrode include (Ref. 89):
   a. anterior thigh
   b. posterior thigh
   c. upper arm
   d. buttock
   e. over a bony prominence
   f. abdomen
   g. midback

Q26. List four pieces of information relative to the use of electrosurgery that should be documented. (Ref. 94)

____

____

____

____

NOTES

Association of Operating Room Nurses (AORN). (1995). *Standards and recommended practices.* Denver, CO: AORN.

Atkinson, L.J. (1992). *Berry & Kohn's operating room technique* (7th ed.). St. Louis: Mosby Year Book.

ECRI. (1992, March). Understanding the fire hazard. *Technology for perioperative nurses* (Vol. 1). (1). Plymouth Meeting, PA.: ECRI.

Patterson, P. (1993, June). OR exposure to electrosurgery smoke a concern. *OR Manager*, *9*(6), 6–7.

Phippen, M., & Wells, M. (1994). *Perioperative nursing practice.* Philadelphia: W.B. Saunders.

Tucker, R., & Randle, V. (1995, July). Laparoscopic electrosurgical complications and their prevention. *AORN Journal*, *62*(1), 51–71.

Tucker, R.D., Voyles, C.R., & Silvis, S.E. (1992, July/August). Capacitive coupled stray currents during laparoscopic and endoscopic electrosurgical procedures. *Biomedical Instrumentation & Technology*, *26*, 303–311.

ADDITIONAL READING

Patterson, P. (1993). Hazards of electrosurgery in laparoscopy overlooked. *OR Manager*, *9*(3), 1–3.

Wicker, C.P. (1991). *Working with electrosurgery.* Harrogate, England: National Association of Theatre Nurses.

Appendix 8–A

Chapter 8 Post Test

1. In natural hemostasis the protein fibrinogen is converted to ___________ that forms the basic structure of a clot. (Ref. 5)

2. Thrombin, gelatin sponge, and ties are examples of artificial methods of hemostasis. List four additional artificial methods. (Ref. 7)

   ____

   ____

   ____

   ____

3. It is a fluffy white material made from purified bovine dermis. (Ref. 11)
   a. thrombin
   b. microfibrillar collagen
   c. gelatin sponge

4. It is a specially treated gauze or cotton used to control oozing of blood in areas that are difficult to control by other methods of hemostasis. (Ref. 10)
   a. gelatin sponge
   b. styptic
   c. oxidized cellulose

5. It absorbs 45 times its weight in blood and is used to control capillary bleeding. (Ref. 9)
   a. gelatin sponge
   b. thrombin
   c. oxidized cellulose

6. List two types of injury that a patient could sustain from improper tourniquet use. (Ref. 22)

   ____

   ____

7. The pneumatic tourniquet should be tested and inspected prior to use. What is tested? (Ref. 28)

   ____

   ____

8. The length of the tourniquet cuff should (Ref. 29):
   a. wrap around the extremity so the ends of the cuff meet
   b. wrap around the extremity so there is overlap of 6 or more inches
   c. wrap around the extremity so there is an overlap of 3 to 6 inches

9. Before the tourniquet is applied the extremity should be padded with ___________. (Ref. 30)

10. The tourniquet should be applied (Ref. 31):
    a. at the most proximal point
    b. at the most distal point

11. What risk to the patient is there if prep solutions are allowed to pool under the tourniquet? (Ref. 32)

    ____

    ____

12. The maximum length of time for tourniquet inflation has not been determined; however, 2 hours for an arm and 2½ hours for a leg are usual inflation times. (Ref. 34)

    True False

13. Reinflating a pneumatic tourniquet over an area already engorged with blood creates a risk for what type of injury. (Ref. 37)

    ____

14. The nurse should periodically report to the surgeon the length of time the tourniquet has been inflated. (Ref. 35)

    True False

15. In addition to documentation as to whether the desired patient outcome was achieved, list four other pieces of information that should be documented regarding tourniquet use. (Ref. 39)

    ____

    ____

    ____

    ____

16. The purpose of electrosurgery is to ______ or ______body tissue using a high radio frequency current. (Ref. 41)

17. Why are solid state electrosurgery units sometimes referred to as "Bovie" machines? (Ref. 45)

    ____

    ____

18. What is the purpose of the active electrode? (Ref. 46)

    ____

    ____

19. In a ground-referenced generator the dispersive electrode is connected or grounded to earth. Should there be an interruption in the ground connection (Ref. 48):
    a. the current could seek an alternate path and cause the patient to sustain a severe burn
    b. the machine would automatically shut itself off

20. An advantage of bipolar surgery is (Ref. 59):
    a. the ability to perform electrosurgery with increased hemostasis
    b. current does not disperse throughout the patient
    c. the ability to perform electrosurgery without a separate dispersive electrode

21. Dispersive electrodes are often referred to by many names. Give two other names for the dispersive electrode. (Ref. 60)

____

____

22. The active electrode (Ref. 56, 67, 68):
   a. delivers current to the operative site
   b. channels current back to the generator
   c. may be used to desiccate or fulgurate

23. Explain why a return electrode-monitoring electrosurgery unit system is safer than the isolated electrosurgery unit system and the ground-referenced system. (Ref. 49)

____

____

____

24. Capacitive coupling can occur in laparoscopic surgery (Ref. 78):
   a. when insulation on the active electrode is intact
   b. only if the dispersive electrode is not adequately adhered to the patient
   c. when stray current from the active electrode couples with other conductive surgical instrumentation

25. The patient undergoing laparoscopic surgery may sustain an injury from an active electrode (Ref. 72, 73, 74):
   a. and the injury will not be detected until after discharge
   b. from nonintact insulation on an active electrode instrument
   c. from direct coupling

26. Fire is a hazard associated with use of electrosurgery. (Ref. 81, 82, 83)

   True False

27. The desired patient outcome is that the patient will experience no injury as a result of the use of electrosurgery. List two criteria that may be used to evaluate whether this outcome has been achieved. (Ref. 86)

____

____

28. Why should the active electrode be maintained in a holster when on the sterile field? (Ref. 89)

____

____

29. Identify two sites/areas where the dispersive should *not* be placed. (Ref. 89)

____

____

30. During a procedure where the patient is repositioned, what intervention should the nurse take to ensure patient safety? (Ref. 89)

____

31. The active electrode should not be operated very close to a pacemaker because it may interfere with the pacemaker's functioning. (Ref. 91)

    True False

32. Describe an action that may be taken to reduce risk to personnel of the potential health hazards associated with plume. (Ref. 84)

    ____

    ____

Appendix 8–B

Competency Checklist: Hemostasis—Tourniquet

Under observer's initials enter initials upon successful achievement of competency. Enter N/A if competency is not appropriate for institution.

NAME ____________________________________

	OBSERVER'S INITIALS	DATE
1. Assembles equipment:		
a. Webril	________	________
b. tourniquet	________	________
c. Esmarch	________	________
d. other	________	________
2. Assesses skin condition on extremity.	________	________
3. Appropriate size cuff selected.	________	________
4. Tourniquet inspected and tested:		
a. cuff	________	________
b. console	________	________
c. tubing	________	________
d. connections	________	________
e. electrical cords	________	________
f. power source/amount of gas in tank	________	________
g. cleanliness	________	________
5. Cuff applied:		
a. over padding	________	________
b. proximal point of limb selected (of maximum circumference)	________	________
6. Tourniquet inflated and deflated upon surgeon instructions.	________	________
7. Length of inflation reported at agreed upon intervals.	________	________
8. Pressure gauge checked during procedure for fluctuations in pressure.	________	________
9. Documentation of:		
a. skin assessment under cuff before and after tourniquet application	________	________

	OBSERVER'S INITIALS	DATE
b. location of cuff	________	________
c. time of inflation and deflation	________	________
d. tourniquet identification number	________	________
e. identification of person who applied the cuff	________	________

OBSERVER'S SIGNATURE INITIALS

______________________________ ________

ORIENTEE'S SIGNATURE

____

Appendix 8–C

Competency Checklist: Electrosurgical Equipment

Under observer's initials enter initials upon successful achievement of competency. Enter N/A if competency is not appropriate for institution.

NAME ______________________________

	OBSERVER'S INITIALS	DATE
1. Equipment assembled:		
a. electrosurgical generator	______	______
b. active and dispersive electrode	______	______
c. foot pedal	______	______
2. Generator:		
a. inspected for frayed cords and loose connections	______	______
b. alarm checked and setting is audible	______	______
3. Skin is assessed for integrity prior to application of dispersive electrode.	______	______
4. Dispersive electrode:		
a. appropriate size chosen	______	______
b. inspected for adequate adhesive/gel	______	______
c. positioned over large muscle mass (not positioned over bony prominence, excessively hairy site, large metal prosthetic implant)	______	______
d. contacts skin uniformly	______	______
e. areas close to electrocardiographic electrodes avoided	______	______
5. Active electrode:		
a. inspected for insulation defects	______	______
b. inspected for loose connections	______	______
c. housed in protective container/holster on the field	______	______
6. Power settings confirmed with surgeon.	______	______
7. Equipment positioned to cause tension at connection sites (generator close to patient).	______	______
8. Trouble-shooting:		
a. surgeon repeatedly requests higher settings		
–all connections checked	______	______
–adherence of dispersive electrode checked	______	______

	OBSERVER'S INITIALS	DATE
b. alarm sounds		
–all connections checked	________	________
–adherence of dispersive electrode checked	________	________
9. Following procedure, skin integrity at dispersive electrode site is assessed for integrity; assessment documented.	________	________

OBSERVER'S SIGNATURE INITIALS

______________________________ __________

ORIENTEE'S SIGNATURE

____

CHAPTER 9

Prevention of Injury—Use and Care of Basic Surgical Instrumentation

Learner Objectives

At the end of Prevention of Injury—Use and Care of Basic Surgical Instrumentation, the learner will

- identify potential patient injury that is related to failed surgical instrumentation
- identify desired patient outcome that is related to surgical instrumentation
- describe the basic categories and functions of surgical instrumentation
- list six conditions that should be checked during the inspection of instruments
- describe the process for the care and cleaning of basic surgical instrumentation
- describe nursing responsibilities related to the care and handling of surgical instrumentation

Lesson Outline

I. **BASIC SURGICAL INSTRUMENTATION**
   A. Overview
   B. Potential Injury—Desired Patient Outcomes
      1. Nursing Diagnosis
      2. Outcome Criteria

II. **CATEGORIES OF INSTRUMENTATION**
   A. Dissectors
   B. Clamps
      1. Hemostatic Clamps
      2. Occluding Clamps
      3. Grasping/Holding Clamps
      4. Grasping Forceps
   C. Retractors
   D. Suction
   E. Other

III. **CARE AND HANDLING**
   A. Manufacture
   B. Inspection
   C. Cleaning
   D. Guidelines for Care and Cleaning

IV. **NURSING RESPONSIBILITIES RELATED TO SURGICAL INSTRUMENTATION**

Chapter 9

Prevention of Injury—Use and Care of Basic Surgical Instrumentation

BASIC SURGICAL INSTRUMENTATION

Overview

1. Surgical instrumentation dates back to 10,000 B.C. when stone knives were used to perform surgery. Trephined skulls dating to the Neolithic era provide evidence that surgery was performed long before sophisticated surgical instrumentation was developed. Some early surgical implements included sharpened flints that were used for circumcision and sharpened animal teeth that were used for blood letting.
2. Until the 1700s instruments were made by blacksmiths, cutlers, and armorers. In the eighteenth and nineteenth centuries, when surgery gained recognition as a scientific discipline, skilled craftsman—silversmiths, wood turners, coppersmiths, and steel workers—began to make surgical instruments.
3. Instruments were made to individual specifications and often incorporated finely carved ornate wooden or ivory handles. They were generally cased in velvet-lined boxes.
4. The advent of anesthesia in the 1840s permitted surgeons to work slowly and deliberately and also generated the need for more precise and varied surgical instrumentation. With the concurrent acceptance of instrument sterilization, wooden and ivory handles were replaced by all-metal instruments that were capable of being sterilized.
5. The development of stainless steel in the 1900s further enhanced the manufacturer's ability to make precise surgical instruments, and instrument making evolved into a highly skilled occupation. The majority of surgical instruments continue to be manufactured from stainless steel, although titanium, vitallium, and other metals are also used.
6. Advances in surgery, particularly minimally invasive endoscopic surgery, combined with the discoveries of new materials has led to the development of many precise, sophisticated, complex, delicate, and very expensive surgical instruments. Use, cleaning, care, and processing of surgical instrumentation demands that knowledgeable personnel with critical thinking skills are available to determine the specific care and handling that is appropriate and necessary for specific instrumentation.
7. Inappropriate care and handling of instrumentation can result in patient injury, delays in surgery, and costly instrument repairs or replacements.

Potential Injury—Desired Patient Outcome

Nursing Diagnosis

8. Nursing diagnoses pertinent to the patient who is undergoing surgery are high risk for injury related to use of surgical instrumentation and high risk for infection related to use of surgical instrumentation.
9. Potential injury to a patient can include unintended injury to tissue, such as tearing, that is caused by an instrument that does not perform as expected, or the retention of a foreign body caused by a portion of an instrument that breaks off inside the patient and that is not retrieved. A patient may also incur an infection or a foreign-body

reaction from an improperly cleaned or sterilized instrument. An instrument that is inappropriately processed may leave a toxic residue that can harm a patient.

Outcome Criteria

10. At the end of surgery the patient should be free from infection. The patient should also be free from injury related to . . . extraneous objects, or . . . physical hazards (Association of Operating Room Nurses [AORN], 1995a, pp. 125–26).
11. When a patient sustains an injury or incurs an infection during surgery it is sometimes difficult or impossible to trace the exact cause. As an example, a postoperative infection may result from poor aseptic technique, poor surgical technique, inadequate skin preparation, improperly cleaned and processed instrumentation, or a combination of any of the above.
12. Outcome criteria to evaluate whether the patient sustained an infection or injury related to surgical instrumentation may include the same criteria that are used for the evaluation of proper aseptic technique. Although all appropriate measures for cleaning, care, and processing of instrumentation may have been accomplished, the patient still may not meet the outcome criteria because of factors unrelated to instrumentation.
13. If an instrument was inadequately processed, and a toxic residue results, the effect of that residue may not be measurable for some time and a cause-and-effect relationship may never be established. This does not negate the necessity to take all requisite steps to protect the patient from injury that could possibly be related to instrumentation.
14. The following criteria provide the best indication that instrument practices coupled with correct aseptic practices were adequate to protect the patient.
15. Postoperatively the patient should demonstrate
    - no evidence of unintended impaired tissue integrity, such as excessive swelling or discoloration, at the surgical site
    - no evidence of retained instrument or instrument part upon instrument count or subsequent X-ray
    - no evidence of pain, excluding incision pain
    - no evidence of infection

CATEGORIES OF INSTRUMENTATION

Dissectors

16. Dissecting instruments are used to cut or separate tissue. Such instruments may be sharp or blunt.
17. Scalpels and scissors are examples of sharp dissectors. Scalpels consist of a handle and a blade (see Figure 9–1). The handle has a groove at the tip for attaching the blade. This makes it possible to change the blade as needed during the procedure. Scalpel handles are available in a variety of sizes.
18. Blades are commercially prepackaged and are sterile. They are dispensed to the sterile field by the circulating nurse and contained on a magnetic mat or other receptacle designed to prevent accidental injury. At the end of surgery all blades are placed on the needle mat and the mat is disposed of in a specially designated sharps containers.
19. To prevent accidental injury to the scrub person, blades are firmly grasped with a needle holder while they are attached to the knife handle. They are not held in the hand during attachment. Scalpels are handed to the surgeon with the cutting edge facing away from the surgeon's palm. The safest technique is to pass scalpels to and from the surgeon in an emesis basin.

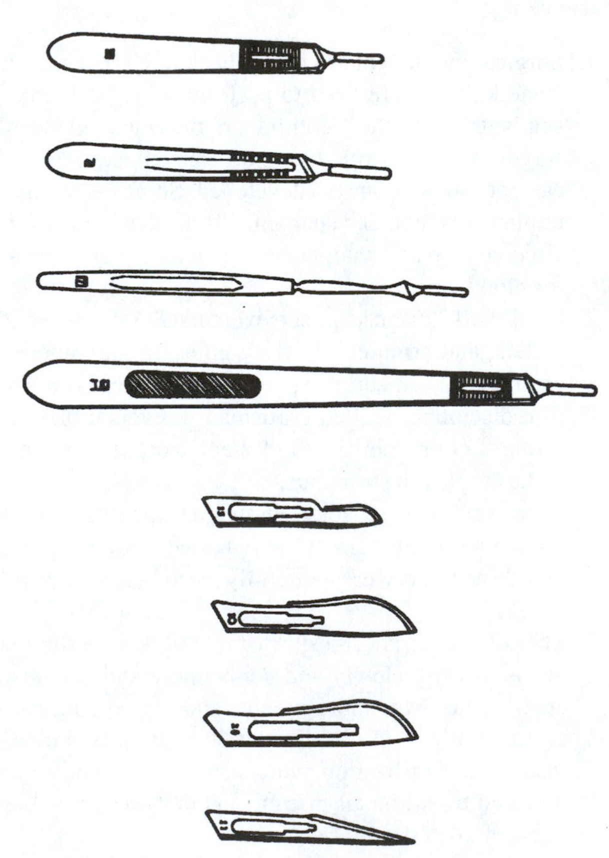

Figure 9–1 Scalpel Handles and Blades. *Source:* Courtesy of Bard-Parker Blades, Becton Dickinson, Franklin Lakes, New Jersey.

20. Scissors are manufactured in many different sizes and styles. Mayo and Metzenbaum scissors are used often and are contained in most general surgery instrument sets (see Figure 9–2). Mayo scissors have either a straight or curved tip. Curved Mayo scissors are used to cut heavy, tough tissue. Straight-tipped Mayo scissors are used for cutting sutures. Metzenbaum scissors have a rounded tip, are more delicate than Mayo scissors, and are used to cut or dissect delicate tissue. These scissors open and close in the same manner as household scissors. For more delicate surgeries, such as plastic, micro, or eye surgery, a spring-action scissor in which the jaws are held open may be used. In a spring-action scissor a single movement pressing the spring together causes the jaws to close.
21. Examples of other sharp dissectors are osteotomes, chisels, and rongeurs that are used for bone; curettes that are used for bone and soft tissue; and periosteal elevators that are used to separate tissue from bone or from other tissue.
22. Blunt dissectors are the back end of a knife handle, a small peanut-shaped sponge, or a folded 4 x 4-inch gauze attached to an instrument. Curettes and elevators may also be blunt.

Clamps

23. Clamps are instruments that are designed to hold tissue or other materials (see Figure 9–3). They are provided in a wide variety of shapes and sizes. The tips may be straight, curved, or angled. Some clamps are fine and delicate. Others are sturdy and appear more substantial.
24. Overall design is similar for all clamps. The design includes finger rings for holding the instrument, shafts of varying length, a joint (either a screw or box lock) that joins the two halves of the instrument and permits opening and closing, a ratchet at the distal end for locking the instrument in a closed or partially closed position, and a distal tip or jaw, the design of which determines the instrument's use.

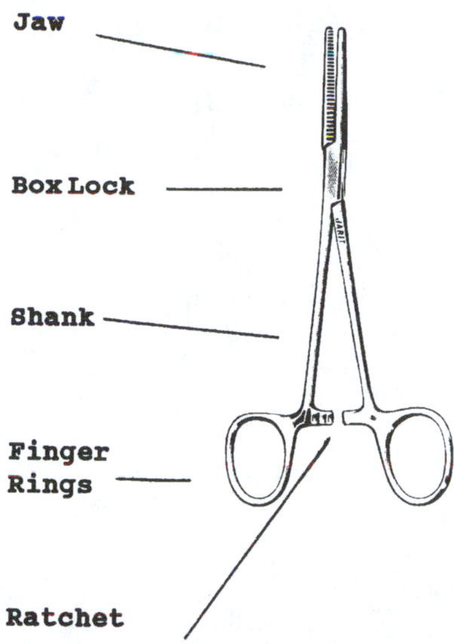

Figure 9–3 Clamp. *Source:* Courtesy of Jarit Instrument Company, Hawthorne, New York.

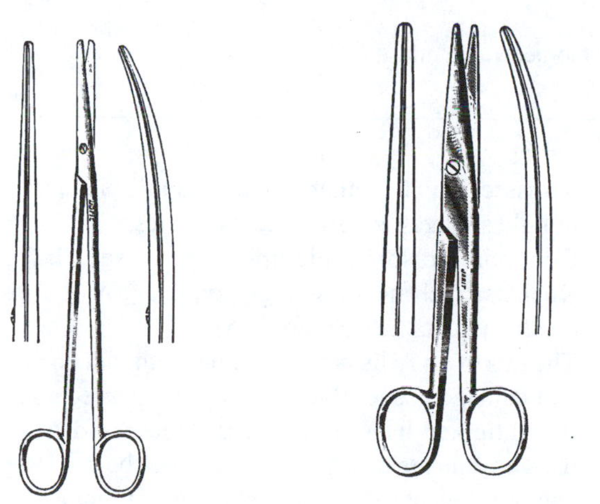

Figure 9–2 Scissors: Metzenbaum and Mayo (side views showing straight and curved jaws). *Source:* Courtesy of Jarit Instrument Company, Hawthorne, New York.

Hemostatic Clamps

25. Hemostatic clamps, commonly referred to as hemostats, are used to control bleeding. The clamping jaws of the instrument are horizontally serrated. This allows the clamp to compress the vessel with enough force to stop bleeding. The serrations also prevent the clamp from slipping off the tissue.
26. Common hemostats are mosquitos, Criles, Kellys (Rochester Peans), tonsils (Schnidts), and mixters (see Figure 9–4). Mosquitos are small clamps that may be curved or straight. They are most often used to clamp small bleeders in the superficial layers of tissue. Criles are curved and slightly longer and heavier than mosquitos. Tonsil clamps are curved and longer than Criles. They are used where additional length is needed. Kellys are straight or curved and are heavier than Criles or Tonsils clamps. The tip of a mixter is in the shape of a right angle. Longer mixters are useful for clamping and separating tissue in the abdominal cavity. Shorter mixters are

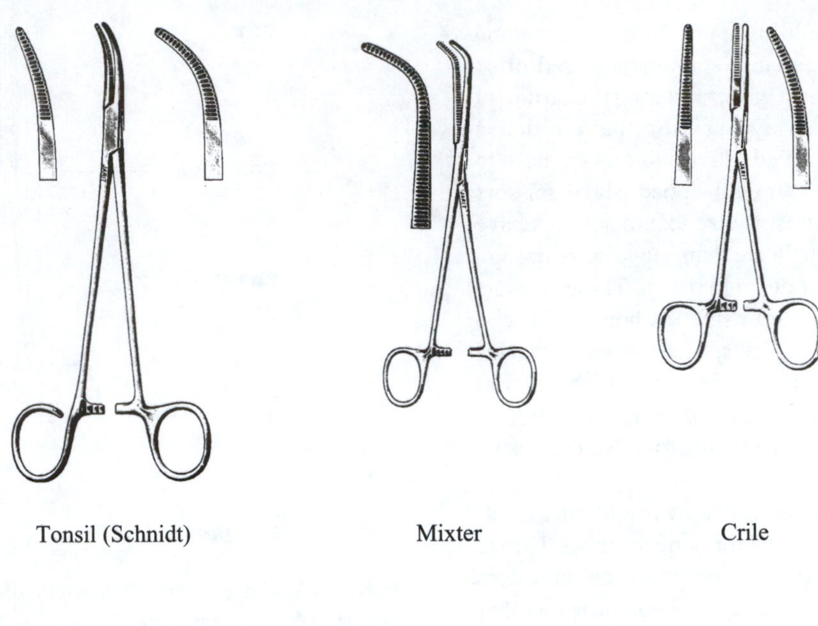

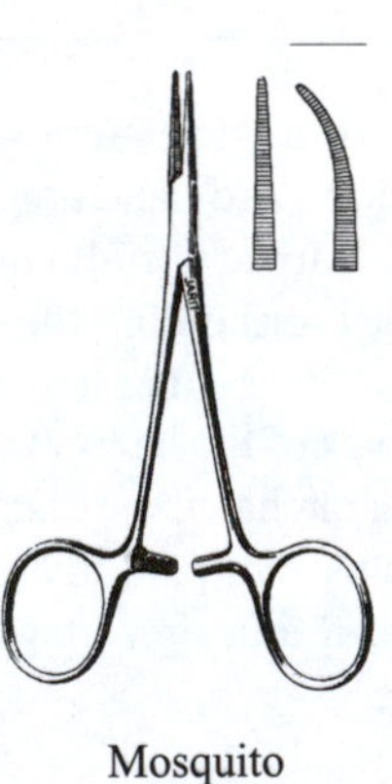

Figure 9–4 Hemostats. *Source:* Courtesy of Jarit Instrument Company, Hawthorne, New York.

often used to separate tissue during surgery on vasculature that is not deep within the body.

Occluding Clamps

27. Occluding clamps are used to clamp tissue, such as bowel or blood vessels, where prevention of leakage and minimization of tissue trauma is desired. The serrations on occluding clamps are vertical, close together, and arranged in multiple rows.

Grasping/Holding Clamps

28. Grasping or holding clamps are used on tissue for retraction and as aids during dissection and suturing. They allow the surgeon to hold tissue with one hand and suture or dissect with the other. Some grasping clamps are used to hold sponges, suture needles, or ties.
29. Common grasping clamps are Allises, Babcocks, Kochers (Ochsners), sponge forceps, towel clips, and needle holders (see Figure 9–5).
30. The tips of an Allis have multiple teeth that do not crush and damage tissue. Babcocks have a curved and fenestrated tip and have no teeth. Babcocks and Allises are used on delicate tissue. A Babcock can be used to grip or enclose delicate structures such as a fallopian tube or ureter. A Kocher has transverse serrations and a single heavy tooth at its tip and is useful for grasping tough tissue. Sponge forceps can be used to hold tissue, but most often are used to hold a folded 4 × 4-inch gauze

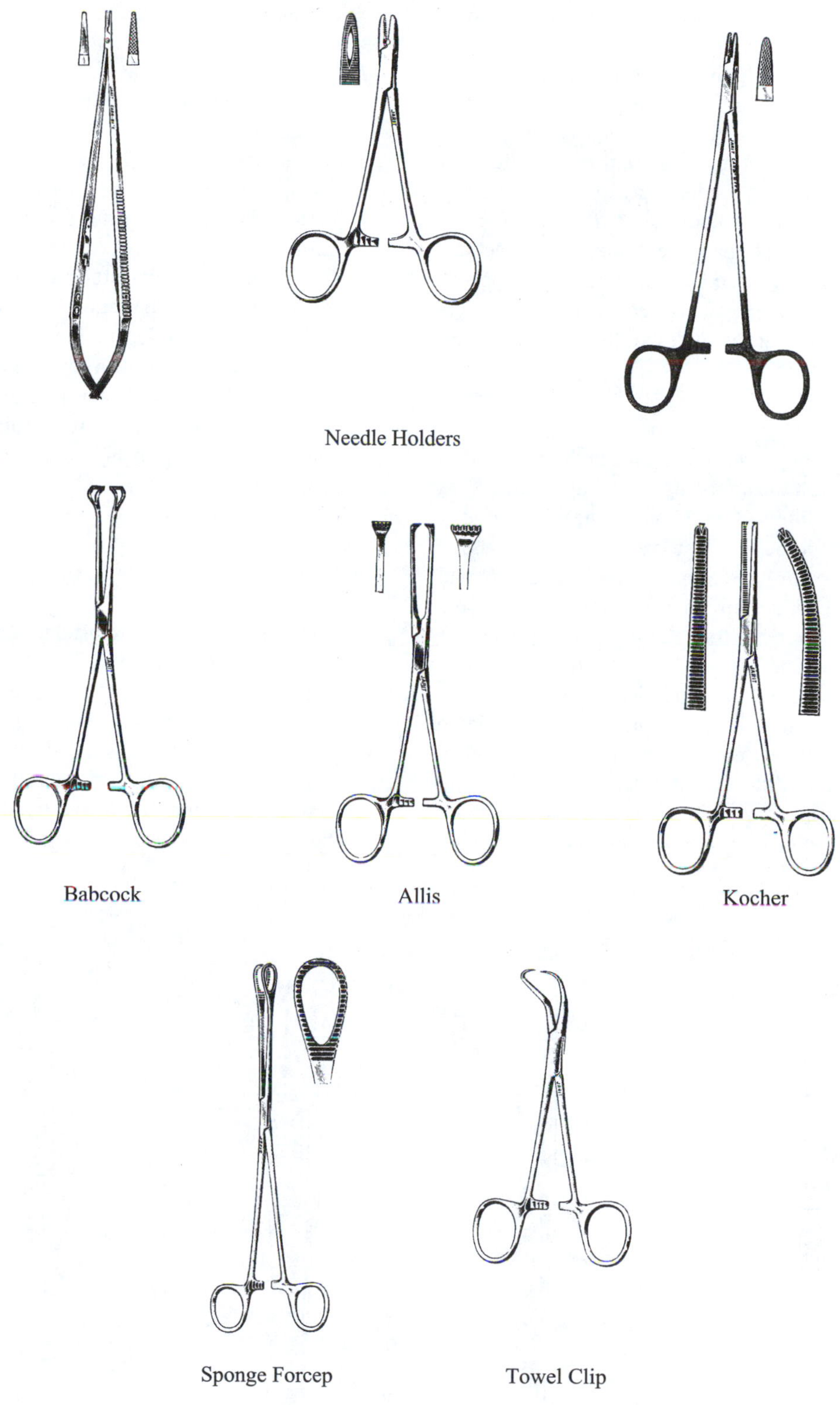

Figure 9–5 Common Needleholders and Grasping Clamps. *Source:* Courtesy of Jarit Instrument Company, Hawthorne, New York.

sponge that can be used to blot or sponge fluids or blood or to retract tissue. Towel clips are used to secure towels around the operative site and to hold drapes in place. Towel clips may have sharp tips that penetrate drapes or blunt tips that do not. Needle holders are designed to hold a needle securely in place so that the needle does not rotate or slip. Needle holders may or may not have a locking ratchet. Needle holders used for very fine sutures include a spring action rather than a ratchet action. The needle is held in place by a single movement that presses the spring together between the surgeon's fingers. When the pressure is released, the jaws open and the needle is released.

Grasping Forceps

31. Grasping and holding instruments that are not shaped as clamps are referred to as forceps or pickups (see Figure 9–6). They are used to lift and hold tissue. The surgeon frequently holds forceps in one hand to hold the tissue while using the other hand to cut, coagulate, or separate the tissue. Forceps are similar to tweezers. They have two arms and a spring action. A single movement that presses the arms together results in the tips of the forceps approximating. Forceps may have vertical or horizontal serrations, may vary in length, and are available with or without one or more teeth on the tip. Toothed forceps are used to hold thick tissue, such as skin, that may require extra grip. Nontoothed forceps hold more delicate tissue and cause minimal trauma.

Retractors

32. Retractors are designed to facilitate visualization of the operative field while preventing trauma to the surrounding tissue.
33. Retractors are available in various sizes and shapes. Some retractors require that the surgeon or assistant hold them while exerting pressure; others are self-retaining.
34. Common non–self-retaining retractors are rakes, Richardsons, Deavers, Army-Navys, Parkers, malleables (ribbons), and loops (see Figure 9–7).
35. A Weitlaner and a Balfour with a blade are examples of commonly used self-retaining retractors (see Figure 9–8). Some self-retaining retractors attach to the operating table and support blades of various length and configuration.

Suction

36. Suction instruments are used to remove blood and other fluids from the operative field.
37. Frazier, Yankauer, and Poole suctions may be included in a basic instrument set (see Figure 9–9).
38. A Frazier-tip suction is a right-angle tube with a small diameter. It is used where capillary bleeding and small amounts of fluid are encountered and maintains a dry field without the use of sponges. Some Frazier suctions

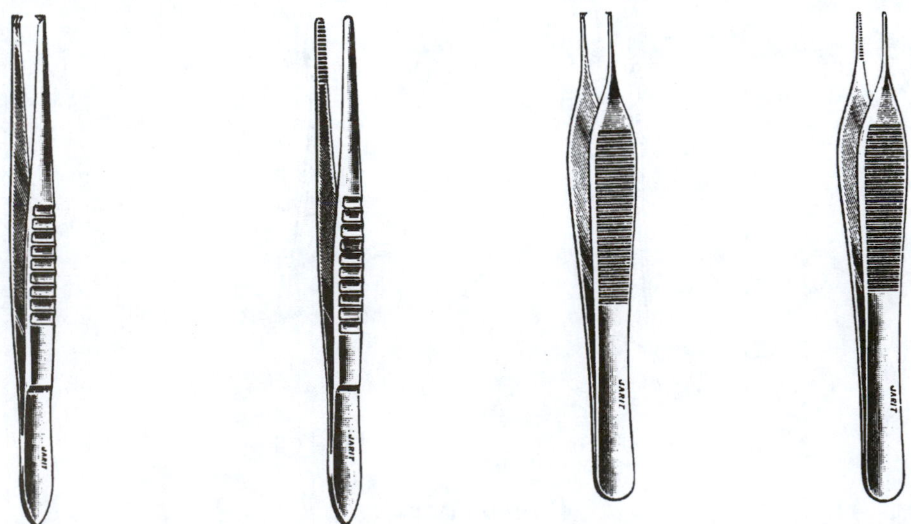

Figure 9–6 Tissue Forceps with and without Teeth. *Source:* Courtesy of Jarit Instrument Company, Hawthorne, New York.

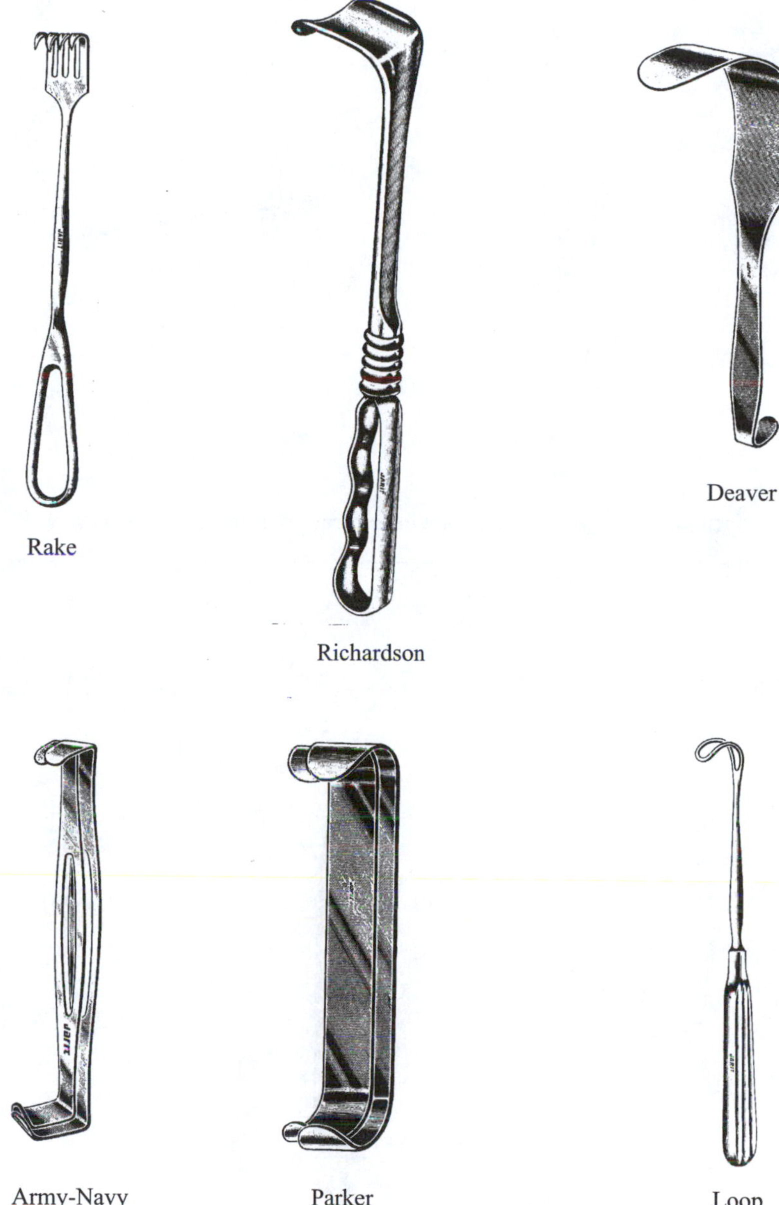

Figure 9–7 Handheld Retractors. *Source:* Courtesy of Jarit Instrument Company, Hawthorne, New York.

incorporate an active electrode into the tip so that it may be used to coagulate tissue as well as suction.

39. A Yankauer suction is an angled tube that is used in most general surgeries including those involving the mouth and throat.
40. A Poole suction is a straight tube with an outer perforated shield that acts as a filter. Poole suction is used where large amounts of blood or fluid collect and where the surgical area is deep.

Other

41. In addition to the instruments identified above, there are thousands of other surgical instruments, many of which are dedicated to a particular surgical specialty. Drills of various types are available for orthopedic, neuro, and ear, nose, and throat (ENT) surgery.
42. The phenomenal growth in minimally invasive surgery has led to the development of a wide variety of rigid and

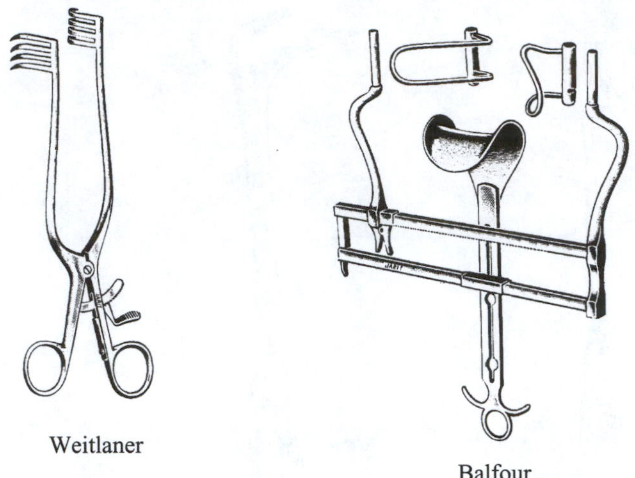

Figure 9–8 Self-Retaining Retractors. *Source:* Courtesy of Jarit Instrument Company, Hawthorne, New York.

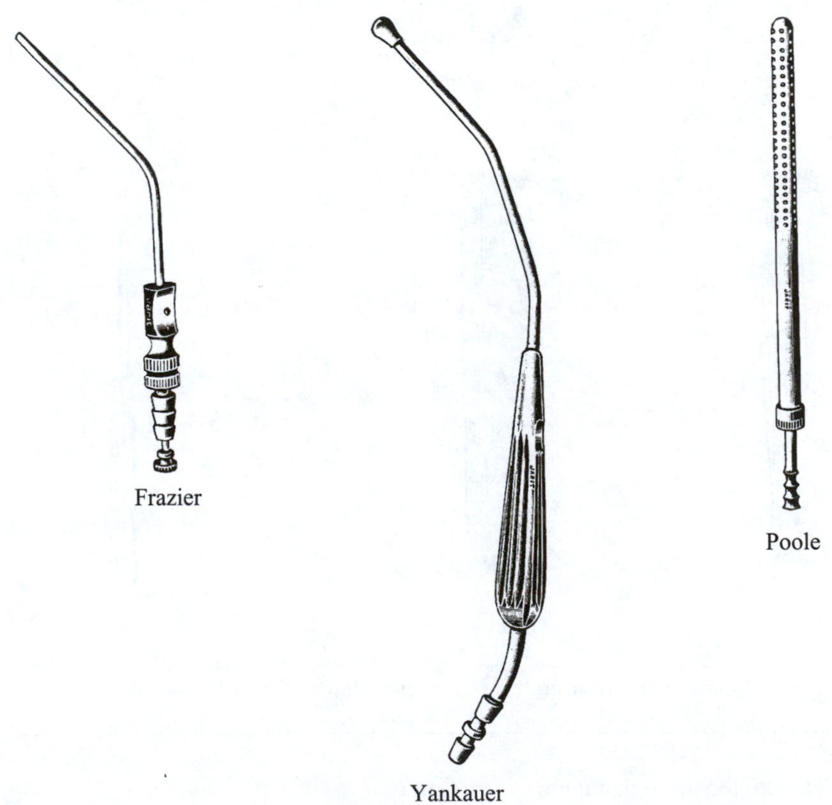

Figure 9–9 Suction Instruments. *Source:* Courtesy of Jarit Instrument Company, Hawthorne, New York.

flexible endoscopes and accessory instruments. Rigid scopes that have become commonplace in the operating room are cystoscopes, hysteroscopes, arthroscopes, and laparoscopes.

43. Flexible fiberoptic scopes, though more commonly used in endoscopy suites, are increasingly being developed for operating room procedures and in many suites are routinely used.

Section Questions

Q1. Most surgical instruments are made of (Ref. 5):
a. titanium
b. stainless steel
c. vitallium

Q2. List two injuries that the surgical patient is at risk for related to instrumentation that is not properly cared for. (Ref. 9)

____

____

Q3. When a patient incurs an infection following surgery, the cause is easily identified. (Ref. 11)

True False

Q4. To attach a blade to a knife handle, the scrub person grasps the blade firmly with the thumb and forefinger and slides the blade parallel to the handle into the grooves at the top of the handle. (Ref. 19)

True False

Q5. Metzenbaum scissors (Ref. 20):
a. are intended to dissect delicate tissue
b. are intended to cut suture
c. have a straight tip
d. have a rounded tip
e. are used to cut heavy, tough tissue

Q6. Grasping or holding instruments are useful (Ref. 28)
a. for retraction
b. during dissection
c. as an aid in suturing

Q7. Match the instrument name with the description. (Ref. 30)

a. Kocher	_____	fenestrated tip, used to enclose delicate structures
b. Allis	_____	transverse serrations, single heavy tooth
c. Babcock	_____	multiple teeth at tip, does not crush tissue
d. sponge forcep	_____	designed to hold folded 4 × 4-inch gauze pad

Q8. A Weitlaner and a Balfour with blade are self-retaining retractors. (Ref. 35)

True False

Q9. ____________, ____________, and ____________ are the names of suction instruments. (Ref. 37, 38, 39, 40)

CARE AND HANDLING

Manufacture

44. The great majority of basic instruments are made from stainless steel, which is composed of iron ore and varying amounts of carbon and chromium. Carbon provides the necessary hardness to the steel and chromium provides a stainless, corrosion-resistant quality. Most stainless-steel instruments are made with alloys that are high in carbon and low in chromium.
45. There are more than 80 different types of stainless steel. The quality of stainless steel varies according to its composition. It is classified according to the amount of carbon and chromium that it contains. High quality stainless steel resists rust and corrosion, has good tensile strength, and maintains a keen edge. The stainless steel selected for instrument manufacture is determined by the intended use of the instrument and desired flexibility and malleability.
46. Raw steel is converted into sheets that are milled, ground, or lathed into instrument blanks that are forged, die-cast, molded, or machined into specific instrument pieces of various shape and size. Excess metal is trimmed and the pieces are hand assembled, ground, and buffed. The instrument is then heat treated, or tempered, to achieve desired spring, temper, and balance. Balance and temper provide the flexibility that is necessary to withstand the stress of repeated use.
47. After an inspection that may include X-ray or fluoroscopy to expose any defects, the instrument is subjected to a finishing process to protect the surface and to minimize corrosion. In the finishing process, referred to as passivation, the instrument is immersed in a nitric-acid-bath solution that removes carbon steel particles and promotes the formation of a chromium oxide coating on the surface. Removal of the carbon particles may leave behind tiny pits that must be polished away. The final step is polishing, which creates a smooth surface on which a continuous layer of chromium oxide forms. Passivation and polishing essentially close the instrument pores and prevent corrosion. The chromium oxide layer continues to form when the instrument is exposed to the atmosphere and when it is subjected to the oxidizing agents contained in cleaning agents.
48. Three types of instrument finish are bright, highly polished; satin or dull; and ebony. The highly polished finish resists surface corrosion. It is shiny and reflects light that, on occasion, may distract the surgeon or obscure visibility.
49. The satin finish eliminates glare and is slightly more susceptible to corrosion.
50. The ebony finish is black and also eliminates glare. The black surface is useful in laser surgery to prevent reflection of the laser beam.
51. The term *stainless steel* is a misnomer. Although stainless steel resists corrosion and staining, over time and with repeated use, some spotting and/or staining will occur. The degree of spotting, staining, or corrosion is dependent on how instruments are used, cleaned, processed, and cared for.
52. Instruments made with titanium have a bluish finish. They are primarily manufactured for use in microsurgical procedures. Titanium is stronger and lighter than stainless steel and more corrosion resistant.
53. There are three types of joints used in the manufacture of instruments that are composed of two halves. These are the screw, the box lock, and a semibox joint. In the screw joint, a screw is used to secure the two halves of the instrument. In the box-lock joint one arm of the instrument is passed through a slot in the other arm. In the semibox joint the two halves can be separated.

Inspection

54. Instruments should be inspected prior to, during, and after surgery.
55. The inspection process is an ongoing process with the bulk of inspection taking place after decontamination and prior to assembly into sets in preparation for sterilization. Instruments should be inspected to ensure that they are clean and in proper working condition. Instruments that fail inspection should be removed and sent for repair.
56. Inspection should include the following:
    - Clamps, scissors, and forceps are checked to ensure that tips are even and that they approximate. Tips should be in alignment and should not overlap.
    - To be in perfect alignment the serrations on the jaws of the clamps must mesh perfectly. To test how well the serrations mesh, clamps are fully closed and held up to a light. If the serrations mesh perfectly, no light will be visible between the jaws. Misalignment of hemostatic clamps is a common problem often caused by misuse of the instrument
    - Instruments that feature a tooth or teeth at the tips are checked to ensure that they approximate and open freely. Tips that are not aligned properly will stick and release will be sluggish.
    - Ratchets and hinges on hinged instruments must close easily and hold firmly. If the jaws of clamps spring open during use they may be misaligned, the ratchet teeth worn, or the shanks may be bent or have insuffi-

cient tension. To test the ratchet teeth, the instrument is closed on the first ratchet tooth, held by the box lock and the ratchet portion tapped against a solid surface. If the instrument springs open, the ratchets are faulty. A clamp that springs open when clamped on a blood vessel presents the potential for patient injury.

- Joints and hinges are checked to ensure that they move easily and are not stiff. Stiff joints may indicate inadequate cleaning, need for lubricant, or a defective instrument.
- Box locks are inspected for cracks and looseness. Excessive play in the box lock indicates an alignment problem. Clamps with loose box locks will not hold tissue securely. Cracked box locks are a sign of impending breakage.
- Scissors must be smooth and sharp. Blades are inspected for burrs and chips. Scissors with burrs and chips will not cut cleanly and can cause trauma to tissue. Tips of Mayo and Metzenbaum scissors should cut through four layers of gauze with little resistance.
- Edges of sharp instruments, such as osteotomes, chisels, and ronguers, should be inspected for chips, nicks, or dents.
- Needle holders should hold the needle securely without slipping or rotation. Testing is accomplished by securing a needle in the jaws and locking the instrument in the second ratchet tooth. If the needle can be easily moved by hand, the holder is worn and needs repair.
- If plated instruments are in use, they must be inspected for chips that can harbor microorganisms and worn spots that can rust during autoclaving. (Although most instruments are made of stainless steel, a few plated instruments remain in use. Plated instruments are made by putting a chromium, cadmium, nickel, or silver coating directly on forged steel.)
- Rigid scopes should be held to the light and the lens observed for clarity. A cloudy lens may indicate a leak in the lens seal and a subsequent accumulation of moisture inside. A partially blocked view may indicate a crack in one of the internal glass lenses.
- Flexible endoscopes should be inspected for obvious external defects to the outer sheath. The lens should be held to the light while observing the distal end for tiny black spots. Black spots indicate a broken fiber, and broken fibers result in decreased light transmission.
- Instruments are inspected to determine that all parts are present and that the instrument is intact. Pins and screws that are loose can cause an instrument to malfunction and a part can be lost inside a patient.
- Instruments with insulation are inspected to verify that all insulation is intact. Insulation cracks or flaws can lead to inadvertent patient burn and serious injury. Insulation should always be checked by the scrub person before he or she permits use of the instrument in surgery.

57. Instruments should be inspected by the scrub person just prior to surgery. Although time may permit only a cursory inspection, this is sometimes sufficient to detect a defective instrument that could cause patient injury.
58. During surgery the surgeon may detect an instrument malfunction that is not immediately visible and only noticed when the instrument is used. In this event, the instrument should be set aside and identified as needing repair.

Cleaning

59. Instruments contaminated with blood, body fluids, or tissue should be rinsed during and immediately following the procedure. When blood and other debris is permitted to dry on an instrument it can harden in joints and become trapped in lumens or serrations or between scissor blades, which can cause malfunction, facilitate rusting and pitting, and can make final cleaning more difficult.
60. During the procedure, instruments are kept free of gross soil by wiping with a sponge moistened with sterile water. Instruments with a lumen are kept open and free of debris by irrigating the lumen with sterile water (AORN, 1995b, p. 197). The scrub person should be provided with a syringe for this purpose. This is a particularly important step in the cleaning process, according to J. Allen, as there have been reported cases of patient infection related to inadequate cleaning of endoscopic lumens (cited in Klaick, 1995, p. 24).
61. Debris and organic material should not be permitted to dry on instruments. Material that has dried may be difficult to remove, particularly within lumens, and may remain attached to an instrument during washing and sterilization, thus creating the potential for patient infection or foreign-body reaction.
62. Instruments should be cleaned as soon as possible after surgery in a washer-sterilizer or washer-decontaminator. In the presence of gross debris, some precleaning may be necessary. Instruments may be presoaked in a proteolytic enzymatic detergent, according to the instrument and the detergent manufacturer's recommendations. Microsurgical, eye, and other very delicate instruments should be hand cleaned.
63. If a washer-sterilizer or washer-decontaminator is not available, instruments may be hand washed.
64. Personnel who are responsible for washing instruments should be attired in protective gloves, waterproof aprons, and face shields.

65. Following washing, instruments are placed in an ultrasonic cleaner. Ultrasonic cleaning uses sound waves to remove debris from all parts of the instrument. Ultrasonic cleaning is not microbicidal and is used only after processing in a washer-sterilizer or washer-decontaminator or, in the absence of these, after hand washing. Following ultrasonic cleaning, instruments are rinsed to remove loose debris, and instruments with movable parts are lubricated with an antimicrobial water-soluble lubricant. The lubricant is used according to the manufacturer's instructions.
66. Some cleaning equipment is designed to wash, decontaminate, provide ultrasonic cleaning, and lubricate.
67. Lensed instruments, flexible scopes, powered drills, and instruments that cannot tolerate high temperatures or immersion in water are not processed in a washer-sterilizer, washer-decontaminator, or ultrasonic cleaner. These are cleaned according to the manufacturer's instructions. For some specialized instruments such as flexible endoscopes, specialized cleaning equipment is available.

Guidelines for Care and Cleaning

68. Guidelines for care and cleaning of instruments are as follows:
    - Instruments are used only for the purpose for which they were designed. Misuse can readily result in improper alignment, dull blades, and cracking of joints or tips.
    - During use, instruments are kept clean by wiping and frequent rinsing in sterile distilled water.
    - Instruments are handled gently and individually or in small lots.
    - Instruments are carefully put into the splash basin. They are not tossed. Entangled instruments can become misshapen or damaged.
    - Lighter, more delicate instruments are placed on top of heavy, less delicate instruments. Delicate instruments can easily be damaged by the weight of heavy metal instruments.
    - Following a surgical procedure, instruments are promptly cleaned. Prolonged exposure to blood and saline can cause corrosion and pitting of stainless steel. Instruments are washed and rinsed in water, not in saline. To reduce the potential for spotting that is caused by alkaline mineral deposits, demineralized or distilled rinse water is preferred.
    - During cleaning, all hinges and joints are opened to expose box locks and serrations where blood and debris may be concealed.
    - All instruments with removable parts are disassembled for cleaning.
    - A noncorrosive, low-sudsing, free-rinsing detergent with as neutral a pH as possible is used for washing instruments. A high-sudsing detergent may not be completely removed during rinsing and can cause spotting and staining. A neutral pH is recommended because alkaline detergents can stain instruments and acid detergents can cause pitting.
    - During manual washing, only soft brushes are used to clean serrations and joints. Steel wool, scouring powder, and other abrasives are not used for cleaning. These can cause scratches and remove protective finishes.
    - Only water-soluble lubricants are used. Oil-based lubricants leave a residue that is not water soluble and can compromise the sterilization process by preventing steam contact during the steam sterilization process.

NURSING RESPONSIBILITIES RELATED TO SURGICAL INSTRUMENTATION

69. Responsibility for the care and handling of instruments is shared by operating room and central service personnel. Instruments are usually purchased on operating room request and processed in the central service department. Perioperative nurses who order and use surgical instruments have a responsibility to be knowledgeable about instrument care and handling even if they are not responsible for implementation of the cleaning and sterilization process.
70. The complexity of instrumentation, diversity of materials, high cost, and potential for patient injury require that the nurse know what special handling is required and what cleaning and sterilization are appropriate. Often the person assigned to care for the instrument receives this information from the nurse. In addition, urgent need for a particular instrument or instrument set may necessitate the nurse's implementing or directing the cleaning and sterilization process. The ultimate responsibility of the perioperative nurse is to provide for patient safety. Proper care and handling of instruments are deterrents to patient injury.

Section Questions

Q10. Instruments with an ebony finish are particularly useful in ____________ surgery. (Ref. 50)

Q11. The term *stainless steel* is a misnomer. The degree of spotting, staining, or corrosion that a stainless-steel instrument may sustain is dependent on how instruments are (Ref. 51):
a. used
b. subjected to diseased tissue
c. processed
d. cared for

Q12. What would someone be inspecting a clamp for while holding it up to the light in a closed position? (Ref. 56)

____

____

Q13. Tips of Mayo and Metzenbaum scissors should be sharp enough so that the tips cut through _____ layers of gauze with little resistance. (Ref. 56)

Q14. Describe how a rigid scope should be checked prior to use. (Ref. 56)

____

____

Q15. Cleaning of lumens is very important to patient safety. Inadequate cleaning can lead to what type of patient injury? (Ref. 60)

____

Q16. List three pieces of personal protective attire that should be worn when cleaning contaminated instruments. (Ref. 64)

____

____

____

Q17. Ultrasonic cleaning is (Ref. 65):
a. the use of sound waves to remove debris
b. used prior to placing instruments in a washer-decontaminator
c. followed by rinsing
d. an excellent method of destroying pathogenic microorganisms

Q18. Instruments are cleaned in (Ref. 68):
a. water
b. saline
c. low-sudsing detergent with neutral pH
d. alkaline detergent
e. acidic detergent

Q19. Why is it important that oil-based lubricants never be used to lubricate instruments? (Ref. 68)

____

____

NOTES

Association of Operating Room Nurses (AORN). (1995a). Patient outcomes: Standards of perioperative care. *Standards and recommended practices.* Denver, CO: AORN.

Association of Operating Room Nurses (AORN). (1995b). Recommended practices for care of instruments, scopes, and powered surgical instruments. *Standards and recommended practices.* Denver, CO: AORN.

Klaick, S. (1995). Cleaning endoscopes: The basics. *Infection Control & Sterilization Technology*, *1*(6), 24–30.

ADDITIONAL READINGS

Spry, C. (1994). Care and handling of surgical instruments. In Tight, S. (Ed.), *Instrumentation for the operating room* (pp. 1–8). St. Louis: Mosby Year Book.

Storz Instrument Co. (1991). *The care and handling of surgical instruments.* St. Louis: Storz Instrument Company.

Appendix 9–A

Chapter 9 Post Test

1. List two potential patient problems that can arise if instruments are improperly handled and cared for. (Ref. 9)

   ____

   ____

2. All postoperative wound infections are the result of improperly cleaned instruments or poor aseptic technique. (Ref. 11)

   True False

3. Describe the safest technique for passing scalpels to and from the surgeon. (Ref. 19)

   ____

   ____

4. The two types of scissors used most often in general surgery are ____________ and ____________. (Ref. 20)

5. A periosteal elevator is used to ____________. (Ref. 21)

6. Clamps used to control bleeding are often referred to as ____________. (Ref. 25)

7. A ____________ is a grasping clamp with a single tooth at its tip and is used to grasp tough tissue. (Ref. 30)

8. A _____ forcep is most appropriate to hold the skin while suturing. (Ref. 31)
   a. toothed
   b. nontoothed

9. What is the purpose of a Deaver, Richardson, and Army-Navy? (Ref. 32, 34)

   ____

10. Most stainless-steel instruments are made with alloys that are high in carbon and low in chromium to provide hardness and resistance to corrosion. (Ref. 44)

    True False

11. Instruments used primarily in microsurgical procedures and that have a bluish finish are made from ____________. (Ref. 52)

12. Describe a method to check a needle holder to determine if it is working properly. (Ref. 56)

    ____

    ____

13. What instrument flaw can cause a patient to sustain a burn? (Ref. 56)

    ____

14. Instruments should be kept clean during surgery by rinsing or wiping with saline. (Ref. 60)

    True False

15. Lensed instruments may be cleaned in either a washer-decontaminator or an ultrasonic cleaner. (Ref. 67)

    True False

16. Match the instrument to the description. (Ref. 22, 25, 30, 31, 34, 35)

a. hemostat	_____ blunt dissector
b. small peanut-shaped sponge	_____ controls bleeding
c. Kocher	_____ non–self-retaining retractor
d. Richardson	_____ grasps tough tissue
e. Weitlaner	_____ two arms with spring action
f. forceps	_____ self-retaining retractor

Appendix 9–B

Competency Checklist: Instrumentation—Care and Handling

Under observer's initials enter initials upon successful achievement of competency. Enter N/A if competency is not appropriate for institution.

NAME ____________________________________

	OBSERVER'S INITIALS	DATE
1. Instrument inspection, prior to procedure:		
a. tips approximate	________	________
b. serrations mesh	________	________
c. ratchets hold securely	________	________
d. opens and closes easily	________	________
e. cutting instruments are sharp	________	________
f. needle holders hold securely	________	________
g. scopes clear	________	________
h. electrode insulation intact	________	________
2. Instruments handled carefully (placed, not tossed into basin).	________	________
3. Instruments cleaned periodically during procedure (rinsed, wiped, irrigated).	________	________

OBSERVER'S SIGNATURE INITIALS

____________________________________ __________

ORIENTEE'S SIGNATURE

____

CHAPTER 10

Prevention of Injury—Wound Management

Learner Objectives

At the end of Prevention of Injury—Wound Management, the learner will

- identify potential patient injury related to wound healing
- identify desired patient outcome related to wound healing
- identify the characteristics of absorbable and nonabsorbable suture material
- describe criteria for the selection of either absorbable or nonabsorbable suture material
- match suture-needle characteristics with intended use
- differentiate between first, second, and third intention wound healing
- describe three types of wound closure
- list the nursing responsibilities related to wound closure

Lesson Outline

I. NURSING DIAGNOSIS
- A. Potential Injury
- B. Desired Patient Outcomes/Criteria

II. SURGICAL WOUNDS
- A. Surgical Wound Classification
- B. Wound Healing
  1. Primary, Secondary, and Tertiary Intention
  2. Process of Wound Healing

III. SUTURE MATERIAL
- A. Classification of Suture Material
  1. Absorbable Suture
  2. Nonabsorbable Suture
  3. Suture Diameter
- B. Suture Package Information

IV. SURGICAL NEEDLES
- A. Needle Characteristics
- B. Needle Attachment

V. OTHER WOUND CLOSURE DEVICES
- A. Stapling Devices
- B. Skin Tapes
- C. Drains

VI. NURSING RESPONSIBILITIES RELATED TO WOUND MANAGEMENT

CHAPTER 10

Prevention of Injury—Wound Management

NURSING DIAGNOSIS

Potential Injury

1. An appropriate nursing diagnosis for patients undergoing surgery is high risk for injury (compromised or interrupted wound healing) related to wound closure.
2. Patients are also at high risk for infection related to wound closure.
3. Wound dehiscence and wound evisceration are complications of wound healing. Wound dehiscence is the partial or complete separation of the wound edges after wound closure. Wound evisceration is the actual protrusion of the abdominal viscera through the incision. Although the incidence of either is relatively uncommon, it is a risk for patients who undergo abdominal surgery.
4. In patients under 30 years of age, wound dehiscence is rare. Occurrence in patients over 60 who undergo laparotomy is 5%. Overall occurrence is 1% to 3% according to W.L. Way (cited in Long, 1993, p. 462).
5. There are many factors that determine the patient's risk for injury related to wound closure. Dehiscence or evisceration that occurs on days 1 to 3 postoperatively is usually the result of inadequate wound closure. Occurrences after the third postoperative day are often the result of excessive vomiting or coughing, infection, distention, or dehydration. A patient with a preexisting condition such as obesity, diabetes, malignancy, immunocompromise, dehydration, or malnourishment with hypoproteinemia may experience delayed or complicated wound healing. Wound separation that occurs 2 or more weeks postoperatively is generally a result of one or more of the above conditions.
6. Aseptic technique, suture materials, and surgical technique also influence wound healing. The majority of surgical wound infections are initiated along or adjacent to suture lines (Atkinson, 1992, p. 385). A break in aseptic technique as well as poor surgical technique can contribute to wound infection. Suture materials vary in their ability to prevent infection.

Desired Patient Outcomes/Criteria

7. The desired outcomes for the patient who undergoes surgery is freedom from injury related to wound closure and freedom from infection related to wound closure. Evaluation criteria include absence of
   - dehiscence or evisceration
   - excessive scar formation
   - wound site infection, including abscess, serous drainage, cellulitis, fever 72 hours postoperatively, redness, and pain or swelling 72 hours postoperatively

SURGICAL WOUNDS

Surgical Wound Classification

8. Surgical wounds are classified as clean (class I), clean contaminated (class II), contaminated (class III), and dirty or infected (class IV). Wound classification is provided by the Centers for Disease Control.

9. A clean wound is one in which the gastrointestinal (GI), genitourinary, or respiratory tract is not entered. No inflammation is encountered and there is no break in aseptic technique. Examples of clean surgical procedures include hernia repair, carpal tunnel repair, total joint replacement, and cataract extraction.
10. Approximately 75% of all surgical wounds fall into this category. Most are elective surgeries and are not predisposed to infection (Ethicon, 1994).
11. The risk for infection for a class I procedure is between 1% and 5% nationally.
12. A clean contaminated wound is one in which the GI, genitourinary, or respiratory tract is entered under planned, controlled means. No spillage occurs and no infection is present. Examples of clean contaminated procedures include cholecystectomy, cystoscopy, colon resection, and bronchoscopy.
13. The risk of infection for a class II procedure is between 3% and 11% nationally (Groah, 1996, pp. 129–133).
14. A contaminated wound is one in which nonpurulent inflammation, gross spillage from the GI tract, a traumatic wound, or a major break in aseptic technique is encountered. Examples of contaminated procedures include gunshot wound, colon resection with GI spillage, appendectomy with inflamed but not ruptured appendix, and rectal procedures.
15. The risk for infection for a class III procedure is between 10% and 17% nationally.
16. A dirty or infected wound is one in which an old traumatic wound with dead tissue exists or an infectious process is present. Examples of dirty or infected procedures include colon resection for ruptured diverticulitis, appendectomy for ruptured appendix, and amputation of a gangrenous appendage.
17. The risk for infection for a class IV procedure is 27% or higher nationally (Fernsebner, 1986, p. 893).

Wound Healing

Primary, Secondary, and Tertiary Intention

18. Surgical wounds may heal by primary, secondary, or tertiary intention.
19. Wounds heal by primary intention when minimal tissue damage occurs, aseptic technique is maintained, tissue is handled gently, and all layers of the wound are approximated. The wound generally heals quickly with minimal scarring.
20. Wounds heal by secondary intention when the wound cannot be sutured and is left open. An example is an ulcer where the edges cannot be sutured together. The wound heals from the bottom upward and is characterized by a red beefy appearance. Granulation tissue forms in the wound and gradually fills in the defect. The wound heals slowly and there is considerable scarring. Because the wound is open there is a greater risk for infection than if the wound were closed.
21. Wounds heal by tertiary intention when the wound is not sutured until several days after initial surgery. Extensive tissue loss from injury, or debridement of dirty or infected tissue, may result in a wound that cannot be closed at the time of the procedure. The open wound begins to heal and has gained sufficient resistance to infection to permit closure. The resulting granulation tissue is then sutured together, usually 4 to 6 days after the initial injury or procedure (Ethicon, 1994, p. 11).

Process of Wound Healing

22. Wound healing is generally divided into three overlapping stages, inflammatory, proliferation, and maturation.
23. The first phase of wound healing is the inflammatory stage that begins when the incision is made and extends through the fourth or fifth postoperative day. This stage is marked by hemostasis and phagocytosis. The inflammatory response includes redness, swelling, and pain. Platelets form a clot, fibrin is deposited in the clot, and new blood vessels develop across the sutured wound. A thin layer of epithelial cells bridge and seal the wound.
24. The inflammatory stage is followed by the proliferation stage in which the epithelial cells are regenerated, collagen is synthesized, and new blood vessels form. The new highly vascular tissue is referred to as granulation tissue. The proliferation stage generally lasts 3 to 20 days. Toward the end of this stage the wound begins to take on a raised pinkish scar, and will have gained enough strength to permit suture removal.
25. The final stage of wound healing is the maturation stage that can last more than a year. Collagen continues to be deposited and is remolded, the wound shrinks and contracts, and a thin white scar line is formed (see Figure 10–1).
26. After 6 weeks most wounds will have regained approximately 50% of their original tensile strength (the amount of strength provided by the suture material at the time of wound closure; Wysocki, 1989, p. 508).

SUTURE MATERIAL

27. The word *suture* refers to a strand of material used to tie (ligate) a blood vessel so as to occlude the lumen or sew tissue together. Tissues are sutured together for the purpose of holding them until healing takes place.

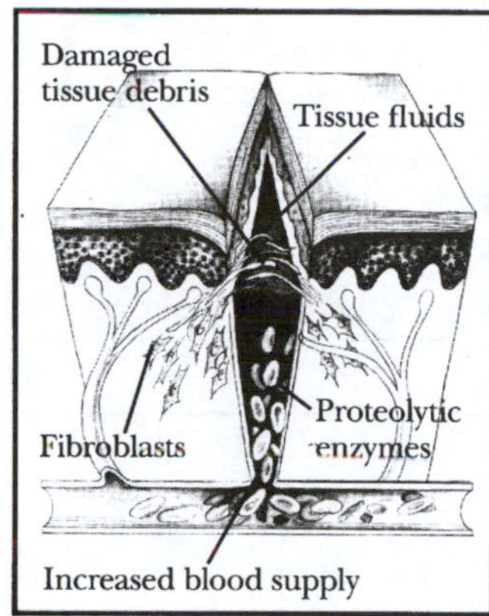

PHASE 1 —
Inflammatory response and debridement process

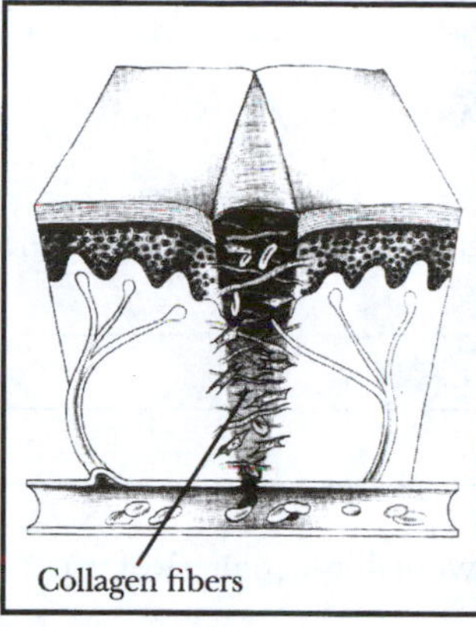

PHASE 2 —
Collagen formation (scar tissue)

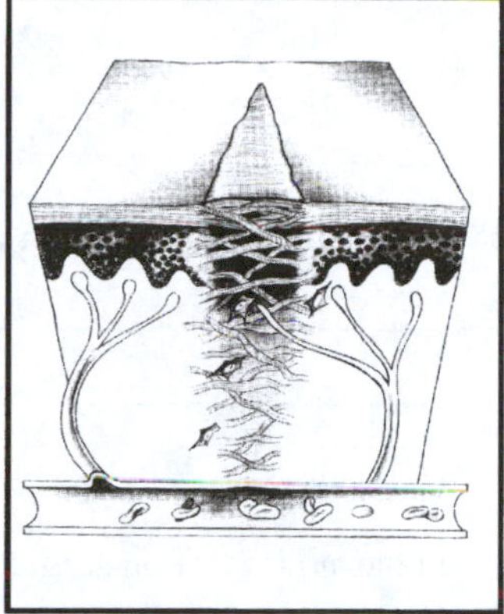

PHASE 3 —
Sufficient collagen laid down

Figure 10–1 Tissue Response to Injury. *Source:* ETHICON, INC., 1996, Somerville, NJ.

28. Desired characteristics of all sutures are sterility, ease of handling, consistent tensile strength appropriate to the suture size, and minimal reactivity in tissue.
29. Suture materials must be sterile when they are placed inside the patient's body. This requires packaging that permits sterile presentation to the field and adherence to aseptic technique, thus maintaining sterility.
30. Tensile strength is the amount of tension or pull that a suture will withstand when knotted before it breaks. The tension or pull is expressed in pounds. Tensile strength determines the amount of wound support that the suture provides during the healing process. Suture tensile strength should be as strong as the tensile strength (ability to withstand stress) of the tissue in which it is placed. As suture diameter decreases, suture tensile strength decreases.
31. Suture should be pliable, elicit minimal drag, slide easily through tissue, tie easily, and hold the knot securely.
32. Because suture material is a foreign body, some tissue reaction is inevitable. The foreign-body reaction will persist until it is either absorbed by the body or encapsulated. Suture is selected that offers the least potential for tissue reaction.
33. The surgeon's choice of suture is influenced by many factors. These are: the surgeon's familiarity with the suture, physical and biological characteristics of the suture material, healing characteristics of the tissue in which it will be placed, presence of infection or contamination, physical condition of the patient, and expected postoperative course of the patient.
34. Although suture selection is the surgeon's responsibility, the perioperative nurse must be familiar with suture material and its appropriate uses in order to plan for surgical procedures and to respond to unanticipated events, such as surgical complications, emergencies, and suture substitutions.

Section Questions

Q1. Inadequate wound closure can result in what injury to the surgical patient? (Ref. 5)

____

____

____

Q2. Suture material has no impact on surgical wound infection. (Ref. 6)

True False

Q3. Surgery to repair an Achilles tendon, where no preexisting inflammation and no break in aseptic technique occurs, would be classified as (Ref. 9)

a. clean
b. clean contaminated
c. contaminated

Q4. Risk of infection for a class II procedure is _____ than the risk for a class I procedure. (Ref. 11,13)

a. lower
b. higher

Q5. The most desirable method of wound healing is by _____ intention. (Ref. 19)

a. primary
b. secondary
c. tertiary

Q6. Inflammation is a natural occurrence in the process of wound healing and extends through the fourth or fifth postoperative day. (Ref. 23)

True False

Q7. Suture removal at the end of the proliferation stage of wound healing is appropriate. (Ref. 24)

True False

Q8. A surgical wound will generally have regained approximately 50% of the strength provided by the suture material at the time of wound closure by (Ref. 26):

a. 1 week
b. 6 weeks
c. 1 year

Q9. Suture selection is influenced by (Ref. 33):

a. healing characteristics of the tissue in which it is placed
b. surgeon's familiarity with the suture
c. biological characteristics of the suture material
d. expected postoperative course
e. patient preference

Classification of Suture Material

35. Standards and classification of suture are set by the United States Pharmacopeia (USP). There are two basic classifications of suture materials: absorbable and nonabsorbable.
36. Absorbable suture is assimilated by the body during the healing process and is considered temporary. Nonabsorbable suture is not assimilated and is considered permanent once it is placed within the body.
37. Other classifications of suture are monofilament and multifilament; coated and uncoated.
38. Monofilament sutures are comprised of a single strand of material. Because they are a single strand, they incur less resistance as they are drawn through tissue and as they are tied. Knots made with monofilament suture have a tendency to loosen and additional throws in the knot are needed to secure it. Monofilament sutures do not harbor bacteria and therefore reduce the potential for a suture-line infection.
39. Multifilament sutures are several strands twisted or braided together. They handle and tie securely and provide greater tensile strength than do monofilament sutures. Multifilament sutures have a certain amount of capillarity. Capillarity allows tissue fluid to be soaked into the suture and carried along the strand. A disadvantage of multifilament sutures is that microorganisms that may be contained in tissue fluid may be carried along the strand into the wound and result in infection. Many multifilament sutures are coated to improve their handling characteristics and to reduce capillarity.
40. Absorbable suture is made of material that is digested by body enzymes or hydrolyzed (broken down by water in tissue fluids). Absorbable suture may be natural or synthetic. Natural absorbable sutures are either gut or collagen.

Absorbable Suture

41. The most common natural absorbable suture is plain or chromatic surgical gut.
42. Plain surgical gut is natural suture made from the submucosa of sheep intestine or serosa of beef intestine. It has limited use and loses its tensile strength within 7 to 10 days. Absorption takes place in approximately 70 days. This means it will take about 70 days for the suture to be absorbed; however, it will only provide support for the wound for 7 to 10 days. Therefore, plain gut suture is used primarily to ligate superficial blood vessels and to suture the subcutaneous tissue layer.
43. Surgical gut that has been treated in a chromium salt solution is referred to as chromic gut. Chromatization renders the gut more resistant to absorption. Chromic gut retains its tensile strength for approximately 3 weeks and enables a wound to heal slowly while providing support. It is absorbed in about 90 days.
44. Collagen suture is made from cattle tendon. It is frequently supplied as a fine suture for eye surgery. It also loses tensile strength in approximately 3 weeks.
45. Plain gut, chromic gut, and collagen sutures are digested by body enzymes through phagocytosis, which results is varying degrees of inflammatory reaction.
46. The rate of decline in tensile strength and absorption of surgical gut is influenced by the type of tissue in which it is used, the condition of the tissue, and the state of health of the patient. If the patient is anemic, malnourished, protein deficient, debilitated, or has an infection, the rate of absorption and the loss of tensile strength may be accelerated.
47. Surgical gut sutures are packaged in a conditioning fluid of alcohol and water. This conditioning fluid keeps the suture pliable. Surgical gut should be handled only when moist; therefore, it should be used immediately upon removal from the package. Gut suture that is removed from the package and allowed to dry will lose its pliability. Moistening it with sterile saline just prior to use will restore pliability. Gut suture should not be immersed or permitted to remain in saline or water because excessive moisture will reduce tensile strength.
48. Synthetic absorbable sutures are made from synthetic polymers of lactic and glycolic acid. They are absorbed through hydrolysis, which causes the polymer chain to break down. Hydrolysis results in less tissue reaction than does enzymatic suture absorption. Synthetic suture is minimally affected by the presence of infection, the type of tissue, or the patient's state of health. Absorption time and loss of tensile strength are predictable.
49. The tensile strength of synthetic absorbable sutures is greater than for natural materials and varies from several weeks to 3 months. Sixty to 70 percent of tensile strength may remain after 3 weeks, and for some suture a 25% tensile strength remains after 6 weeks.
50. Synthetic absorbable sutures that provide the longest wound support times are appropriate for patients who heal slowly, such as the elderly, or patients with acquired immune deficiency syndrome (AIDS), or those receiving radiation therapy.
51. Synthetic absorbable sutures are packed dry and should not be immersed in solutions because this can reduce tensile strength.
52. Examples of synthetic absorbable sutures are Dexon (polyglycolic acid), Vicryl (polyglactin 910), PDS (polydioxanone), Maxon (polyglyconate), and Monocryl (poliglecaprone).

Nonabsorbable Suture

53. Nonabsorbable suture may be made of natural or synthetic materials.
54. Silk and cotton are natural nonabsorbable sutures. Cotton suture is made from cotton fibers that have been combed, aligned, and twisted into a multifilament strand. Because it is somewhat reactive in tissue, it is used very infrequently. Tensile strength is enhanced when the suture is moistened.
55. Surgical silk is a natural material made from thread spun by silkworms in their making of cocoons. The silk strands are twisted or braided and are usually dyed black. Silk loses its tensile strength within 1 year after implantation, and cannot be used where very long-term support is needed, such as in a heart valve. Silk is not totally nonabsorbable and may dissolve after several years. On occasion, a silk suture will migrate to the wound surface. This action is referred to as spitting.
56. Silk is one of the most widely used nonabsorbable sutures and is often used in the gastrointestinal tract. It is pliable and holds the knot securely. Because of its capillarity, silk is treated to resist absorption of body fluids.
57. Nylon, polyester, polyethylene, polybutester, and polypropylene are synthetic polymers used to manufacture synthetic nonabsorbable sutures. Synthetic fibers cause less tissue irritation, retain their strength longer, and have a higher tensile strength than do natural fibers.
58. Nylon suture (Ethilon, Dermalon, Nurolon, and Surgilon) has high tensile strength and is inert in the body. It is smooth and slides easily through tissue. Additional throws in the knot and square ties are necessary to provide knot security. Nylon is often used for skin closure, and because it can be manufactured into very fine strands, it is suitable for ophthalmic surgery and microsurgery.
59. Polyester suture (e.g., Dacron, Mersilene, Ethibond, Tevdek, and Tri-Corn) is closely braided, is available in a variety of sizes, and is usually coated with a specially designed lubricant that reduces drag as the suture is passed through tissue.
60. Polybutester suture (Novafil) is a monofilament suture with more flexibility and elasticity than other synthetic polymers.
61. Polypropylene suture (e.g., Prolene, Surgilene, Dermalene) is an inert monofilament, has good tensile strength, and slides smoothly through tissue. It is available in a variety of sizes including very fine strands. Its use is standard in cardiovascular surgery and other surgeries where prolonged healing is anticipated. Additional throws and square ties are necessary for knot security. Polypropylene suture should be gently stretched before use to eliminate memory and prevent kinking.
62. Stainless-steel suture has the highest tensile strength and is the most inert of all sutures. It is particularly useful where strong permanent wound security is needed, such as the sternum following cardiovascular surgery. Metallic suture is difficult to handle and requires an exacting suture technique.

Suture Diameter

63. Suture diameter ranges from a heavy size 7 to a very fine size 11-0. In decreasing thickness, suture begins with 7 and progresses as follows: 7, 6, 5, 4, 3, 2, 1, 0, 2-0, 3-0, 4–0, . . . 11-0 (see Figure 10–2). Tensile strength decreases as suture diameter decreases. Sutures size 5-0 through 11-0 are finer than a human hair and are often used in microsurgery. They are fragile and must be handled with the utmost care.
64. The majority of suture material used in general surgery have diameters in the 1-0 to 4-0 range.

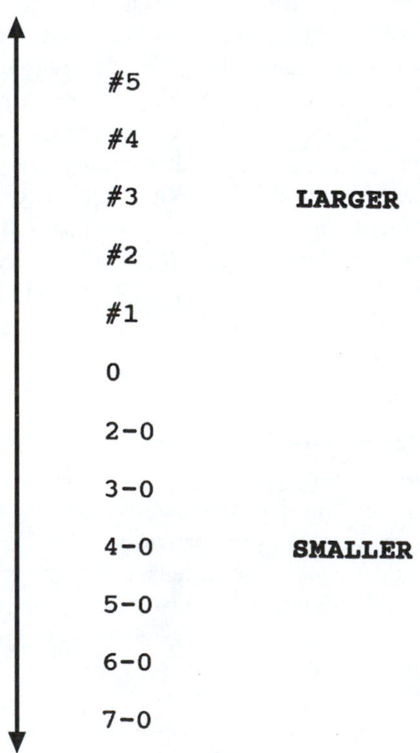

Figure 10–2 Size Progression of Sutures

Section Questions

Q10. Suture that is assimilated by the body during the healing process is classified as (Ref. 36):

____

Q11. Suture that is considered permanent once it is placed within the body is classified as (Ref. 36):

____

Q12. Monofilament suture resists harboring microorganisms. (Ref. 38)

True False

Q13. Explain why capillarity is a disadvantage. (Ref. 39)

____

____

____

Q14. Plain gut is used in tissue where very long-term support is necessary. (Ref. 42)

True False

Q15. Chromic gut is (Ref. 43, 45):
a. absorbed through phagocytosis
b. absorbed in approximately 90 days
c. is not absorbable

Q16. List three patient conditions that may influence the rate of suture absorption and decline in tensile strength. (Ref. 46)

____

____

____

Q17. Surgical gut (Ref. 47):
a. should be allowed to dry before being used for suturing
b. should be moist when used
c. may be moistened with sterile saline prior to use

Q18. List three advantages of synthetic absorbable suture over natural absorbable suture. (Ref. 48)

____

____

____

Q19. Surgical silk suture (Ref. 55):
  a. is made from thread spun by silkworms
  b. is a good choice for heart-valve replacement surgery
  c. is classified as nonabsorbable but may in fact dissolve over time
  d. may spit

Q20. Synthetic nonabsorbable sutures have a greater tensile strength and retain their strength longer than do natural nonabsorbable sutures. (Ref. 57)

True False

Q21. What may be done during the manufacturing process to reduce the drag on polyester-braided suture material? (Ref. 59)

____

____

Q22. A 4-0 suture has less tensile strength and is finer, that is, has a smaller diameter than a 5-0 suture. (Ref. 63)

True False

Suture Package Information

65. Sutures are supplied sterile from the manufacturer in a double envelope package. The inner package contains the sterile suture. The outer package is a see-through peel package designed to permit aseptic delivery of the suture to the sterile field. Some suture material is supplied in a single package that also permits aseptic delivery to the sterile field.
66. Information required by the USP is printed on each suture package. This includes material; trade name; generic name; product number, size, length, and color; number of sutures in the package; description of the needle; whether the suture is braided or monofilament, absorbable or nonabsorbable; coating material if used; manufacturer; date manufactured and expiration date; and compliance with USP standards (see Figure 10–3).
67. Sutures are supplied in boxes containing multiple packages. They are commercially sterilized with ethylene oxide or ionizing radiation. Unused sutures should not be resterilized because packaging materials may not permit resterilization in hospital sterilizing processes without adversely affecting package or product integrity.

SURGICAL NEEDLES

Needle Characteristics

68. Surgical needles are designed to carry suture material through tissue with minimum trauma. They are precision made to prevent excessive bending and still provide some flexibility without breaking. Surgical needles may be characterized by their shape, type of point, size, and how the suture material is attached.
69. The three basic parts of the needle are the point, shaft, and eye.
70. Needle points are tapered, cutting, or blunt (see Figure 10–4). Tapered needles are used in tissue, such as peritoneum or intestine, that offers little resistance to the needle as it is passed through. A taper-point needle is designed so the shaft gradually tapers to a sharp point so as to make the smallest possible hole in the tissue.
71. A cutting-point needle is designed with a razor-sharp tip and is used for tissue that is difficult to penetrate, such as skin or tendon. Cutting needles have cutting edges that extend along the shaft. There are variations of the cutting needle that are used according to surgical preference in selected tissue.
72. Blunt-tip needles have a rounded end and are used in friable tissue, such as the liver or kidney, when neither piercing nor cutting is appropriate.
73. The shaft of the needle may be straight or curved (see Figure 10–5). Curvatures are 1/4, 3/8, 1/2, and 5/8 circle. Selection of needle shape and size is determined by the size and properties of the suture material, nature of the surgery, and the surgeon's preference.

Needle Attachment

74. Suture may be attached to the needle during manufacture or may be threaded at the time of surgery. Suture that is attached during manufacture is referred to as an atraumatic or swaged suture. Needle and suture strand are a continuous unit in which needle diameter and suture diameter are matched as closely as possible. Atraumatic suture eliminates the need for threading. The large majority of sutures are atraumatic.
75. A modification of the permanently swaged suture is the controlled-release suture, sometimes referred to as a "pop off." Needle and suture are one continuous unit; however, they may be separated by means of a light tug. Controlled-release sutures facilitate rapid interrupted suturing techniques.
76. Suture may be attached to a needle with a round, oval, or square eye (see Figure 10–6). It is threaded in much the same manner as a household needle.
77. A French-eyed needle has a slit from the inside of the eye to the end of the needle. Suture is forced, rather than threaded, through this slit (see Figure 10–7).
78. Use of an eyed needle necessitates two strands of suture being pulled through tissue. This bulk causes tissue trauma and for this reason most surgeons prefer the eyeless atraumatic suture.

OTHER WOUND CLOSURE DEVICES

Stapling Devices

79. Stapling devices are available for approximation of internal tissues and for skin closure (see Figure 10–8). Staples are made of stainless steel or titanium. Stapling devices are designed for stapling specific tissue and are not interchangeable. Staples may be applied individually, as in skin or fascia staplers, where clips or staples are delivered one at a time. Stapling devices that deliver multiple staples simultaneously are used in intestinal and thoracic surgery.

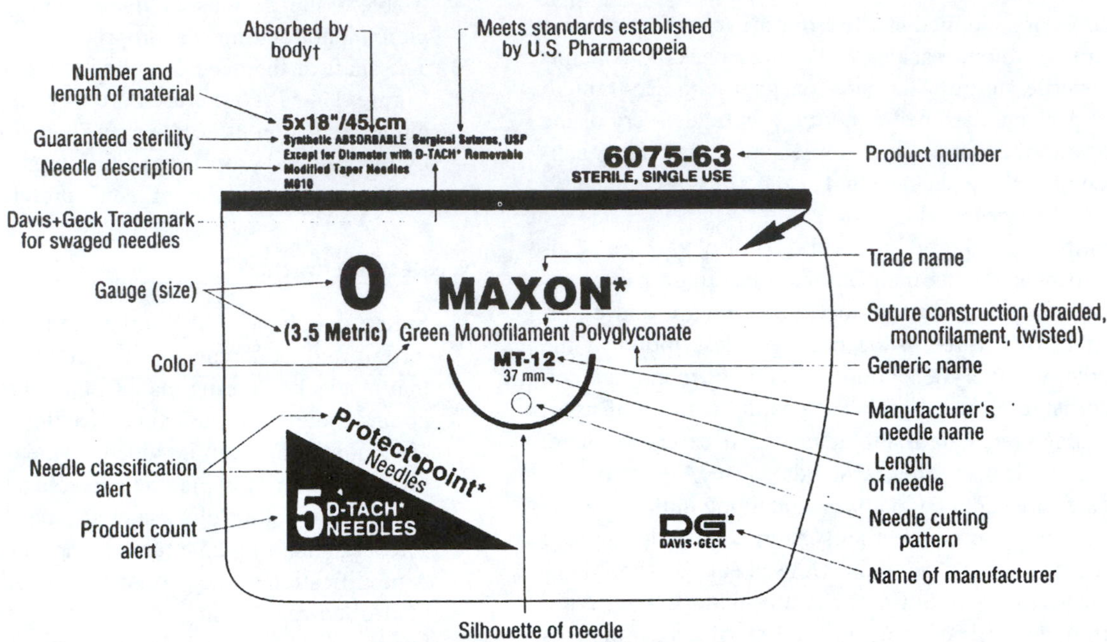

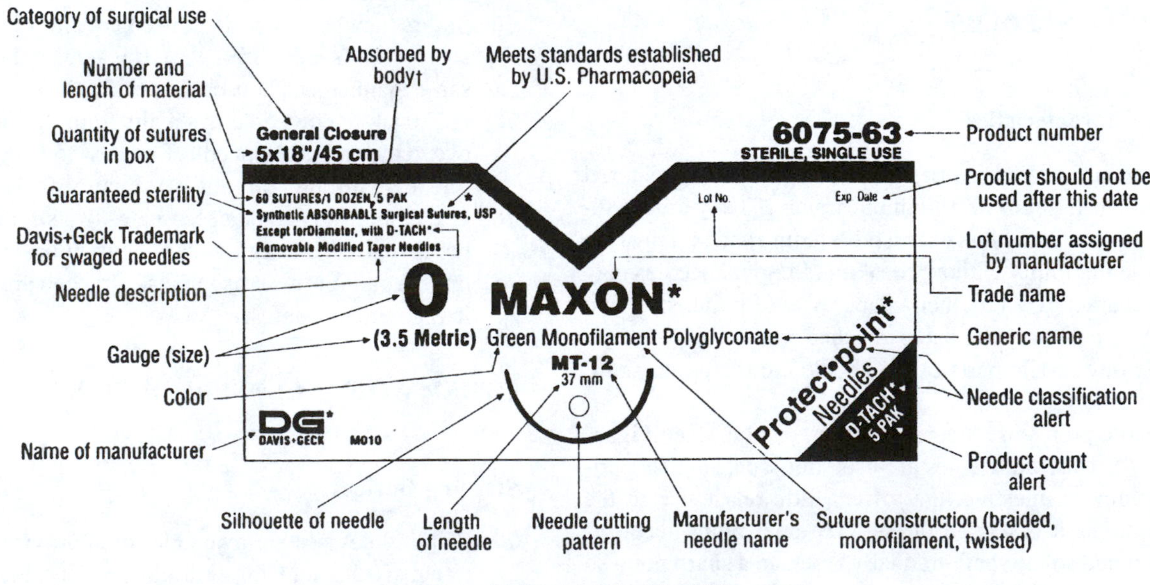

Figure 10–3 Suture Packet Information. *Source:* Courtesy of Davis and Geck, St. Louis, Missouri.

POINT/BODY SHAPE	APPLICATIONS
Conventional Cutting 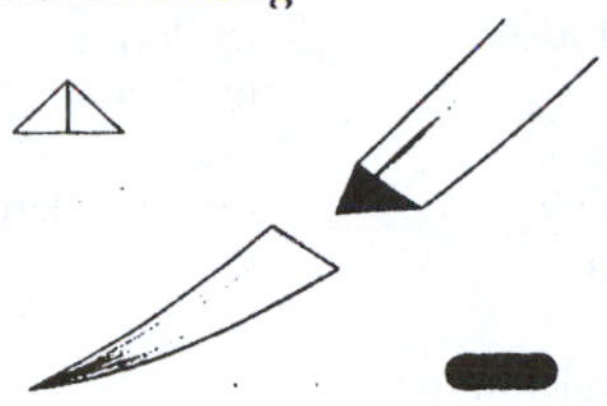	ligament nasal cavity oral cavity pharynx skin tendon
Reverse Cutting 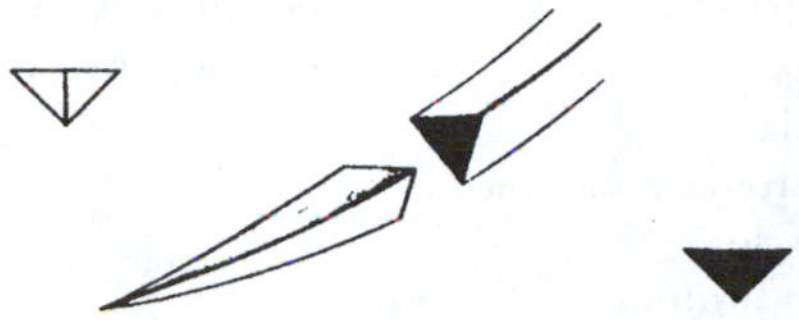	fascia ligament nasal cavity oral mucosa pharynx skin tendon sheath
MICRO-POINT Reverse Cutting Needle 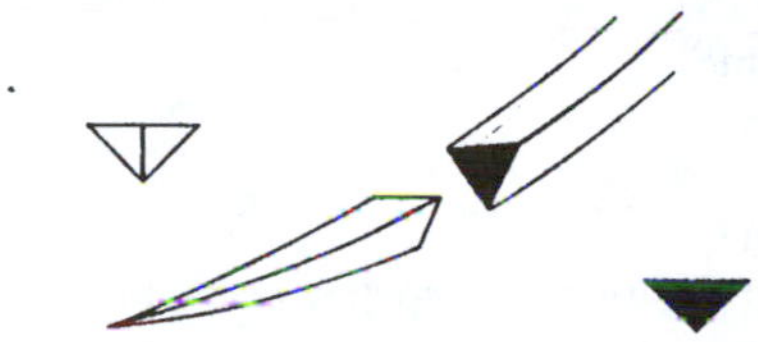	eye
Precision Point Cutting 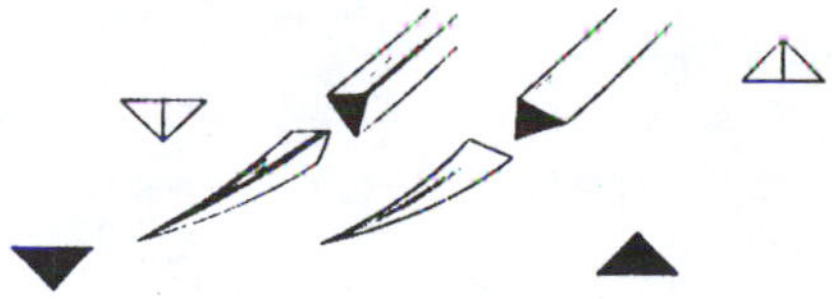	skin (plastic or cosmetic)
Side-cutting Spatula 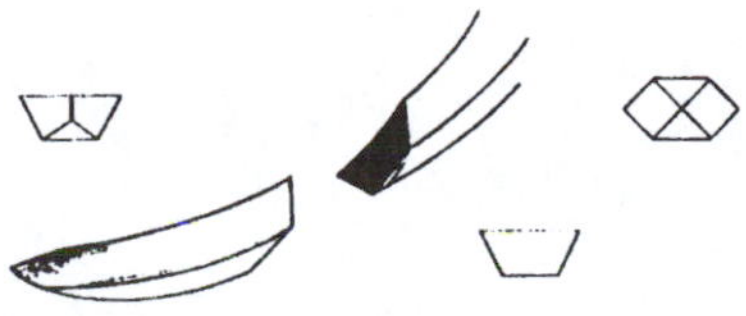	eye (primary application) microsurgery ophthalmic (reconstructive)

continues

Figure 10–4 Needle Points and Body Shapes with Typical Applications. *Source:* Reprinted with permission from ETHICON, INC., 1996, Somerville, NJ.

POINT/BODY SHAPE	APPLICATIONS
TAPERCUT Surgical Needle	bronchus calcified tissue fascia ligament nasal cavity oral cavity ovary perichondrium periosteum pharynx tendon trachea uterus vessels (sclerotic)
Taper	aponeurosis biliary tract dura fascia gastrointestinal tract muscle myocardium nerve peritoneum pleura subcutaneous fat urogenital tract vessels
Blunt	blunt dissection (friable tissue) fascia intestine kidney liver spleen cervix (ligating incompetent cervix)
CS ULTIMA Ophthalmic Needle	eye (primary application)
PC PRIME Needle	skin (plastic or cosmetic)

Figure 10–4 continued

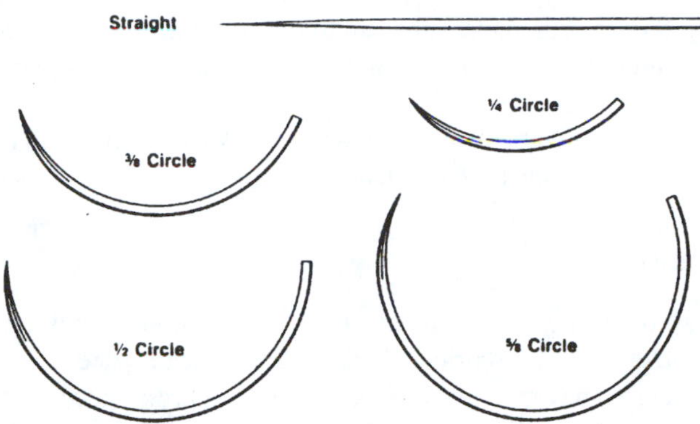

Figure 10–5 Needle Shapes. Surgical needles vary in shape, size, type of point and body, and how suture is attached (swaged or threaded). *Source:* Reprinted with permission from *Perspectives on Sutures*, p. 52, © 1978, Davis and Geck.

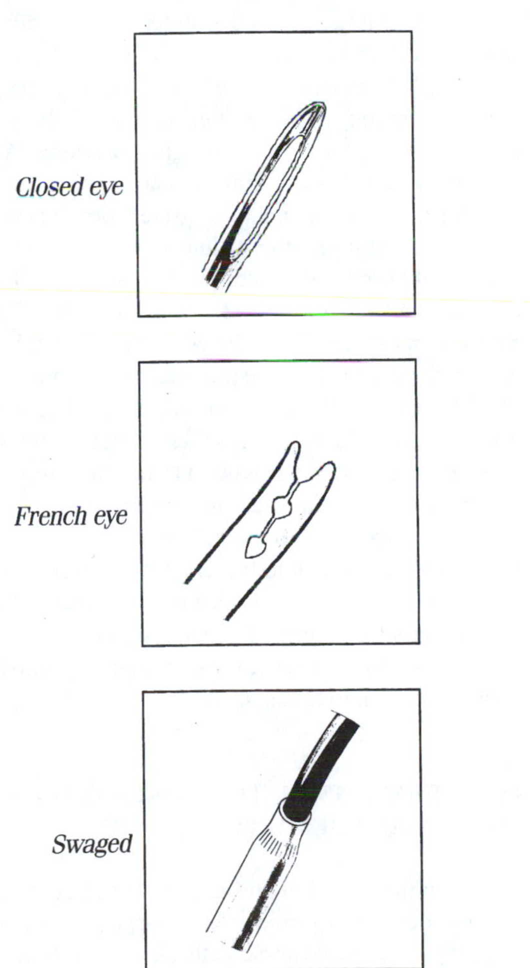

Figure 10–6 Needle Attachments. *Source:* Reprinted with permission from ETHICON, INC., 1996, Somerville, NJ.

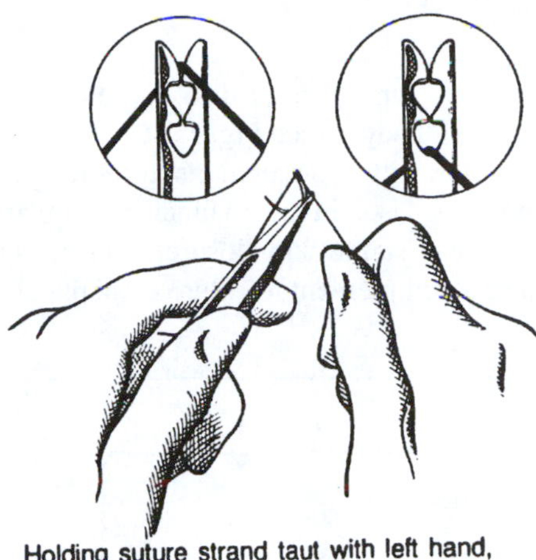

Figure 10–7 Threading a French-eyed Needle. *Source:* Reprinted with permission from *Perspectives on Sutures*, p. 52, © 1978, Davis and Geck.

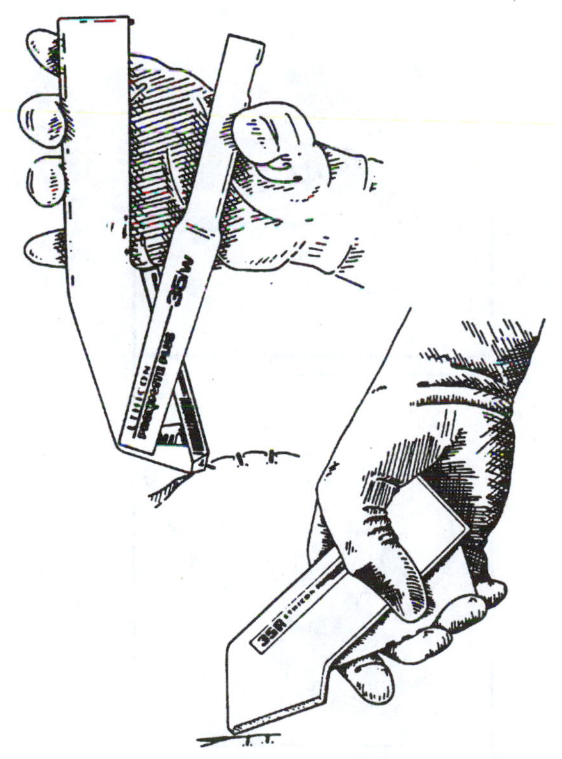

Figure 10–8 Skin Stapler. *Source:* Reprinted with permission from ETHICON, INC., 1996, Somerville, NJ.

Skin Tapes

80. Adhesive skin tapes are used to approximate surgical incision wound edges (see Figure 10–9). They are used in conjunction with subcuticular sutures to approximate incision edges. Used in this manner they are an alternative to suture or staple skin closure. Skin tapes may also be used as a complement to suture or staple closures.

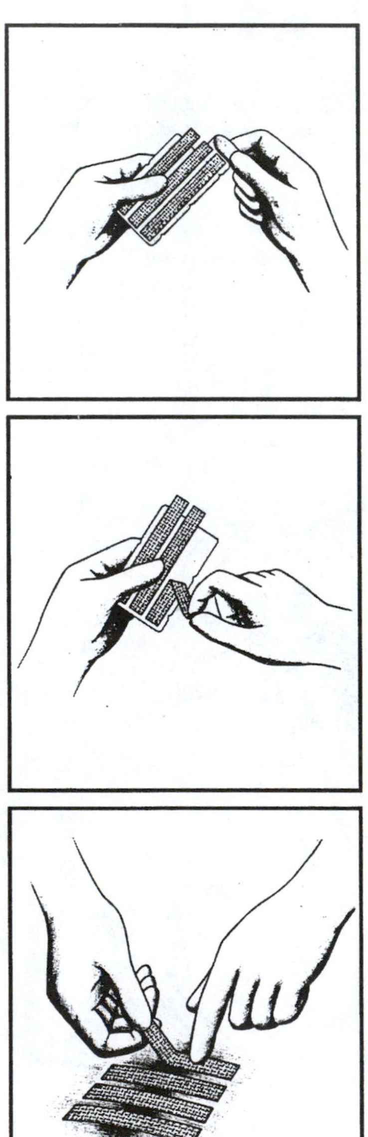

Figure 10–9 Skin Tapes. *Source:* Reprinted with permission from ETHICON, INC., 1996, Somerville, NJ.

81. Skin-closure tapes are used to replace skin staples or sutures that have been removed several days postoperatively.
82. Skin tapes are available in widths of ⅛, ¼, ½ inch and in lengths from 1½ to 4 inches.

Drains

83. Some surgical wound closures will incorporate a drain. Drains are used primarily to obliterate dead space where tissue may not have been adequately approximated or to remove foreign or harmful materials (present or anticipated) that might lead to complication (Gruendemann & Fernsebner, 1995, p. 444). Wounds that are anticipated to produce fluid sufficient to place undue stress on closure may be drained.
84. Three types of drains are gravity, self-contained, and sump.
85. The most commonly used gravity or capillary action drain is a Penrose. A Penrose drain is simple lumen drain made from rubber or silicone. The external end of the drain empties because of gravity or capillary action. Drainage is captured in the surgical dressing. A disadvantage of the Penrose drain is that it provides a pathway for microorganisms to migrate from the surrounding environment into the wound.
86. Commonly used self-contained drains are the Hemovac and the Jackson Pratt (see Figure 10–10). Drainage flows from the end inside the wound through tubing that exits adjacent to the incision site and is attached to a closed reservoir. The reservoir is collapsed before being attached to the drain. The resultant negative pressure directs drainage out of the wound to fill the reservoir. The reservoir may be emptied and negative pressure reinstated to collect additional drainage.
87. Sump drains are double lumened. One lumen provides for the passage of filtered air into the wound, the other permits passage of drainage material from the wound. In the presence of copious drainage the sump pump may be connected to an external suction.

NURSING RESPONSIBILITIES RELATED TO WOUND MANAGEMENT

88. Although the selection and use of wound-closure material and devices is primarily the surgeon's responsibility, the perioperative nurse with a knowledge and understanding of suture and needle characteristics can help prevent patient injury. For example, a cutting needle used in a vascular procedure, where a taper point is de-

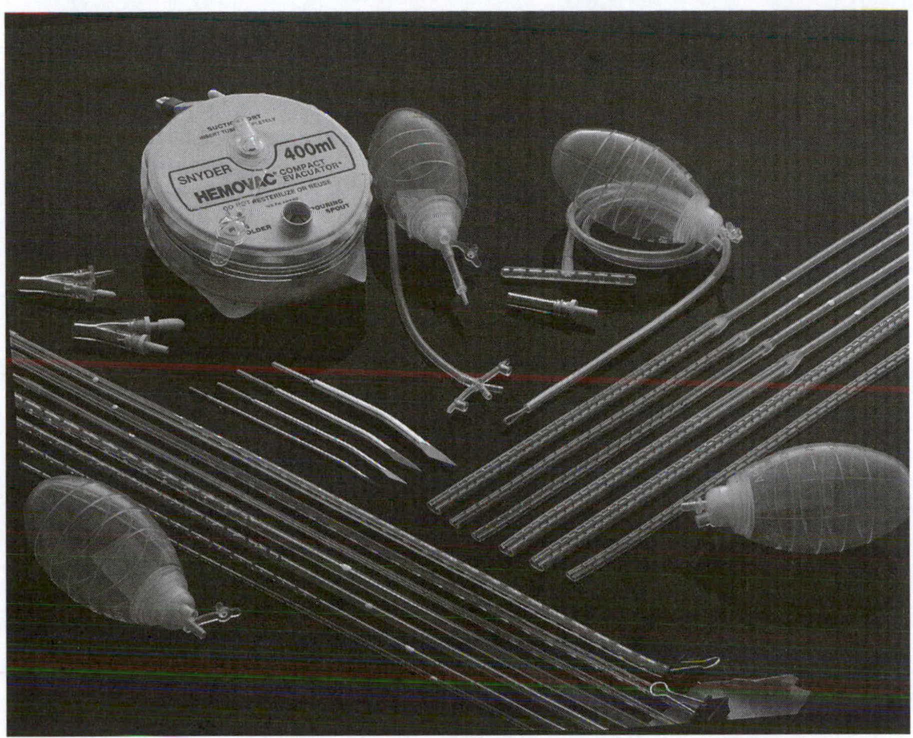

Figure 10–10 Self-Contained Wound Drainage Systems. *Source:* Courtesy of Zimmer, Inc., Dover, Ohio.

sired and anticipated, can cause trauma to the patient and result in additional bleeding; and an absorbable suture used where permanent wound support is desired can result in wound separation.

89. The more knowledgeable the nurse is regarding wound closure materials and devices, the more quickly the surgeon's needs can be anticipated and the length of surgery can thus be kept to a minimum. Also, the less likely it becomes that inappropriate materials and devices that can compromise patient safety will be utilized.
90. Careful handling and maintenance of suture is necessary to prevent the compromise of suture integrity and to ensure adherence to aseptic technique. One or two sutures should be prepared for immediate use, i.e., threaded and/or loaded on a needle holder before the start of surgery. The remainder should be kept in their packets until anticipated in order to maintain sterility.

Section Questions

Q23. List three types of surgical needle points. (Ref 70)

____

____

____

Q24. Name the needle point most appropriate for suturing liver tissue. (Ref. 72)

____

Q25. Needles to which suture is permanently attached are referred to as ____________ or ____________. (Ref. 74)

Q26. Describe a disadvantage to using an eyed needle that must be threaded. (Ref. 78)

____

____

Q27. Explain the two primary purposes of a wound drain. (Ref. 83)

____

____

Q28. Describe the benefit of a Hemovac or Jackson Pratt drain over a Penrose drain. (Ref. 85, 86)

____

____

Q29. The perioperative nurse's knowledge and understanding of wound closure material can help prevent patient injury. Explain an instance of how this is possible. (Ref. 88, 89, 90)

____

____

NOTES

Atkinson, L. (1992). *Berry & Kohn's operating room technique* (7th ed.). St. Louis: Mosby Year Book.

Ethicon. (1994). *Wound closure manual*. Somerville, NJ: Ethicon, Inc.

Fernsebner, B. (1986). Infection control survey: Identifying compliance with guidelines. *AORN Journal*, *3*, 893.

Groah, L. (1996). *Perioperative nursing* (3rd ed.). Stamford, CT: Appleton & Lange.

Gruendemann, B., & Fernsebner, B. (1995). Wound closure. In *Comprehensive perioperative nursing*. Boston: Jones and Bartlett Publishers.

Long, B. (1993). Postoperative intervention. In B. Long, W. Phipps, & V. Cassmeyer (Eds.), *Medical surgical nursing*. St. Louis: Mosby Year Book.

Wysocki, A. (1989). Surgical wound healing: A review for perioperative nurses. *AORN Journal*, *49*(2), 508.

Appendix 10–A

Chapter 10 Post Test

1. List two potential patient injuries related to wound closure. (Ref. 3)

____

____

2. The majority of surgical wound infections are initiated along or close to the suture line. (Ref. 6)

True False

3. Match the columns. (Ref. 9, 12, 14, 16)

wound classification		surgery type
a. class I	_____	amputation of a gangrenous foot
b. class II	_____	cataract extraction
c. class III	_____	bilateral inguinal hernia repair
d. class IV	_____	removal of an inflamed appendix
	_____	bronchoscopy

4. When a wound cannot be sutured together following surgery it is left open to heal from the bottom upward and is filled in with granulation tissue. This is referred to as wound healing by (Ref. 20):
   a. primary intention
   b. secondary intention
   c. tertiary intention

5. The amount of pull that a suture will withstand when knotted before it breaks is defined as _________ strength. (Ref. 30)

6. Suture that is assimilated by the body during the healing process is classified as __________. (Ref. 36)

7. What may be done to multifilament suture during manufacture to reduce capillarity? (Ref. 39)

____

____

8. Monofilament suture (Ref. 38):
   a. resists capillarity
   b. tends to loosen and requires extra throws in the knot to secure it
   c. incurs more resistance than multifilament suture when drawn through tissue

9. The rate of absorption of gut suture is affected by (Ref 46):
   a. the patient's state of health
   b. the presence of infection
   c. the type of tissue in which it is placed
   d. the condition of the tissue in which it is placed

10. Synthetic absorbable suture is absorbed by (Ref. 48):
    a. the action of enzymes
    b. hydrolysis

11. Nylon suture (Ref. 58):
    a. is often used in surgery of the GI tract
    b. is often used for skin closure
    c. can be provided in fine sutures suitable for ophthalmic surgery
    d. is absorbed by enzymes

12. Where prolonged healing is anticipated, such as in cardiovascular surgery, and minimal reactivity is desired, appropriate suture material is (Ref. 61):
    a. chromic gut
    b. Vicryl
    c. Prolene
    d. silk

13. The suture strand with the smallest diameter is (Ref. 63):
    a. 4-0
    b. 6-0
    c. 2-0
    d. 2

14. List five items of information that may be obtained from the suture package. (Ref. 66)

    ____

    ____

    ____

    ____

    ____

15. A taper needle is most appropriate for suturing (Ref. 70):
    a. skin
    b. liver
    c. intestine
    d. peritoneum

16. What is an atraumatic suture? (Ref. 74)

    ____

    ____

17. A stapling device may be used to close fascia. (Ref. 79)

    True False

18. A Penrose drain permits leakage of drainage onto dressings and provides a pathway for migration of microorganisms. (Ref. 85)

    True False

19. The perioperative nurse may utilize knowledge about wound closure materials to (Ref. 88, 89):
    a. anticipate needed suture
    b. help to minimize surgery time
    c. help prevent injury to patient tissue

CHAPTER 11

Prevention of Injury—Anesthesia

Learner Objectives

At the end of Prevention of Injury—Anesthesia, the learner will

- identify potential patient injury related to anesthesia
- identify desired patient outcomes related to anesthesia
- discuss the role of the perioperative nurse during the administration of anesthetic agents and technique
- describe assessment factors relative to the selection of anesthetic agents and technique
- describe malignant hyperthermia and its treatment
- describe four patient monitoring devices and the rationale for their use
- differentiate depolarizing and nondepolarizing neuromuscular blocking agents
- describe techniques of general and regional anesthesia and conscious sedation
- match commonly used anesthetic agents and their actions

Lesson Outline

I. POTENTIAL INJURY—DESIRED PATIENT OUTCOME
- A. Nursing Diagnoses
- B. Desired Patient Outcomes
- C. Outcome Criteria
- D. Overview of Nursing Responsibilities

II. PREANESTHESIA
- A. Assessment Data
- B. American Society of Anesthesiologists Classification
- C. Patient Teaching
- D. Patient Instructions
- E. Selection of Anesthetic Agents and Technique

III. ANESTHESIA TECHNIQUES—OVERVIEW

IV. PREMEDICATION
- A. Goals
- B. Medications/Protocols

V. MONITORING
- A. Practice Recommendations and Standards
- B. Monitoring Devices
  1. Precordial or Esophageal Stethoscope
  2. ECG
  3. Pulse Oximetry
  4. Blood Pressure
  5. Temperature
  6. Capnography

VI. GENERAL ANESTHESIA
- A. Inhalation Agents
- B. Anesthesia Machine
- C. Intravenous Agents
  1. Barbiturate Induction Agents
  2. Nonbarbiturate Induction Agents
  3. Dissociative Induction Agent
  4. Narcotics
  5. Tranquilizers-Benzodiazepines
  6. Neuromuscular Blockers (Muscle Relaxants)
- D. Stages of Anesthesia
- E. Preparation for Anesthesia—Nursing Responsibilities
- F. Sequence for General Anesthesia—Nursing Responsibilities

VII. MALIGNANT HYPERTHERMIA
- A. Overview
- B. Treatment
- C. Nursing Responsibilities

VIII. INTRAVENOUS CONSCIOUS SEDATION
- A. Overview
- B. Nursing Responsibilities

IX. REGIONAL ANESTHESIA
- A. Overview
  1. Spinal
  2. Epidural and Caudal
  3. Intravenous Block (Bier Block)
  4. Nerve Block
  5. Local Infiltration
  6. Topical
- B. Regional Anesthesia—Nursing Responsibilities

CHAPTER 11

Prevention of Injury—Anesthesia

POTENTIAL INJURY—DESIRED PATIENT OUTCOME

1. A little over a hundred years ago anesthesia technique was a crude open-drop ether administration. Depth of anesthesia and physiologic response were inconsistent and poorly controlled. The risk of complication was high. The recent development of sophisticated anesthesia and airway management techniques, new anesthetic agents, refined preanesthesia assessment, and technologically advanced monitoring devices have all made delivery of anesthesia a highly refined process and have dramatically reduced the associated risk.
2. The number of anesthetics administered yearly in the United States is estimated to be 25 million. Studies indicate that death as a complication of anesthesia is 1 per 20,000 to 1 per 85,000 (Meeker & Rothrock, 1995, p. 145).

Nursing Diagnoses

3. Although the death rate associated with anesthesia is extremely low, the risk of complication remains. Anesthetic agents can compromise ventilation, perfusion, and cardiac output, and can alter hypothalamic thermoregulation. Appropriate nursing diagnoses for the patient undergoing anesthesia are high risk for injury (untoward drug reaction or interaction, compromised airway, alteration in cardiac output, electrolyte or fluid imbalance, ineffective breathing pattern, alteration in thought process, and ineffective thermoregulation or hypothermia) related to anesthesia. Other diagnoses may be appropriate based on the patient's condition as identified during assessment.
4. The type of anesthesia, the anesthetic agents employed, the surgical procedure, and the patient's preanesthesia physiological condition all impact the degree of risk for the above conditions. For example, the ambulatory patient who undergoes a minor surgical procedure with local anesthetic or conscious sedation is at minimal risk for hypothermia compared to the patient who undergoes open abdominal surgery with general anesthesia where anesthetic agents cause dilation of blood vessels and the nature of the procedure exposes the patient's gut to room temperature.

Desired Patient Outcomes

5. The desired outcome for the patient who undergoes anesthesia is successful recovery and a return to the preanesthesia physiological state, including normal temperature, unimpeded air exchange, adequate ventilation, maintenance of cardiac output and fluid volume, electrolyte and fluid balance, absence of allergic reaction, and unimpaired thought processes.
6. The time frame in which these desired outcomes is expected to be achieved will vary according to the procedure, anesthetic agents, and anesthesia technique (i.e., local, regional, or general). For example, in the immediate postoperative period, the patient may or may not be expected to breathe unassisted. Goals for when independent breathing should be expected to occur are determined by the patient's preexisting respiratory condition, the intent of the anesthesia care provider, the anesthetic agents employed, and the nature of the surgery.

Outcome Criteria

7. There are several postanesthesia scoring systems used to evaluate the patient's recovery. The most common is the Aldrete postanesthesia scoring system that is used to evaluate the recovery of patients who have received general anesthesia. It evaluates patient activity, respiration, circulation, and oxygen saturation. Points are assigned to patient responses, and discharge from the postanesthesia care unit is dependent on the patient's achieving an acceptable score (see Exhibit 1–1).
8. The acceptable score varies with institutional policy, anticipated recovery, and unit to which the patient is discharged. A patient being transferred from the postanesthesia-care unit to a step-down unit may not require as high a score as does a patient who is returning to a regular unit. For obvious reasons, a patient who is discharged on the same day of surgery must achieve a high score.

Overview of Nursing Responsibilities

9. Anesthesia may be administered by a certified registered nurse anesthetist (CRNA) or an anesthesiologist. A CRNA is a registered nurse with 2 years of anesthesia training. An anesthesiologist is a medical doctor with at least 4 years of anesthesia training after medical school.
10. Preoperatively the CRNA or anesthesiologist will perform a patient assessment, determine the anesthetic agents to be employed, and in collaboration with the surgeon and patient, will select the anesthetic technique. Intraoperative responsibility includes delivery of anesthesia with all the necessary physiological support throughout the procedure and through transport to the postanesthesia-care unit. Postoperatively the CRNA or anesthesiologist evaluates the patient's readiness for discharge and writes a discharge order.
11. Primary responsibility for assisting the anesthesiologist or nurse anesthetist rests with the perioperative nurse in the circulating role. In situations where conscious sedation is administered by the surgeon, and an anesthesiologist or nurse anesthetist is not present, the responsibility for patient monitoring increasingly belongs to the perioperative nurse.
12. Overall responsibilities of the perioperative nurse during anesthesia delivery include but are not limited to
    - Preanesthesia assessment: In addition to the assessment performed by the CRNA or anesthesiologist, the perioperative nurse performs a patient assessment. Information that is obtained serves as a safety check to ensure that significant patient data are known to the surgical team. The information also provides guidelines for anticipating problems, for the course of treatment, and for recovery.
    - Patient support: Emotional support is provided in the preoperative period. Emotional support may consist of answering questions, providing a reassuring touch, and/or remaining close to the patient. Physiological support that is provided throughout the perioperative period is accomplished by applying patient monitoring devices, interpreting monitoring data, being alert to patient physiological status and changes, and implementing interventions, such as providing oxygen or preparing and administering intravenous fluids as appropriate. Assistance is given to the anesthesia care provider by anticipating and providing needed equipment and pharmacological agents in a timely manner. The perioperative nurse accompanies the patient to the postanesthesia-care unit and provides physiological and emotional support as needed. In the postoperative period the perioperative nurse may assist both the anesthesia care provider and the postanesthesia-care unit nurse to stabilize the patient in the unit.
    - Communication: Data obtained during the patient assessment are communicated to and verified with the anesthesia care provider prior to delivery of anesthesia. In addition to the documentation requirements of the institution, the perioperative nurse gives a report to the postanesthesia care-unit nurse that provides information necessary to prepare for the reception of the patient and the patient's recovery from anesthesia. Report to the postanesthesia care nurse should include at least the following:
        1. patient name and age
        2. surgical procedure
        3. surgeon and anesthesiologist
        4. anesthetic agents/technique
        5. intraoperative medications
        6. estimated blood loss
        7. fluid and blood administration
        8. urine output
        9. response to surgery/anesthesia
        10. lab results
        11. chronic and acute health history
        12. drug allergies
        13. expected problems/suggested interventions
        14. discharge plan

      The perioperative nurse may share responsibility for report with anesthesia personnel and must be knowl-

Exhibit 11–1 Aldrete Score

Activity	Able to move four extremities voluntarily on command Able to move two extremities voluntarily on command Able to move no extremities voluntarily on command	2 1 0
Respiration	Able to breathe deeply and cough freely Dyspnea or limited breathing Apneic	2 1 0
Circulation	BP + 20 of preanesthetic level BP + 20–49 of preanesthetic level BP + 50 of preanesthetic level	2 1 0
Consciousness	Fully awake Arousable on calling Not responding	2 1 0
O_2 Saturation	Able to maintain O_2 saturation > 92% on room air Needs O_2 inhalation to maintain O_2 saturation > 90% O_2 saturation < 90% even with O_2 supplement	2 1 0

Source: From Aldrete, A.J., and Wright, A. *Anesthiology News*, *18* (11): 17, 1992. In Litwack, K. (Ed.), *Post Anesthesia Care Nursing*. St. Louis: Mosby Year Book, Inc., 1995.

edgeable of patient status in the above entities and be able to communicate the information to the postanesthesia care-unit nurse.

- Patient teaching: In preparation for anesthesia, the perioperative nurse will provide and reinforce information regarding routines, preanesthesia preparations, instructions for the day of surgery, and procedure-specific postoperative instructions.

13. In many institutions, particularly in small rural facilities, the perioperative nurse provides care throughout the recovery period as well as preoperatively and intraoperatively. In many facilities, however, staffing variances and limited resources have resulted in the need for perioperative nurses to demonstrate competence in postanesthesia care as well as in perioperative nursing. The field of postanesthesia nursing is a specialty in itself and requires significant specialty training. Perioperative nurses who have responsibility for the recovery phase must be skilled in this specialty. Even where responsibility does not include postanesthesia care, the perioperative nurse must be skilled in the use of monitoring equipment and in the interpretation of the data. The perioperative nurse must also be familiar with anesthetic agents and techniques in order to anticipate patient events, quickly implement nursing interventions, and assist the anesthesia care provider.

Section Questions

Q1. The risks associated with anesthesia delivery have been dramatically reduced with the advent of (Ref. 1):
- a. technologically advanced monitoring systems
- b. sophisticated airway management devices
- c. new anesthetic agents
- d. improved monitoring of waste anesthetic gases
- e. refined patient assessment

Q2. Death as a direct result of anesthesia is approximately 1 out of every 10,000 patients. (Ref. 2)

True False

Q3. An appropriate nursing diagnosis for the patient who undergoes anesthesia is high risk for injury such as (Ref. 3):
- a. compromised airway
- b. altered self-image
- c. altered cardiac output
- d. altered thought process
- e. ineffective thermoregulation

Q4. List five desired patient outcomes for the patient who undergoes anesthesia (Ref. 5):

____

____

____

____

____

Q5. The name of the common postanesthesia scoring system that is used to evaluate the recovery of the patient who has received general anesthesia is (Ref. 7):

____

Q6. When conscious sedation is administered in the absence of an anesthesiologist or CRNA, the responsibility for monitoring may appropriately belong to the perioperative nurse. (Ref. 11)

True False

Q7. Relative to anesthesia, the perioperative nursing responsibilities may include (Ref. 12):
- a. patient assessment
- b. patient support
- c. patient data communicated to the anesthesiologist
- d. patient data communicated to the postanesthesia care provider
- e. blood and blood products administered
- f. patient teaching

Q8. In addition to patient name and age, list seven pieces of information that the perioperative nurse should include in the report to the postanesthesia care nurse. (Ref. 12)

____

____

____

____

____

____

____

PREANESTHESIA

Assessment Data

14. In preparation for surgery and anesthesia the patient may be required to undergo assessment and preoperative testing several days prior to surgery. Diagnostic testing may include a chest X-ray; an electrocardiogram (ECG); blood chemistry, including a clotting profile; urine analysis; and other tests as deemed necessary by any of the physicians who are attending to the patient's care. The choice of diagnostic studies is determined by the patient's medical and surgical history, the results of the physical examination, and the intended surgical procedure.
15. At the time of preoperative testing, the patient may be interviewed and examined by the anesthesia care provider who may request additional laboratory and diagnostic testing. During preoperative testing, a perioperative nurse may also interview, assess, and prepare the patient for surgery.
16. The trend today is toward minimal preoperative testing and the healthy patient may require no laboratory or diagnostic procedures. There is a lack of evidence that routine laboratory testing impacts patient outcomes and for this reason most diagnostic testing today is patient and procedure specific.
17. With the continuing movement to ambulatory surgery, the patient may not be seen by the anesthesia care provider or perioperative nurse until the day of surgery. Preoperative instructions may be provided by the nurse who is present at the time that the decision for surgery is made, however. Instructions may also be reinforced by telephone by a perioperative nurse a day or so prior to surgery.
18. Guidelines from the American Society of Anesthesiologists, coupled with institutional requirements, may require an ECG and chest X-ray for patients over a certain age who will undergo general anesthesia or conscious sedation. Preoperative diagnostic requirements will vary according to institutional policy and anesthesia care-provider preference.
19. During preoperative assessment, the perioperative nurse will review the patient's chart and previously obtained assessment data, and assess the patient's readiness for surgery. In addition to the nursing assessment data that are relevant to planning intraoperative care, particular attention is given to data that are significant to anesthesia.
20. Information should be solicited about coexisting disease, history of asthma, previous surgeries, anesthetics, and complications. Family history with anesthetics should be investigated. Such data may provide information suggestive of possible adverse reactions, such as malignant hyperthermia, that can be prevented.
21. Current medications and drug allergies must be noted. This information is critical to prevent drugs that may react unfavorably with current medications or that will cause an allergic reaction from being administered to the patient. Allergies to contrast dyes, iodine solutions, adhesive tape, and latex should also be noted, as should any history of drug and chemical abuse.
22. The patient should be checked for cracked lips, lacerations in or around the mouth, loose or chipped teeth, and dentures. This is important for patients who will undergo general anesthesia and intubation.

23. Female patients of childbearing age should be assessed to determine whether or not they are pregnant. Often this will necessitate a urine pregnancy test.
24. Smoking history is important because smoking may contribute to postoperative pulmonary complication in patients who receive general anesthesia. However, the benefits of smoking cessation of as little as 12 hours have been demonstrated and patient teaching should encourage cessation for as long as possible prior to surgery (Brooks-Braun, 1995, p. 343).
25. Diagnostic testing that was previously ordered should be checked to ensure that the tests were actually performed and that the results are on the chart. In the event that abnormalities are noted, the perioperative nurse should confirm that all team members are aware of the test results.

American Society of Anesthesiologists Classification

26. The anesthesia care provider will assign the patient a physical status in accordance with the American Society of Anesthesiologists (ASA) classification. Patients may be assigned a value from I to VI as follows:

Class I patients	healthy, no organic disease
Class II patients	mild systemic disease (e.g., obesity, controlled hypertension)
Class III patients	severe systemic disease (e.g., poorly controlled hypertension or history of myocardial infarction)
Class IV patients	severe systemic disease that is a constant threat to life (e.g., renal or cardiac failure
Class V patients	moribund and not expected to survive—surgery performed as a last recourse (e.g., ruptured aneurysm)
Class VI	brain dead—organs harvested

This classification system is useful in determining the anesthesia technique to be employed. For example, some institutional policies do not permit class III patients to undergo surgery under general anesthesia as an ambulatory surgery patient, and class III and above patients must have an anesthesiologist or CRNA present during surgery even where anesthesia technique is conscious sedation only.

Patient Teaching

27. Patient teaching is ideally initiated at the time that the decision is made to have surgery. Instruction in preoperative routines, expected outcomes, and day-of-surgery instructions may be given in the physician's office or the clinic where the decision for surgery was made. Teaching and/or reinforcement should occur when and if the patient is instructed to report for a presurgical examination or diagnostic workup. Teaching during the presurgical workup may be initiated by a nurse other than the perioperative nurse. In some facilities, the postanesthesia care-unit nurse initiates preoperative teaching in preparation for anesthesia and reinforces the instructions with a phone call the night before surgery. The patient who is already hospitalized may be instructed by the nurse on the patient's unit.
28. Regardless of where the teaching was accomplished, or who was responsible for preanesthesia instructions, the perioperative nurse should reinforce teaching just prior to surgery and should verify that the patient is in compliance with instructions for the day of surgery.

Patient Instructions

29. Preanesthesia instructions will vary according to the intended surgical procedure and patient condition, and must be individualized. Instructions should include but not be limited to the following:
    - postoperative routines—length of surgery, expected recovery time, postoperative anesthesia care and routines
    - preoperative preparation (if indicated)—preoperative shower or enema
    - preoperative medications—medications to be taken on the day of surgery, both routine and single-dose medications (On occasion specific medications will be ordered for a period prior to surgery, and other medications that the patient routinely takes will be held.)
    - food and liquid intake—traditionally, patients receiving general anesthesia have been instructed to take nothing by mouth (NPO) for 6 to 8 hours prior to surgery. With the loss of a protective airway reflex under general anesthesia a patient who vomits or regurgitates incurs a high risk of aspiration pneumonitis. Aspiration of even a small amount of acid from the stomach can cause severe pneumonitis. A pH of 2.5 and a volume of 0.4 mL is considered an amount that exposes the patient to risk. Ongoing studies, however, indicate that extended periods of fasting do not guarantee an empty stomach (Roth, 1995, p. 214). Current protocols generally restrict solid food intake to 6 to 8 hours before surgery with liquids permitted up to 2 to 3 hours before. NPO restrictions will vary with patient age (infant and young child restrictions are generally

shorter), institutional protocol, and anesthesia care provider preference.

Selection of Anesthetic Agents and Technique

30. Many factors influence the selection of anesthetic agents and technique. Each patient is unique and an assessment must be made to determine those drugs that best meet the surgical requirements and that provide for the patient's well-being. Factors that are considered include, but are not limited to the following:
    - age
    - medical history
    - current physical status
    - intended surgical procedure and expected length of recovery from anesthesia
    - patient preference
    - surgeon preference/requirements
    - anesthesia care provider preference and expertise
    - patient's previous anesthesia/recovery experience
    - whether surgery is elective or emergent
    - considerations for postoperative pain management

ANESTHESIA TECHNIQUES—OVERVIEW

31. Anesthesia may be general, regional, local, or intravenous (IV) conscious sedation.
32. General anesthesia depresses the central nervous system. The patient is unconscious and reflexes are obtunded. Physiologic status is controlled by the anesthesia care provider. This state is characterized by amnesia, analgesia, and muscle relaxation.
33. IV conscious sedation is also referred to as monitored anesthesia care, anesthesia standby, or local standby. In IV conscious sedation the patient is given a local anesthetic at the site of surgery. Medications are administered to provide sedation, systemic analgesia, and depression of the autonomic nervous system. This anesthesia technique may require the presence of an anesthesia care provider. The decision as to whether an anesthesia care provider is needed is based on the patient's condition, ASA classification, the procedure, and institutional policy.
34. IV conscious sedation may be administered to ill patients who cannot tolerate general anesthesia. IV conscious sedation is also appropriate for healthy patients who undergo a minor procedure and who do not require the presence of an anesthesia care provider.
35. In the absence of an anesthesia care provider, the perioperative nurse has the responsibility for monitoring the patient. Institutional policy, in conjunction with the nurse practice act, determines whether the responsibility for intravenous drug administration belongs to the nurse, the surgeon, or both.
36. Regional anesthesia blocks the conduction of pain impulses from a specific region of the body. The patient is awake but does not feel pain during surgery. In regional anesthesia a major nerve block, such as spinal, epidural, or orbital, is anesthetized. Regional anesthetics, such as lidocaine (Xylocaine), bupivacaine (Marcaine), chloroprocaine (Nesacaine), and tetracaine (Pontocaine) are used. Because the patient is awake, additional agents may be administered to reduce anxiety and provide sedation.
37. Local anesthesia is actually a form of regional anesthesia; however, only a small localized area is infiltrated using an anesthetic such as lidocaine (Xylocaine) or bupivacaine (Marcaine).

PREMEDICATION

Goals

38. The practice of preoperative medication is controversial and protocols vary between institutions and anesthesia care providers. Current practices support the evaluation of each patient's needs prior to ordering and administering medications, rather than relying on standard medication protocols.
39. At one time it was standard practice to medicate the patient in preparation for anesthesia and surgery. Today it is not unusual for the patient to receive no preoperative medication. This is particularly true for ambulatory surgery patients where premedication may prolong recovery and delay discharge. In addition, residual effects of medication cannot be monitored after discharge.
40. Goals of premedication may include one or more or all of the following:
    - reduction of anxiety
    - sedation
    - analgesia
    - amnesia
    - prevention of nausea and vomiting
    - reduction in gastric volume and acidity
    - facilitation of induction
    - reduction in potential for allergic reaction
    - decrease of secretions

Medications/Protocols

41. Oral premedications are usually given 60 to 90 minutes prior to surgery with IV agents requiring 30 to 60 minutes. Some agents, such as sodium citrate (Bicitra) and metoclopramide (Reglan) used to promote gastric emp-

tying and lower stomach pH, fall outside these guidelines. These are given 15 to 30 minutes before induction (Litwack, 1995, p. 118).

42. Depending on the desired outcome, the following agents are appropriate for use in the preoperative period:
43. Benzodiazepines—midazolam (Versed), diazepam (Valium), lorazepam (Ativan)—Reduce anxiety, provide sedation and some amnesia.
44. Barbiturates secobarbital—(Seconal), pentobarbital (Nembutal)—Provide sedation with minimal cardiac or respiratory depression.
45. H_2 receptor blocking agents—ranitidine (Zantac, Glaxo), cimetidine (Tagamet), famotidine (Pepcid)—Raise gastric pH and reduce the risk of and complications from aspiration.
46. Nonparticulate antacid—sodium citrate (Bicitra)—Raises gastric pH.
47. Dopamine antagonist—metoclopramide (Reglan)—Increases gastric emptying. Agents that raise pH or increase gastric emptying are particularly useful for patients at high risk for aspiration. Conditions that suggest high risk for aspiration include:
    - morbid obesity
    - old age
    - pregnancy
    - history of hiatal hernia with reflux
    - uncertain NPO status with the need for emergency surgery
    - history of diabetes with gastroparesis
    - history of partial bowel obstruction
    - history of peptic ulcer disease
48. Anticholinergics—atropine, scopolamine, glycopyrrolate (Robinul)—Decrease oral and tracheobronchial secretions and prevent bradycardia that can occur during parasympathetic stimulation or with certain anesthetic agents during induction.
    - These drugs are particularly useful with patients who exhibit excessive salivation problems that put them at risk for aspiration. They are also appropriate for toddlers and young children because they have a tendency to increase salivation up to tenfold when oral mucous membranes are stimulated (Litwack, 1995, p. 118).
    - Anticholinergics, once given routinely as a preoperative medication, are now ordered only for selected patients. Patients who are given anticholinergics may complain of a very dry mouth. A moistened 4 × 4-inch gauze pad can be provided to moisten lips and tongue and provide patient comfort.
49. Antiemetics—droperidol (Inapsine)—Given to prevent nausea and vomiting. These are particularly useful for patients who report a history of nausea and vomiting after anesthesia and surgery. Approximately 20% to 30% of patients do experience postoperative nausea and vomiting (Gruendemann & Fernsebner, 1995, p. 447). Droperidol (Inapsine) also provides some sedation. An untoward reaction to droperidol is dysphoria or heightened anxiety and restlessness.
50. Narcotics—meperidine (Demerol), fentanyl (Sublimaze), morphine—Provide relief from pain. Morphine and meperidine (Demerol) are respiratory depressants and occasionally cause nausea and vomiting. Narcotics are primarily indicated in patients who are experiencing pain. Patients who have received narcotics must be closely observed for adequate ventilation.
51. It is not uncommon for patients who anticipate general anesthesia to mistakenly believe that the premedication they received should have put them to sleep for the surgery. Patients may be anxious because they are still awake. It is important to provide reassurance by informing patients that they will be given additional anesthetic agents for surgery, will be asleep, and will not feel pain.
52. Fear of the unknown, fear of having to relinquish control, and fear of never awakening are some of the concerns expressed by patients in the preoperative period. Perioperative nurses need to be aware of patients' fears, take the time to listen, stay close to the patient, and provide emotional support and reassurance. The period just prior to surgery may be the most stressful for the patient and is a time when the presence of a nurse is crucial to alleviate anxiety.

MONITORING

53. Patient monitoring is essential during anesthesia to detect physiologic changes in response to both the anesthesia and the surgical procedure. Ongoing monitoring is critical to providing appropriate and timely interventions in order to maintain satisfactory physiologic status.
54. The degree of monitoring that is required is determined by the intended procedure and the patient's history and state of health. As a minimum, monitoring for all surgical patients should include ECG, blood pressure, heart rate, and pulse oximetry. When general anesthesia is administered, end tidal volume carbon dioxide, oxygen analysis of anesthesia gases, and temperature monitoring are added.

Practice Recommendations and Standards

55. The Association of Operating Room Nurses (AORN) has adopted practice recommendations for the nurse

who monitors the patient receiving local anesthesia and the patient receiving conscious sedation. The AORN recommendations state that monitoring should include (AORN, 1995, p. 217):

- blood pressure
- cardiac rate and rhythm
- respiratory rate
- oxygen saturation
- skin condition
- mental status/level of consciousness

56. The American Society of Anesthesiologists has standards for basic intraoperative monitoring. Qualified anesthesia personnel shall be present in the room throughout the conduct of all general anesthetics, regional anesthetics, and monitored anesthesia care. During all anesthetics, the patient's oxygenation, ventilation, circulation, and temperature shall be continually monitored (cited in Meeker & Rothrock, 1995, p. 150).
    - Oxygenation—to ensure adequate oxygen concentration in the inspired gas and the blood during all anesthetics.
    - Ventilation—to ensure adequate ventilation of the patient during all anesthetics.
    - Circulation—to ensure the adequacy of the patient's circulatory function during all anesthetics.
    - Body temperature—to aid in the maintenance of appropriate body temperature during all anesthetics.

Monitoring Devices

57. Monitoring devices may be invasive or noninvasive. Noninvasive monitoring devices do not penetrate a body orifice.
58. Examples of noninvasive monitors are ECG electrodes, blood pressure cuffs, and pulse oximeters. Invasive monitors are introduced beneath the skin or mucosa or do enter a body cavity. Examples of invasive monitors are an arterial line and central venous catheter.
59. The choice of monitoring device is determined by the intended procedure, the patient's history and state of health, the anesthesia care provider, the surgeon's judgment, and anticipated postoperative management.
60. Complex, critical, and extensive surgical procedures as well as complex health problems will require extensive monitoring and will employ a combination of invasive and noninvasive monitors. Examples where invasive monitoring is appropriate are in cardiac surgery, in surgeries or in patients where repeated blood samples will be required, and in patients in whom wide variations in blood pressure are anticipated. The healthy patient who undergoes a simple procedure will require noninvasive monitoring only.
61. The perioperative nurse must have a knowledge of monitoring equipment and the ability to interpret data. In situations where the entire responsibility for monitoring rests with the perioperative nurse, such as with local anesthesia or conscious sedation, monitoring competence is especially critical. In these situations, many institutions have supplementary monitoring competency requirements that must be met before the perioperative nurse is permitted to monitor independently. However, even where an anesthesiologist or CRNA is present, the perioperative nurse must be able to recognize normal and abnormal physiologic responses, to administer oxygen and pharmacologic therapy, and to anticipate and assist in pharmacologic and emergency interventions.
62. There are several monitors that are considered standard for patients who receive general anesthesia.

Precordial or Esophageal Stethoscope

63. A stethoscope taped to the patient's chest or an esophageal stethoscope placed within the patient's esophagus provides the capability for continuous auscultation of the chest in order to monitor cardiac rate and rhythm and breath sounds.

ECG

64. ECG monitoring is essential to detect changes in cardiac rate and rhythm and to detect dysrhythmia and myocardial ischemia. Myocardial ischemia in the perioperative period may lead to myocardial infarction postoperatively. Early detection and identification of cardiac irregularities permit timely and specific interventions that can prevent further complications.
65. ECG leads should be placed on clean, dry skin surfaces, and adherence should be checked.

Pulse Oximetry

66. Pulse oximetry measures the oxygen saturation of arterial hemoglobin, which is an indication of the oxygen transfer at the alveolar-capillary level. A photodetector with one end attached to the pulse oximeter is placed on a vascular bed, such as a finger, toe, or an ear lobe. The photo detector consists of a light source side and a receptor side. Two different wavelengths (a red and an infrared) are transmitted through the tissue from the light source side of the photodetector. The receptor side of the photodetector measures the optical density of light that is passed through tissue. Optical density is influenced by the amount of oxygen in the hemoglobin. The

absorption of light for each color indicates the ratio of saturated blood to unsaturated blood.

67. Oxygen saturation readings should be near 100% and readings below 90% are generally indicative of significant hypoxemia. Hypoxemia may lead to cardiac arrest. Pulse oximetry permits the prompt recognition of pending hypoxemia and possible prevention. In the event of decreased oxygen saturation, the perioperative nurse must be prepared to provide ventilatory support and to administer oxygen.
68. Satisfactory oxygen saturation readings from pulse oximetry are not a guarantee that tissues are being adequately perfused with oxygen. Other factors such as hemoglobin level must also be considered. Hemoglobin carries oxygen; however, the hemoglobin may be saturated with oxygen and there may still be insufficient hemoglobin for transport to tissues.
69. Bright lights can interfere with photodetector performance. Exposure to surgical and fluorescent light should be avoided by placing the finger or toe with the attached probe under a blanket or drape.
70. Intravascular dyes, such as methylene blue, will impair the photodetector ability to measure O_2 saturation. Conditions causing vasoconstriction, such as Raynaud's disease or severe peripheral vascular disease, can also hinder an accurate reading (Messina, 1994, p. 229).
71. Photodetectors should not be placed or secured so tightly that localized tissue ischemia results.

Blood Pressure

72. Blood pressure measures pressure in the heart during contraction and relaxation. Blood pressure monitoring may be accomplished manually or with an automatic monitor that takes readings at preset intervals. Automatic monitors that measure blood pressure and cardiac rate, and display rhythm, are considered standard equipment in the operating room and postanesthesia-care unit. These monitors are also incorporated into all general anesthesia delivery machines.
73. Care must be taken to prevent IV lines from being compressed with a blood-pressure cuff. The site of cuff application should be periodically inspected to ensure that adequate deflation has taken place between readings. Extended inflation periods may lead to neurological injury.

Temperature

74. Anesthetic agents affect the patient's temperature by dilating blood vessels and by inhibiting the temperature-regulating mechanism in the hypothalamus. Patient exposure, open surgery, and irrigating fluids that cool also affect body temperature. Hypothermia can reduce the effectiveness of certain anesthetic agents, lead to shivering, and adversely affect pulse oximetry readings.
75. Temperature may be monitored with an external patch thermometer or a more accurate internal esophageal or rectal probe.
76. Warm prep solutions prior to surgery and/or use of a forced-air warming blanket throughout the procedure may decrease the risk of hypothermia (McCormack, 1995, p. 44). Other interventions to maintain normal body temperature include limiting patient exposure and use of warm irrigation fluids.

Capnography

77. Capnography measures the percentage of carbon dioxide exhaled during mechanical ventilation. Capnography is useful as a check to ascertain endotracheal rather than esophageal intubation, and to detect acute changes in metabolic function that indicate the possibility of hypothermia or malignant hyperthermia.
78. Most capnography units provide a digital display of end tidal CO_2 and a waveform readout of expired CO_2 partial pressure versus time.

Section Questions

Q9. To avoid possible missed diagnoses there is a trend today to perform an increasing number of diagnostic tests in preparation for surgery. (Ref. 16)

True False

Q10. All patients who are scheduled for general anesthesia, regardless of their age, should have a preoperative ECG. (Ref. 18)

True False

Q11. During assessment, the following should be noted (Ref. 20, 21, 22):
a. allergies to drugs
b. allergies to tape
c. family history with anesthesia
d. current medications
e. history of substance abuse
f. loose teeth

Q12. Preoperative teaching (Ref. 27, 28, 29):
a. may be performed by the postanesthesia care nurse
b. may be performed by the perioperative nurse
c. should be reinforced just prior to surgery
d. should include medications to take on the day of surgery
e. should include expected recovery time
f. may be performed in the surgeon's office

Q13. Aspiration pneumonitis is a possible consequence of the aspiration of less than 5mL of stomach contents. (Ref. 29)

True False

Q14. General anesthesia is characterized by amnesia, analgesia, and muscle relaxation. (Ref. 32)

True False

Q15. Medications administered during conscious sedation are intended to provide (Ref. 33):
a. muscle relaxation
b. sedation
c. analgesia

Q16. IV conscious sedation should be reserved for healthy patients only. (Ref. 34)

True False

Q17. Spinal anesthesia is an example of regional anesthesia. (Ref. 36)

True False

Q18. An example of a local anesthetic is (Ref. 37, 43, 47):
a. lidocaine (Xylocaine)
b. diazepam (Valium)
c. metoclopramide (Reglan)

Q19. List four goals of preoperative medication. (Ref. 40)

Q20. Patients who are pregnant are at a higher risk of aspiration than patients who are not pregnant. (Ref. 47)

True False

Q21. Anticholinergic drugs, such as atropine, are particularly useful for toddlers as a preoperative medication to reduce oral secretions. (Ref. 48)

True False

Q22. What is the purpose of the drug droperidol (Inapsine)? (Ref. 49)

Q23. Monitoring for all patients should include oxygen saturation and ECG. (Ref. 54, 55)

True False

Q24. Explain the purpose of an esophageal stethoscope. (Ref. 63)

Q25. Pulse oximetry (Ref. 55, 56, 66, 67, 68, 69):
a. measures arterial hemoglobin oxygen saturation
b. should read 80% or higher
c. should be monitored on every patient who undergoes anesthesia
d. permits prompt recognition of pending hypoxemia
e. readings that are above 90% are a guarantee that the patient's tissues are being adequately perfused with oxygen
f. may be faulty in the presence of bright lights

Q26. List three factors during surgery under anesthesia that put the patient at risk for below-normal temperature. (Ref. 74)

Q27. Measuring the percentage of carbon dioxide exhaled during mechanical ventilation is a useful means to check that the endotracheal tube is properly placed. (Ref. 77)

True False

GENERAL ANESTHESIA

79. Effective general anesthesia includes amnesia (sleep and/or hypnosis), analgesia, and skeletal-muscle relaxation. Because different anesthetic agents produce different amounts of these responses, it is usual for more than one agent to be administered.
80. Inhalation and intravenous injection are methods used to deliver general anesthetic agents.

Inhalation Agents

81. Nitrous oxide (N_2O), halothane (Fluothane), enflurane (Ethrane), isoflurane (Forane), desflurane (Suprane), and sevoflurane are the most commonly used inhalation anesthetic agents (see Table 11–1). They enter the system by inhalation and are removed by lung ventilation.
82. Nitrous oxide is a sweet-smelling gas that acts rapidly but lacks potency. It is nonirritating, produces few aftereffects, and recovery is rapid. Because it is a relatively weak anesthetic agent, it is often used as a supplement to other inhalation agents and narcotics. In combination with oxygen alone, it is sufficient only for minor procedures that do not produce intense pain.
83. For major procedures, nitrous oxide is used with other agents to potentiate the anesthetic state.
84. A major precaution with the administration of nitrous oxide is to prevent too high a concentration, which can lead to hypoxia.

Table 11–1 Inhalation Agents

Agent	*Use*	*Advantages*	*Disadvantages*
Oxygen	Sustain life		
Nitrous oxide	Induction of anesthesia; maintenance of anesthesia	Rapid induction and recovery; few aftereffects; nonirritating to respiratory tract	Poor relaxation, insufficient potency for general surgery, hypoxia a potential hazard
Halothane (Fluothane)	Maintenance of anesthesia; may be used for induction	Rapid smooth induction; nonirritating to respiratory tract; useful for patients with bronchial asthma; pleasant odor	Potential toxicity to liver; cardiovascular depressant—hypotension, bradycardia, sensitizes myocardium to catecholamines; may cause ventricular arrhythmias if epinephrine used; affects body temperature control—hypothermia
Enfurane (Ethrane)	Maintenance of anesthesia; may be used for induction	Rapid induction and recovery; minimal aftereffects; potentiates nondepolarizing muscle relaxants; provides some relaxation; pharyngeal and laryngeal reflexes obtunded	Slightly irritating odor; decreased blood pressure and respirations with deepening anesthesia; abnormal electroencephalographic pattern at high concentrations
Isoflurane (Forane)	Maintenance of anesthesia; may be used for induction	Rapid induction and recovery; minimal aftereffects, obtunds laryngeal and pharyngeal reflexes; good relaxation, potentiates all muscle relaxants; protects heart against catecholamine-induced arrhythmias; cardiovascular system remains stable	Expensive, profound respiratory depressant
Sevoflurane	Maintenance of anesthesia; may be used for induction	Most rapid induction and emergence; no ether smell; easy to breathe; protects heart against myocardial irritability	Metabolizes to inorganic fluoride; raises fluoride level in patients with renal disease—unknown consequences; mild and transient chills, fever, nausea; contraindicated in patients susceptible to malignant hyperthermia
Desflurane (Suprane)	Maintenance for short period	Rapid emergence, good relaxation	Irritating to respiratory tract; can cause transient increase in heart rate and blood pressure

85. Halothane, enflurane, isoflurane, and sevoflurane are liquid anesthetics that are vaporized as they pass through a vaporizer on the anesthesia machine. They are inhaled.
86. Halothane is sweet smelling, is nonirritating to the respiratory tract, and is a bronchodilator. Induction and recovery are rapid. It is often used with children.
87. Halothane is also a cardiopulmonary depressant, and side effects include bradycardia, peripheral vasodilation, hypotension, and decreased tidal volume.
88. Halothane has a significant depressant effect on the hypothalamus, which controls body temperature, thus making the patient unable to regulate body temperature to compensate for environment temperature. As a result, if the room is cold, the patient may shiver during emergence from halothane inhalation. Hypothermia is a possible complication.
89. Halothane can sensitize the myocardium to catecholamines and cause ventricular arrhythmia to occur if epinephrine is used as a local injection for vasoconstriction. Therefore, when halothane is used, even small doses of epinephrine are administered with extreme caution.
90. There is a question as to whether the metabolites of halothane affect liver function; therefore, it is generally not given to patients with known liver disease or to patients who will require several surgical procedures within a short period of time.
91. Enflurane provides rapid induction and rapid emergence. Heart rate is not generally affected. Enflurane provides good muscle relaxation and potentiates other muscle relaxants.
92. Enflurane decreases blood pressure, and hypotension is a common occurrence.
93. Isoflurane provides excellent relaxation and potentiates muscle relaxants. Induction and emergence are rapid. The cardiovascular system remains stable and electrocardiographic abnormalities are not associated with isoflurane inhalation.
94. Isoflurane does not sensitize the myocardium to catecholamines and therefore epinephrine may be used for local vasoconstriction.
95. Isoflurane causes peripheral vasodilation. Hypotension is common at induction; however, blood pressure rapidly returns to normal.
96. Desflurane provides good relaxation and offers rapid onset and emergence. A transient increase in cardiac rate and blood pressure may occur. It cannot be used for induction because of its pungent odor, which can cause gagging and laryngospasm.
97. Sevoflurane is a relatively new inhalation agent and allows a more rapid induction and emergence than other inhaled anesthetic agents (Mathias, 1995, p. 36). Because sevoflurane is not irritating to the respiratory tract and does not irritate the myocardium, it may replace halothane as the inhalation of choice for children. Its rapid induction and emergence may also promote use for ambulatory surgery procedures.

Anesthesia Machine

98. Inhalation agents are directed to the patient from an anesthesia machine.
99. Oxygen, nitrous oxide, and air are supplied through hoses from a central source within the health care facility or from cylinders attached to the machine. For safety purposes, the hoses and cylinders are color coded and their fittings are not interchangeable. Oxygen cylinders and hoses are color coded green, nitrous oxide is blue, and air is yellow.
100. Flowmeters attached to the machine measure the amount and flow of nitrous oxide and oxygen being delivered to the patient. The anesthesia care provider selects the ratio of oxygen and nitrous oxide. Flowmeters are also color coded.
101. Another safety feature is a shutoff device that prevents nitrous oxide from being delivered if oxygen is not also delivered.
102. The anesthesia machine is equipped with an oxygen flush button that allows 100% oxygen to be delivered to the patient.
103. The anesthesia machine includes a vaporizer for vaporizing and delivering liquid anesthetics (halothane, enflurane, isoflurane, and sevoflurane).
104. Oxygen and other anesthetic inhalation agents may be mixed and directed to and from the patient through corrugated rubber or plastic tubes. These tubes are joined with a built-in Y connector that may be attached to a face mask or an endotracheal tube. Anesthetic gases are directed to the patient through a one-way valve in one tube, and expired gases are returned through the other tube. A reservoir bag, similar to a balloon, is part of this delivery system. When this reservoir bag is manually compressed, oxygen and inhalation agents may be forced into the lungs and the patient's ventilation may be controlled.
105. As the expired gases are returned from the patient, the carbon dioxide passes through a carbon-dioxide system and is absorbed. Oxygen is added to the remaining exhaled gases, and these are returned to the patient for rebreathing.
106. Anesthesia machines are equipped with a scavenger system that controls the collection of excess expired

gases, which are then eliminated through a suction line.

107. Studies indicate that the presence of nitrous oxide, as well as other anesthetic gases in the atmosphere, presents a serious health hazard to operating room staff. The Occupational Safety and Health Administration has set limits of exposure for anesthetic gases. Every effort must be made to prevent the escape of these gases into the atmosphere.
108. Nitrous oxide limits are as follows:
    - nitrous oxide—25 parts per million (ppm) over an 8-hour time-weighted average
    - halothane—0.5 ppm when used in combination with nitrous oxide, 2 ppm when used alone, per hour
109. The level of anesthetic waste gases is periodically tested to determine an institution's compliance with OSHA regulations. The perioperative nurse should be aware of OSHA limits and testing results.
110. In addition to required periodic testing to monitor the amount of waste gas in the operating room, anesthetic gases should be shut off except during delivery to the patient. Routine testing of anesthesia equipment for leaks and reviews of anesthesia technique can help prevent overexposure.

Intravenous Agents

111. Intravenous agents are introduced directly into the circulatory system, usually through a peripheral vein in the arm or hand.
112. Intravenous agents are most often used as a supplement to inhalation agents.
113. Unlike inhalation agents, which can be easily removed from the system by ventilating the lungs, intravenous agents must be metabolized by the liver or kidneys and excreted.

Barbiturate Induction Agents

114. Barbiturates are used for induction of anesthesia. The most commonly used barbiturates are thiopental sodium (Sodium Pentothal), sodium thiamylal (Surital), and methohexital sodium (Brevital). They are short acting and result in a rapid progression from sedation to loss of consciousness. They do not provide analgesia.
115. Barbiturates are potent respiratory depressants and initial transient apnea is expected. For this reason, before barbiturates are administered, preparations are made to provide oxygen and to assist or control the patient's ventilation.
116. Barbiturates also depress the cardiovascular system, and a degree of hypotension can be expected.
117. Barbiturates are commonly used for induction.

Nonbarbiturate Induction Agents

118. Most recently, the drug propofol (Diprivan) has achieved popularity as an induction and maintenance agent. It is a hypnotic-sedative agent that produces rapid induction.
119. Propofol is delivered in a milky white intralipid emulsion. This medium supports microbial growth, and outbreaks of infection have been associated with its use (Bennett et al., 1995, pp. 147–154). Propofol must be used within 6 hours of preparation, and handling requires strict aseptic technique. The patient may experience pain upon injection. Recovery from propofol is more rapid than with barbiturates. There are minimal aftereffects and less incidence of postoperative nausea and vomiting.

Dissociative Induction Agent

120. Ketamine hydrochloride (Ketalar) is a dissociative agent that produces a catatonic state and provides amnesia and analgesia. The patient will breathe unassisted, may move, and may appear to be awake. However, an anesthetized state has been achieved and surgery may be performed without patient response. Ketamine is rapidly metabolized, and patients emerge quickly from its effects.
121. Ketamine may be given intravenously or intramuscularly. It is useful for diagnostic procedures and procedures where it is desirable to have the patient breathe unassisted. It is sometimes used for children who undergo short procedures that do not require muscle relaxation.
122. Because ketamine is a dissociative agent, patients may experience hallucination postoperatively. This is more common in adults and may be minimized when diazepam or droperidol is given. A quiet, darkened area for recovery is advised.

Narcotics

123. Narcotics may be used preoperatively as a premedication or intraoperatively during induction and maintenance.
124. The narcotics meperidine hydrochloride (Demerol), and morphine sulfate are frequently used premedications.
125. Narcotics that are used intraoperatively are fentanyl (Sublimaze), sufentanil (Sufenta), and alfentanil

(Alfenta). Fentanyl is 80 to 100 times more potent than morphine, and sufentanil is more potent than fentanyl.

126. Small doses of narcotics are used intraoperatively as adjuncts to other drugs and to provide relief from pain in the early postoperative period.
127. Narcotics provide profound analgesia with little influence on blood pressure, cardiac rate, and cardiac output. They are of particular value in cardiac surgery.
128. Narcotics are respiratory depressants and patients who have received high doses of narcotics intraoperatively must be closely monitored to ensure that they are breathing adequately. A patient who has received a high dose of narcotic intraoperatively may appear to be awake and alert postoperatively but may suddenly begin to hypoventilate and lose consciousness.

Tranquilizers-Benzodiazepines

129. Tranquilizers commonly used intraoperatively are diazepam (Valium), midazolam (Versed), and droperidol (Inapsine).
130. Tranquilizers are used for induction and as adjuncts to other anesthetic agents. Their use permits lower doses of other agents.
131. Diazepam produces amnesia, midazolam provides excellent amnesia, and droperidol is an antiemetic agent.
132. Flumazenil (Romazicon) is an important drug that is used to reverse the effects of benzodiazepines. It reverses sedation and respiratory depression without cardiovascular effects. Patients who are reversed must be closely monitored because flumazenil may lose it effect sooner than the underlying benzodiazepine and hypoventilation can then occur.

Neuromuscular Blockers (Muscle Relaxants)

133. Muscle relaxants (see Table 11–2) commonly used intraoperatively are succinylcholine (Anectine and Quelicin), tubocurarine chloride (curare), pancuronium bromide (Pavulon), atracurium besylate (Tracrium), mivacurium (Mivacron), rocuronium bromide (Zemuron), and vecuronium bromide (Norcuron).
134. Two primary indications for neuromuscular blockers are: (1) to relax the jaw and larynx in order to facilitate controlled breathing and tracheal intubation, and (2) to increase muscle relaxation to permit ease of tissue handling during surgery.
135. Muscle relaxants have varying onset and duration of effect. Intubation is accomplished with neuromuscular blockers that have rapid onset and are short acting.
136. Neuromuscular blockers paralyze the neuromuscular junction and block impulses from motor nerves to skeletal muscle. The patient becomes paralyzed. Neuromuscular blockers are depolarizing or nondepolarizing.
137. Succinylcholine is a depolarizing muscle relaxant. When it reaches the neuromuscular junction it acts like acetylcholine, producing a depolarization of the membrane at the motor end plate. The depolarization causes a muscle contraction that is followed by a neuromuscular block. The drug prevents repolarization, and the muscle remains relaxed and paralyzed. The muscle contractions are sometimes obvious and appear similar to twitching. This twitching, referred to as fasciculation, progresses in cephalocaudal sequence as the drug circulates through the patient's body.
138. Succinylcholine produces paralysis within seconds and is used for intubation. Because of its rapid onset, it is valuable in emergency situations where rapid intubation is required.
139. Nondepolarizing muscle relaxants block the action of acetylcholine at the neuromuscular junction but do not cause depolarization at the motor end plate so fasciculation does not occur.
140. Nondepolarizing agents have a slower onset than depolarizing agents and their effect lasts longer.
141. The anesthesia care provider continually monitors the patient to determine the amount of paralysis present. The application of a nerve stimulator to a peripheral nerve, such as the ulnar nerve or a branch of the facial nerve, and observing for absence of contractions is helpful in determining the amount of paralysis present.
142. Pyridostigmine (Regonol) or neostigmine (Prostigmin) is used when necessary to reverse the action of nondepolarizing agents.

Table 11–2 Muscle Relaxants

Agent	*Use*	*Advantages*	*Disadvantages*
Depolarizing Muscle Relaxant—Rapid Onset, Short Duration			
Succinylcholine (Anectine, Quelicin)	Intubation Short procedures	Rapid onset; brief duration	Can cause muscle fasciculation, postoperative myalgia; requires refrigeration, contraindicated in patients with recent burn, muscle trauma, or recurrent neuromuscular disorder; can trigger malignant hyperthermia; prolonged effect in patients with serum cholinesterase deficiency
Nondepolarizing Muscle Relaxants—Intermediate Onset, Intermediate Duration			
Atracurium (Tracrium)	Intubation Maintenance of muscle relaxation	No significant cardiovascular effects	Requires refrigeration; slight release of histamine
Vecuronium (Norcuron)	Intubation Maintenance of muscle relaxation	No significant cardiovascular effects; no release of histamine	Must be mixed
Mivacurium (Mivacron)	Intubation Maintenance of muscle relaxation		Expensive; prolonged effect in patients with serum cholinesterase deficiency
Rocuronium (Zemuron)	Intubation Maintenance of muscle relaxation	Provides excellent intubating conditions; rapid onset	May increase heart rate; eliminated via liver, contraindicated in patients with hepatic disease, contraindicated for rapid intubation for cesarean sections
Nondepolarizing Muscle Relaxants—Delayed Onset, Longer Duration			
Tubocurarine (curare)	Maintenance of muscle relaxation		Strong histamine release; autonomic blockade can cause hypotension
Pancuronium (Pavulon)	Maintenance of muscle relaxation	Long duration	Can cause hypertension and increased heart rate

Section Questions

Q28. Nitrous oxide is a useful supplement to other inhalation agents and is seldom used in combination with oxygen alone. (Ref. 82)

True False

Q29. Inhalation agent(s) commonly used for children are (Ref. 86, 97):
a. Halothane
b. Enflurane
c. Isoflurane
d. Desflurane
e. Sevoflurane

Q30. Oxygen cylinders, hoses, and flowmeters are color coded ________________________. Nitrous oxide cylinders, hoses, and flowmeters are color coded ________________________(color). (Ref. 99, 100)

Q31. Explain why is it important that anesthesia delivery machines be equipped with a scavenger system. (Ref. 107)

____

____

Q32. Inhalation and intravenous agents may be used in combination to achieve general anesthesia. (Ref. 112)

True False

Q33. Thiopental sodium (Sodium Pentothal), sodium thiamylal (Surital), and methohexital sodium (Brevital) are barbiturates that are used for induction because they cause rapid loss of consciousness. (Ref. 114)

True False

Q34. Propofol (Ref. 118, 119):
a. is a narcotic
b. is a rapid induction agent
c. provides muscle relaxation
d. may cause pain to the patient upon injection
e. handling requires strict aseptic technique because it is supplied in a medium that supports bacterial growth
f. results in minimal aftereffects

Q35. What adverse reaction might a patient have following ketamine? (Ref. 122)

____

Q36. Narcotics such as fentanyl (Sublimaze) may be administered intraoperatively to provide relief of pain postoperatively. (Ref. 126)

True False

Q37. Explain why patients who have received high doses of narcotics should be closely monitored postoperatively to ensure that they are breathing adequately. (Ref. 128)

____

____

____

Q38. Flumazenil (Romazicon) is a reversal agent for (Ref. 132):
a. narcotics
b. tranquilizers
c. muscle relaxants

Q39. Neuromuscular blockers (Ref. 134, 136):
a. cause paralysis
b. produce sleep
c. are useful for jaw relaxation to facilitate intubation
d. permit ease of tissue manipulation

Q40. Succinylcholine (Ref. 137, 138):
a. is a depolarizing muscle relaxant that causes a muscle contraction followed by a neuromuscular block that results in paralysis
b. can cause fasciculation
c. has a slow onset
d. is useful where emergency rapid intubation is needed

Stages of Anesthesia

143. In 1720, Arthur Guedel integrated the four stages of anesthesia with their signs and symptoms into a system that until recent times was used to estimate the depth of anesthesia. By observing the patient's physiological changes and reflex responses, the depth of anesthesia was determined. The system applied to patients who were not premedicated, breathed spontaneously, and were administered ether.

144. The stages are as follows:
- Stage I, Relaxation—from administration of anesthesia to loss of consciousness. Patient response–dizziness, drowsiness, exaggerated hearing, and a decreased sense of pain.
- Stage II, Excitement—from loss of consciousness to onset of regular breathing. Patient response–irregular breathing, increased muscle tone and involuntary motor activity, thrashing and struggling activity (susceptible to auditory and tactile stimulation).
- Stage III, Surgical Anesthesia—from onset of regular breathing to cessation of respiration. Patient response–regular thoracoabdominal breathing, a relaxed jaw, a loss of pain and auditory sensation, and loss of eyelid reflex.
- Stage IV, Danger—from cessation of respiration to circulatory failure and death. Patient response–pupils that are fixed and dilated, a rapid and thready pulse, and paralyzed respiratory muscles.

145. Because anesthetic agents that are used today quickly bring the patient to stage III, the untoward responses of stage II are seldom seen and Guedel's system is not suitable for evaluating the depth of anesthesia. Perioperative nurses, however, should have an appreciation of the depth of anesthesia. An awareness of the patient's level of anesthesia allows the nurse to plan for and provide safety measures. Recovery from anesthesia occurs in reverse order.

Preparation for Anesthesia—Nursing Responsibilities

146. As much as possible, the room should be made ready and preparations for surgery completed before the patient is brought into the operating room suite. Once the patient is in the room it is important that the circulating nurse be immediately available to provide emotional

support, ensure patient dignity, institute safety measures, and assist the anesthesia care provider.

147. In preparation for induction, nursing responsibilities include transfer of the patient from the stretcher to the operating room table, placement of electrocardiographic leads, application of blood-pressure cuff, placement of the intravenous line, application of the safety strap, and adjustment of the patient's gown and sheets. Because these preparatory activities have the potential for exposing the patient, nursing interventions at this time should focus on maintaining patient dignity. The perioperative nurse must limit exposure of the patient by immediately closing the operating room doors and keeping unnecessary personnel from the room.

148. As preparations are made for anesthesia induction, patients can experience feelings from mild anxiety to acute fear. The perioperative nurse can help allay these feelings by being at the patient's side, by speaking calmly, by answering questions, and by explaining activities. Nonverbal support, such as holding the patient's hand, can be the most supportive intervention.

149. Efforts should be made not to stimulate the patient or interrupt the calming effect of the preoperative medication. All unnecessary noise should be avoided. It is the responsibility of the perioperative nurse to provide and maintain a quiet atmosphere in the operating room; however, all team members must participate in the effort. All unnecessary conversation should be curtailed. The operating room door should remain closed. Instrument counting should not be performed within range of the patient's hearing. Overhearing "blades, "needles," "mosquitoes," and so forth, can be frightening to the patient. Hearing is the most difficult sense to anesthetize (McKinney, 1993, p. 1467). It is the last sensation lost before unconsciousness, and noise should be kept to a minimum.

150. Prior to anesthesia induction, the perioperative nurse should check the suction to ensure that it is turned on and working properly. The suction catheter should be placed within easy reach of the anesthesia care provider.

151. Induction is the period from beginning of anesthesia until the patient loses consciousness and is stabilized at the desired level of anesthesia (Atkinson & Kohn, 1986, p. 223).

152. Induction is a critical time during the administration of anesthesia, and it is essential for patient safety that the perioperative nurse be present and available to assist the anesthesia care provider with suctioning and intubation and, if necessary, to restrain the patient (particularly children).

153. In young children who may not tolerate the placement of an intravenous line, and in patients with a tracheostomy tube, induction is usually begun with an inhalation agent.

Sequence for General Anesthesia—Nursing Responsibilities

154. In patients who have an intravenous line, a typical sequence for general anesthesia might progress as follows:
    - If the patient can tolerate it, a mask is placed over the nose and mouth while the patient breathes 100% oxygen for a few minutes. The oxygenation serves as a safety margin in the event of an airway obstruction or brief period of apnea during insertion of the endotracheal tube.
    - A narcotic and/or a benzodiazepine is injected and ventilation is monitored.
    - A barbiturate (thiopental sodium or thiamylal sodium) or a hypnotic (propofol) is injected to produce sleep. Sleep may be judged by the lack of eyelid movement when the eyelid is stroked. Sleep will usually occur within 1 or 2 minutes.
    - With the mask over the patient's nose and mouth, the anesthesia care provider will ventilate the patient and observe the chest rise. If the chest does not rise, the head and mandible are repositioned until a patent airway is maintained.
    - When it is established that the airway is clear, a paralyzing dose of muscle relaxant is administered to facilitate intubation. (Muscle relaxants with a longer onset may be injected before the patient is asleep as the effect will not occur until after sleep is achieved.)
    - A laryngoscope is used to visualize the vocal cords, and the patient is intubated. (An endotracheal tube is inserted into the trachea.) The perioperative nurse can assist the anesthesia care provider by pulling outwardly on the corner of the patient's mouth to permit better visualization of the vocal cords and placement of the endotracheal tube. The perioperative nurse can also assist by passing the endotracheal tube to the anesthesia care provider so he or she does not have to interrupt visualization to pick up the tube, and by providing a 10-mL syringe to inflate the endotracheal tube cuff.
    - Correct endotracheal tube placement is confirmed (Stein, 1995, p. 797) by:
        1. observing fog in the clear endotracheal tube

2. observing the patient for bilateral chest excursion without epigastric enlargement
3. listening for bilateral breath sounds
4. identifying carbon dioxide expiration through end-tidal monitoring

155. If the patient is not intubated, a combination of inhalation agents will be administered via a mask or laryngeal airway. For short procedures and procedures where paralysis is not necessary, the patient is usually not intubated. The mask is strapped or held over the patient's nose and mouth and connected via anesthesia tubing to the anesthesia machine. The patient may breathe spontaneously, or breathing and delivery of anesthetic agents is accomplished manually by compressing a reservoir bag on the anesthesia machine. This is also referred to as "bagging the patient."
156. The laryngeal mask airway is a relatively new device that provides good airway protection without intubation. It is inserted into the patient's mouth, positioned securely over the larynx, and inflated to keep it securely in place. The patient may breathe spontaneously or the airway can be attached to anesthesia circuitry for mechanical ventilation (see Figure 11–1).
157. If the patient is intubated, the endotracheal tube is inserted directly into the larynx and secured in place by inflating a cuff that is attached to the tube. The endotracheal tube is connected to the anesthesia machine via tubing, and inhalation agents are delivered automatically according to preset parameters.
158. When a barbiturate or hypnotic is given at the start of induction, it will quickly reach the patient's brain and apnea will usually result. The patient's pharyngeal muscles and tongue relax, and airway obstruction can occur. If a clear airway is not maintained, the patient will attempt to breathe as the drug washes out of the brain. The abdominal muscles may strain and pull the diaphragm down, compressing the stomach and causing the patient to regurgitate. If the patient regurgitates and attempts to breathe, he or she can aspirate gastric contents into the lungs with resultant aspiration pneumonia. The perioperative nurse must be prepared to immediately provide suction, turn the patient's head to the side, adjust the table into the Trendelenburg position, and assist the anesthesia provider as needed.
159. Patients who have not been NPO for the required period of time are not given general anesthesia unless it is an emergency situation wherein regional anesthesia is not appropriate. The patient who ate and then became ill, the trauma victim with blood in the stomach, or the patient with a hiatal hernia is at risk for aspiration. Aspiration of stomach contents can prove fatal. The perioperative nurse's first priority is to remain at the patient's side at the head of the table, prepared to assist the anesthesia care provider until intubation is complete and assistance is no longer needed. A suction catheter or tip, a nasogastric tube, an emesis basin, and a towel should be immediately available.

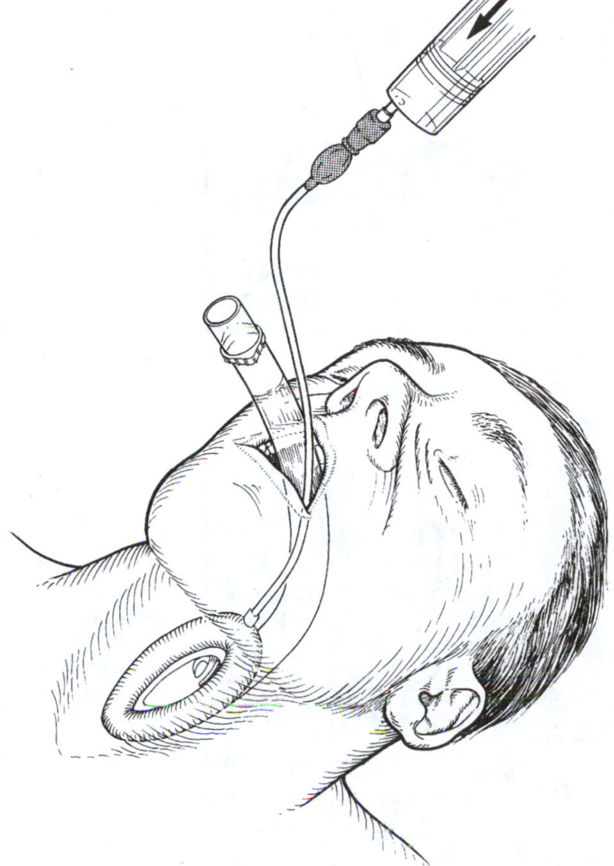

Figure 11–1 Laryngeal Mask. *Source:* Reprinted with permission from ETHICON, INC., 1986, Somerville, NJ.

160. During intubation the perioperative nurse may be asked to assist by firmly pressing the cricoid cartilage posteriorly with the index finger or thumb and forefinger. This maneuver is referred to as the Sellick maneuver. It compresses the esophagus between the cricoid cartilage and the vertebral column. It aids in visualization of the tracheal lumen for intubation and occludes the esophagus to prevent regurgitation. Pressure must begin when the patient is awake and must be maintained until the endotracheal tube is in place and inflated (see Figure 11–2).
161. Once the cuff is inflated, the endotracheal tube is connected to the anesthesia machine from which the inha-

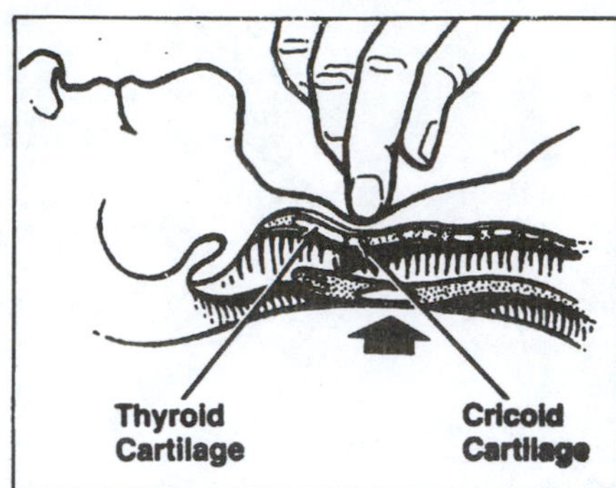

Using the index finger to displace the cricoid cartilage posteriorly thus obstructing the esophagus

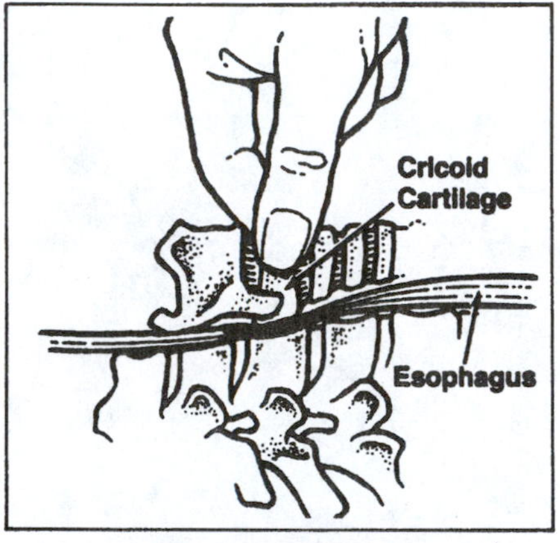

Two-finger technique that obstructs the esophagus between the sixth cervical vertebra and the cricoid cartilage

Figure 11–2 The Sellick Maneuver. *Source:* Courtesy of Gensia Pharmaceuticals, Inc., San Diego, California.

lation agents are delivered and by which ventilation is controlled.

162. General anesthesia depresses the hypothalamus, thus preventing the patient from compensating for the temperature in the room. If the operating room is cold, the anesthetized patient can become hypothermic. Nursing interventions should be directed toward maintaining the patient's body temperature within normal limits. Appropriate interventions include providing a warming blanket, covering the patient with a warm blanket, limiting skin exposure, and supplying warm fluids for irrigation during surgery.
163. Injury that is related to improper positioning is a risk for the anesthetized patient. Patients who are improperly positioned can sustain injury of the integumentary, respiratory, circulatory, or musculoskeletal system. Peripheral nerves, eyes, skin, and digits are especially susceptible to injury. Injury resulting from improper positioning may be temporary or can be permanent.
164. Following the induction of anesthesia, the perioperative nurse should scan the patient from head to foot and, if necessary, take corrective action to ensure that the patient is properly positioned. This is a critical review because once the patient is draped, positioning cannot be visualized.
165. If the patient is moved or repositioned during the procedure, a check should again be made to ensure a safe and proper position.
166. Before repositioning the patient, the perioperative nurse should confer with the anesthesia care provider to determine that the patient can be moved without compromise to the airway and to ventilation, and that he or she is ready to assist in repositioning by guiding and securing the patient's head to prevent accidental extubation or disconnection from the ventilator.
167. During the procedure, the perioperative nurse monitors fluid output and replacement, blood loss, blood and blood product replacement, and the amount of irrigating solution.
168. Emergence from anesthesia, particularly from extubation, is a critical period when the perioperative nurse must be at the patient's side and immediately available to assist the anesthesia care provider.
169. Extubation can initiate bronchospasm or laryngospasm reflex. The airway may become obstructed and vomiting can occur. Airway management and adequate ventilation are priorities. Prior to extubation the perioperative nurse should check to make sure that a suction catheter is within reach of the anesthesia care provider and that suction is turned on and working.

MALIGNANT HYPERTHERMIA

Overview

170. Malignant hyperthermia is an emergency complication of general anesthesia. It is characterized by a rapid rise in temperature, with temperatures rising as high as 109.4°F (43°C).
171. Incidence of malignant hyperthermia is estimated to be 1:250,000 (Donnelly, 1994, p. 393). It is considered to be, according to H. Hein, the leading cause of anesthetic deaths in healthy young adults (cited in Beck, 1994, p. 367). Approximately 10% of patients who experience a malignant hyperthermia episode will die according to G. Gronert and J. Schulman (cited in Donnelly, 1994, p. 393).

172. In patients who experience malignant hyperthermia, the sarcoplasmic reticulum (calcium-storing membrane of the muscle cell) is unable to regulate calcium within the muscle cell in the presence of certain anesthetic agents.
173. When malignant hyperthermia occurs, intracellular calcium increases and the result is sustained contracture of skeletal muscle. The contractions cause muscles to consume higher than normal amounts of oxygen, which then produces lactic acid and heat. The patient's temperature rises rapidly and dramatically. Electrolytes, enzymes, and myoglobin leak from the cells. Hyperkalemia may result and lead to cardiac arrhythmias. The loss of myoglobin can result in renal failure (Donnelly, 1994, p. 395).
174. Symptoms may be multifocal and include sudden inappropriate tachycardia with tachypnea, unstable blood pressure, generalized rigidity, masseter muscle spasm, metabolic and respiratory acidosis, increased end-tidal CO_2, fever, profuse sweating, cyanotic mottling of the skin, and dark unoxygenated blood in the field. Temperature can rise as much as 1.8°F (1°C) every 5 minutes.
175. Tachycardia and increased end-tidal CO_2 are often the first symptoms to appear and may be attributed to causes other than malignant hyperthermia. The classic symptom of fever may occur after the appearance of other symptoms.
176. Certain inhalation agents and depolarizing muscle relaxants are known to be malignant hyperthermia triggers. The inhalation agent fluothane (Halothane) and the muscle relaxant succinylcholine (Anectine and Quelicin) are primary triggering agents. Enflurane, isoflurane, desflurane, and sevoflurane are also contraindicated for patients susceptible to malignant hyperthermia.
177. When succinylcholine is the triggering agent, a sudden severe rigidity of the jaw may be seen following administration of the drug.
178. Depending on the patient and the triggering agent, malignant hyperthermia can occur immediately or as late as 24 hours following the administration of anesthesia.
179. There are multiple causes of malignant hyperthermia; however, inheritance is believed to be a significant factor. Certain muscle disorders, such as Duchenne's muscular dystrophy, have been associated with malignant hyperthermia.
180. Patients who are susceptible to malignant hyperthermia can sometimes be identified through preoperative assessment. Assessment risk factors are
    - personal or family history of malignant hyperthermia or complications arising from anesthesia
    - a family history of suspicious anesthesia experience
    - history of unexplained muscle cramps with fever
    - inherited skeletal muscle disorders
181. If it is suspected that the patient is susceptible to malignant hyperthermia the surgery may be postponed until a skeletal muscle biopsy test is performed to confirm the diagnosis.

Treatment

182. If a patient experiences a malignant hyperthermia episode during surgery, initial treatment is to immediately discontinue all triggering anesthetic agents, hyperventilate with 100% oxygen, administer dantrolene sodium (Dantrium), and rapidly terminate surgery. Dantrolene sodium is a skeletal muscle relaxant that blocks the release of calcium from the sarcoplasmic reticulum that in turn decreases muscle contractions.
183. If it is impossible to terminate surgery, anesthesia is continued with nontriggering agents.
184. Cooling of the patient is achieved by wound irrigation with cold saline, administration of cold intravenous solutions, surface cooling with ice or a cooling blanket, and a cold gastric and rectal lavage.
185. The anesthesia circuit and carbon-dioxide absorbent should be changed to reduce risk from residual triggering agents.
186. Dantrolene sodium is administered at 2.5 mg/kg until the patient responds, or a maximum of 20 doses is given. The patient will generally respond within minutes. Acidosis is treated with sodium bicarbonate.
187. Additional treatment is governed by blood gas, electrolyte, creatine phosphokinase (CPK), lactic dehydrogenase (LDH), and blood-clotting analysis.
188. Following an episode of malignant hyperthermia the patient must be closely monitored for a possible recurrent episode. Dantrolene sodium is continued for 48 hours or more.
189. Every operating room where general anesthesia is administered should have immediate access to dantrolene sodium and a written, readily accessible, protocol for the management of malignant hyperthermia. A cart containing supplies needed to manage a malignant hyperthermia occurrence should be readily available and staff should be familiar with the contents and the treatment protocol.
190. In addition to a posted policy and a cart with necessary supplies, many operating room departments have an

anesthesia machine reserved for use in the event of a malignant hyperthermia episode. Should an episode occur, the reserved anesthesia machine is brought to the room to replace the one in use. This saves time by eliminating the necessity to change the anesthesia circuit and replace the carbon-dioxide absorbent on the existing machine.

191. Dantrolene sodium is supplied in a 20-mg vial and requires 60 mL of sterile water for reconstitution. The water should contain no preservative. Reconstitution of dantrolene sodium is difficult and requires vigorous shaking. The malignant hyperthermia supply cart should contain 36 vials of dantrolene and sufficient sterile water for reconstitution. (Thirty-six vials are required to reach a maximum dose for a 175-pound patient.)

Nursing Responsibilities

192. During the preoperative interview the perioperative nurse should assess the patient for risk factors associated with malignant hyperthermia.

193. The perioperative nurse should be familiar with the malignant hyperthermia protocol and be able to institute prompt and appropriate treatment. Competencies include the ability to
   - assess the patient preoperatively for malignant hyperthermia risk factors
   - prepare the room with appropriate supplies for a patient known to be susceptible to malignant hyperthermia
   - recognize signs and symptoms of malignant hyperthermia
   - rapidly supply and reconstitute dantrolene sodium
   - provide necessary supplies without hesitation
   - assist the anesthesia care provider with intravenous line setup and placement, drug preparation and administration, implementation of laboratory testing, and as otherwise directed
   - cool patient; surface, intravenous, and lavage

194. If the patient is known or considered to be susceptible to malignant hyperthermia, regional anesthesia or only nontriggering anesthetics are administered, and fresh anesthesia circuitry and CO_2 absorbent are used. Other interventions are the preparation of the operating room table with a cooling blanket, transfer of the malignant-hyperthermia cart and supplies into the room, and depending on institutional policy, prophylactic administration of dantrolene sodium.

Section Questions

Q41. Describe two nursing interventions to assist the patient to maintain dignity while in the operating room just prior to anesthesia induction. (Ref. 147)

____

____

Q42. During induction, the perioperative nurse (Ref. 146, 148, 149):
a. may provide significant support by holding the patient's hand
b. must be immediately available to assist the anesthesia care provider
c. should maintain quiet in the room

Q43. The laryngeal mask airway protects the patient's airway without intubation. (Ref. 156)

True False

Q44. In the event that the patient aspirates stomach contents, the perioperative nurse must be prepared to immediately place the table in reverse Trendelenburg position. (Ref. 158)

True False

Q45. The Sellick maneuver is performed (Ref. 160):
a. to occlude the esophagus to prevent regurgitation
b. to visualize the tracheal lumen
c. only by the anesthesia care provider
d. to assist patient ventilation

Q46. Extubation may initiate (Ref 169):
a. bronchospasm
b. laryngospasm
c. vomiting

Q47. Malignant hyperthermia is a disorder of the hypothalamus, which regulates temperature. (Ref. 172, 173, 179)

True False

Q48. The neuromuscular blocker ______________ is a primary triggering agent of malignant hyperthermia. (Ref. 176)

Q49. The treatment drug for malignant hyperthermia is ______________ and it is administered at ______________ mg/kg until the patient responds, or a maximum of 20 doses is given. (Ref. 182, 186)

Q50. Describe two interventions to cool the patient during a malignant hyperthermia crisis. (Ref. 184)

____

____

Q51. Describe two nursing interventions to prepare the room if the patient is considered to be susceptible to malignant hyperthermia. (Ref. 196)

____

____

INTRAVENOUS CONSCIOUS SEDATION

Overview

195. Conscious sedation is a minimally depressed level of consciousness during which the patient retains the ability to maintain a continuous airway and respond appropriately to physical stimulation or verbal commands (Somerson et al., 1995, p. 26).
196. Conscious sedation is frequently employed for diagnostic procedures or minor surgery where the presence of an anesthesiologist is not routinely necessary. Examples of procedures are colonoscopy, incision and drainage of an abscess, vasectomy, and the reduction of a dislocation with a cast application.
197. The goals of conscious sedation are to
    - allay fear and anxiety
    - maintain consciousness and the ability to cooperate
    - elevate pain threshold
    - maintain stable vital signs
    - achieve partial amnesia
    - facilitate prompt return to activities of daily living
198. Each institution should develop criteria to identify which patients are suitable candidates for conscious sedation. Physiological status and psychological maturity should be evaluated.
199. Medications are delivered intravenously. Commonly used agents include midazolam, meperidine, propofol, fentanyl, katamine, diazepam, and fentanyl with droperidol (Stein, 1995, p. 801).
200. Reversal agents include naloxone hydrochloride (Narcan) for narcotics, and flumazenil (Romazicon) for benzodiazepines
201. Desired effects of IV conscious sedation are relaxation, cooperation, and intact protective reflexes. Verbal communication is diminished; the patient breathes unassisted and is easily aroused.
202. Undesirable effects are nystagmus (may be normal with large doses of diazepam), slurred speech, unarousable sleep, hypotension, agitation, combativeness, respiratory depression, airway obstruction, and apnea (AORN, 1995, p. 206)

Nursing Responsibilities

203. The registered nurse who monitors the patient who is receiving IV conscious sedation should have no other responsibilities during the procedure that would leave the patient unattended and compromise monitoring (AORN, 1995, p. 206).
204. The patient who receives IV conscious sedation must be continuously monitored for any reaction to drugs and for physiologic and psychologic changes.
205. In addition to the ability to perform a thorough preoperative assessment, the nurse who is monitoring the patient should have a working knowledge of resuscitation equipment and the function and use of monitoring equipment, and should be able to interpret any data that are obtained (AORN, 1995, p. 207).
206. Necessary knowledge and/or skills include the following:
    - knowledge of anatomy and physiology
    - knowledge of airway management, including the use of oxygen delivery devices and equipment
    - use of monitoring equipment for determining oxygen saturation, blood pressure, cardiac rate and rhythm, respiratory rate, and level of consciousness
    - interpretation of monitoring data
    - knowledge of pharmacology and action of IV conscious sedation agents
    - knowledge of desirable and undesirable effects of IV conscious sedation agents
    - recognition of complications related to IV conscious sedation
    - use of resuscitative equipment
207. Some institutions require advance life-support certification for nurses who monitor patients who receive IV conscious sedation.
208. Patients who are discharged to another unit should be monitored for several hours to ensure the maintenance of a satisfactory level of consciousness, patent airway, and stable vital signs.
209. Ambulatory surgery patients should not be discharged until the following criteria have been met:
    - vital signs are stable
    - airway is patent
    - alert level of consciousness is maintained
    - mobility and sensory functions are intact
    - protracted vomiting is absent
    - surgical site and dressing are satisfactory
210. Patients should be given written postoperative instructions because medications used in IV conscious sedation can diminish their abilities to recall information that has been given verbally.

REGIONAL ANESTHESIA

Overview

211. Regional anesthesia is preferable for patients who require emergency surgery and have a full stomach. It is

also used where general anesthetic agents are contraindicated in patients who have metabolic, renal, or hepatic disease. The respiratory and cardiac systems remain relatively stable with regional anesthesia.

212. Regional anesthesia techniques include spinal, epidural and caudal block, intravenous block, nerve block, local infiltration, and topical administration.

Spinal

213. Spinal anesthesia is obtained when the anesthetic agent is injected into the cerebrospinal fluid in the subarachnoid space. Injection is made through a lumbar interspace usually between L2 and L3, or below, so that the needle is not inserted into the spinal cord, which normally ends at L1–L2. As the anesthetic is absorbed by the nerve fibers, nerve transmission is blocked. Spread of the anesthetic agent and the subsequent level of anesthesia is determined by cerebrospinal pressure, injection site, amount, concentration, and specific gravity of the anesthetic solution, speed of injection, and the position of the patient during and immediately following the injection.
214. Spinal anesthetic solutions are generally a mixture of local anesthetic and dextrose. These solutions settle in accordance with gravity. The block can be directed up, down, or to one side of the spinal cord by adjusting the patient's position. After 10 or 15 minutes the block is set and does not extend further.
215. Agents frequently used for spinal anesthesia are lidocaine (Xylocaine), pontocaine (Tetracaine), and bupivacaine (Marcaine).
216. Spinal anesthesia is used for lower abdominal, pelvic, lower extremity, and urologic procedures, and for cesarean sections.
217. The administration of spinal anesthesia requires patient cooperation. Proper positioning is the key to successful placement of the anesthetic injection. Nursing intervention should be directed toward positioning the patient and providing support during administration of the spinal.
218. Injection of the anesthetic is accomplished with the patient in a sitting or lateral decubitus position. In the sitting position, the patient is assisted to sit on the operating table with the legs over the side and the feet on a stool. The stool should be high enough to cause the patient's knees to be raised above the level of the waist. The patient should be encouraged to arch the back outward and lower the chin to the chest (see Figure 11–3). In the lateral decubitus position the hips, back, and shoulders are aligned parallel with the edge of the table. The patient is instructed to bring the knees up toward the chest and to flex the head and neck. These maneuvers assist in spreading the vertebrae and exposing the desired interspaces to facilitate correct needle insertion.
219. During preparation for spinal anesthesia, the perioperative nurse should help to position the patient, assist the anesthesia care provider as needed, and provide assurance to the patient. The patient in the lateral decubitus position is very close to the edge of the table and safety measures to prevent falling are necessary. The perioperative nurse should remain with the patient, institute measures to prevent falling, and help the patient feel secure.
220. When administering spinal anesthesia, strict attention to asepsis is important in order to prevent entry of pathogens that can cause meningitis into the subarachnoid space.
221. Complications of spinal anesthesia include a rapid drop in blood pressure, nausea and vomiting, total spinal anesthesia, postdural headache, and neurological or integumentary positioning injury.

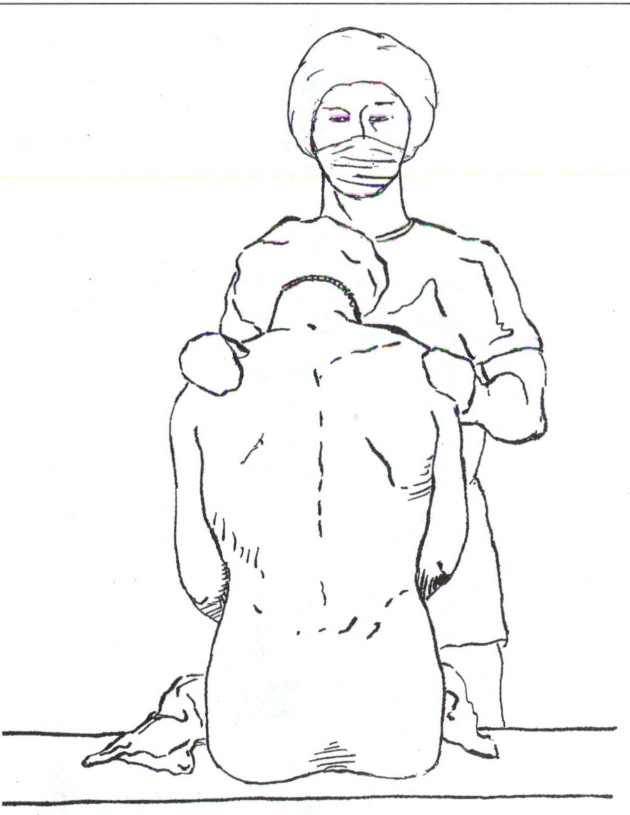

Figure 11–3 Position for Spinal Anesthesia. *Source:* Courtesy of Andrew Maillard.

222. Sudden hypotension is caused by vasodilation when sympathetic nerves that control vasomotor tone are blocked. Peripheral pooling, decreased venous return, and reduced cardiac output can also result. Ephedrine may be administered to restore normotension.
223. Nausea and vomiting can occur as a result of hypotension or as a reaction to sedation medication. Suction should be immediately available and an emesis basin and wet towel should be provided.
224. Total spinal anesthesia occurs when the level of anesthesia becomes so high that paralysis of respiratory muscles results and respiratory distress occurs. This is an emergency situation. Ventilation must be supported and intubation may be required.
225. Patients may experience headache 24 to 48 hours following spinal anesthesia if the dura at the site of injection does not seal itself off and cerebrospinal fluid leaks into the epidural space. The loss of cerebrospinal fluid decreases cerebrospinal pressure, leaves less fluid to cushion the brain, and can cause headache.
226. In most cases, treatment consists of hydration, intravenous or oral caffeine, sedation, and bed rest. If symptoms persist longer than 24 hours a blood patch of the patient's blood may be administered at the puncture site to seal the epidural leak.
227. Neurological or integumentary injuries can occur because the patient's sensory pathways are blocked and improper positioning or pressure cannot be felt.

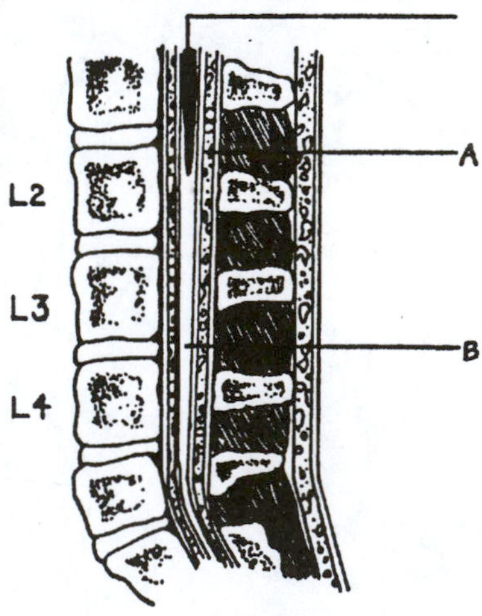

Figure 11–4 Regional Anesthesia Sites. **A.** Epidural anesthesia is achieved by injection of the anesthetic into the epidural space. **B.** Spinal anesthesia is achieved when the anesthetic agent is injected into the cerebrospinal fluid in the subarachnoid space. Injection is made between L2 and L3 or below. *Source:* Courtesy of Jeanne Spry.

Epidural and Caudal

228. Epidural anesthesia is achieved by injection of the anesthetic agent into the epidural space (see Figure 11–4). The agent may be injected through the interspaces of the thoracic or cervical vertebrae; however, the lumbar region is the usual site of injection.
229. Epidural anesthesia is useful in anorectal, vaginal, and perineal procedures and is often used in obstetric surgery.
230. For caudal anesthesia the anesthetic is injected into the epidural space through the caudal canal in the sacrum.
231. Commonly used epidural and caudal anesthetic agents are lidocaine hydrochloride (Xylocaine), bupivacaine (Marcaine), and chloroprocaine (Nesacaine).
232. Epidural anesthesia can be delivered as a single dose, or a small catheter can be left in place for continuous infusion. Continuous infusion is useful for pain management.
233. Anesthetic agents that are injected into the epidural space are not as affected by positioning as in spinal anesthesia.
234. Complications of epidural anesthesia are
    - dural puncture—postdural headache
    - inadvertent subarachnoid injection—total spinal anesthesia
    - inadvertent intravascular injection—extreme hypotension and cardiac arrest

Intravenous Block (Bier Block)

235. Intravenous block involves intravenous injection of a local anesthetic agent into the vein of a tourniquet-occluded extremity. In this procedure an intravenous catheter is inserted into the operative extremity. Two side-by-side tourniquets, or one double-cuffed tourniquet, are applied but not inflated on the extremity. The extremity is elevated and drained of blood with an Esmarch or elastic bandage. The proximal tourniquet or cuff is then inflated and a fixed amount of anesthetic agent is injected. The anesthetic agent infiltrates and is confined to the tissues that are distal to the tourniquet. To alleviate tourniquet pain, the second distal cuff is inflated after the anesthetic agent has taken effect. The proximal cuff is then deflated.
236. After the procedure, the tourniquet is released and the remaining anesthetic is absorbed into the general circulation. If absorption is too rapid, cardiovascular collapse or central nervous system toxicity can occur.
237. This technique is used most often for surgeries of the upper extremity that last an hour or less.
238. Lidocaine (Xylocaine) is used for intravenous block.

Nerve Block

239. In nerve block, the anesthetic agent, usually lidocaine (Xylocaine), is injected into and around a nerve or nerve group that supplies sensation to a small area of the body.
240. Nerve blocks can be used for purposes of surgical intervention but are more commonly used for sustained relief in patients with chronic pain and to increase circulation in some vascular diseases.
241. Nerve blocks can be minor or major. Major blocks involve multiple nerves or a plexus. Minor blocks block a single nerve.
242. Major nerve blocks used in operative procedures are brachial-plexus block for procedures of the arm, orbital block for eye procedures, and cervical block for procedures involving the neck.
243. Common minor blocks are radial and ulnar nerve blocks for procedures of the elbow, wrist, or digits.
244. The perioperative nurse may assist during nerve block by aspirating the needle during placement to check for inadvertent vascular injection. The nurse may also be asked to inject the local anesthetic while the anesthesia care provider secures the placement of the needle.

Local Infiltration

245. Local infiltration involves the injection of the anesthetic agent into subcutaneous tissue at, or close to, the anticipated incision site.
246. Local infiltration is useful for minor, superficial procedures.
247. The most frequently used local anesthetic is lidocaine (Xylocaine). Epinephrine may be added to the lidocaine to cause vasoconstriction, reduce bleeding, and slow absorption of the drug.
248. Toxic reactions from local anesthetics can occur if too rapid an absorption from a vascular site occurs or if there is an inadvertent intravascular injection. Toxic reactions include central nervous system and cardiovascular depression. The nurse needs to be alert to the possibility of a toxic reaction. Initial signs of central nervous system toxicity are restlessness, lightheadedness, visual and auditory disturbances, dizziness, tremors, and convulsions. This may be followed by unconsciousness, apnea, and cardiac arrest. Patients who say that they hear unusual sounds or express a feeling of uneasiness may be experiencing a toxic reaction. Initial treatment consists of establishing and maintaining an airway, assisting or controlling ventilation with oxygen, and administering sedation.
249. It is the responsibility of the perioperative nurse to ensure that resuscitation equipment is available when local anesthetics are administered.
250. During local anesthesia the perioperative nurse should monitor the patient's blood pressure, cardiac rate and rhythm, respiratory rate, oxygen saturation, skin condition, and mental status (AORN, 1995, p. 217).

Topical

251. In topical anesthesia, the anesthetic is applied directly to a mucous membrane or an open wound. Topical anesthesia is often used for nasal surgery, cystoscopy, and procedures of the respiratory tract in which it is advantageous to eliminate cough and laryngeal reflex.
252. Commonly used topical anesthetics are pontocaine (Tetracaine), cocaine, and lidocaine (Xylocaine).
253. Cocaine is used in nasal passages; pontocaine in the eye; and lidocaine in the throat, nose, esophagus, and genitourinary tract.
254. Lidocaine may be supplied as a liquid, liquid spray, or jelly.
255. Topical anesthetics are readily absorbed by mucous membranes and therefore act rapidly. Sudden cardiovascular collapse is possible following the application of topical anesthetic in the respiratory tract. Resuscitation equipment should be immediately available.

Regional Anesthesia—Nursing Responsibilities

256. Responsibilities of the perioperative nurse will vary according to the type of regional anesthesia being administered.
257. Patients who are scheduled to receive regional anesthesia may be apprehensive about being awake during surgery. They may mistakenly believe that their being awake will result in inevitable pain or that they will be unable to avoid observing the surgery. Providing assurance, answering questions, and remaining close to the patient will, in most instances, significantly reduce anxiety. Although usually sedated, the patient should be aware that the nurse is close by and is available to provide support.
258. For some surgeries it is important that the patient be alert and cooperate with the surgeon to facilitate the procedure. The perioperative nurse can provide encouragement, support, and information that the patient needs during these times.
259. Patients who receive regional anesthesia are awake, and conversation in the operating suite should reflect this consideration. Regional anesthesia patients are usually given supplemental tranquilizers and may sleep. However, they are arousable and may be startled by noise or made anxious by inappropriate conversation. It is appropriate to place a sign on the door of the operating suite, stating that the patient is awake. This will serve as a reminder to persons who enter.

260. During placement of the needle for spinal, epidural, caudal, and nerve block, the patient should be protected from unnecessary exposure to prevent embarrassment and cooling. Pillows and blankets should be provided to increase patient comfort.
261. Preparation of the incision site with an antiseptic scrub may necessitate exposing the patient and may cause the awake patient to become embarrassed or anxious. It is important to maintain the patient's dignity and minimize exposure.
262. Every patient receiving some type of regional anesthesia should be monitored. The extent of monitoring and the person responsible for monitoring is determined by the anesthesia technique, the results of preoperative assessment, the surgical procedure, the recognized anesthesia standards and practices, and the institution's policy. Administration of topical and local infiltration anesthetics is the surgeon's responsibility. During spinal, epidural, caudal, intravenous block, and nerve block an anesthesia care provider is present. However, during local anesthesia it is unusual for an anesthesia care provider to be present, and monitoring is the responsibility of the perioperative nurse. The AORN recommended practice for the patient receiving local anesthesia states, "All patients receiving local anesthesia should be monitored by a perioperative nurse for reaction to drugs and for physiological and behavioral changes. . . . The perioperative nurse should have the knowledge, skill, and ability to use and interpret the data from monitoring equipment" (AORN, 1995, pp. 217–218).
263. The nurse who monitors the patient who is receiving local anesthesia must be able to recognize a normal baseline and any changes that occur. Baseline data must include blood pressure, cardiac rate and rhythm, respirations, oxygen saturation, skin condition, and mental status. In addition, a knowledge of the drugs used as well as possible reactions to them is necessary in order for the perioperative nurse to be able to provide appropriate nursing interventions.
264. During local anesthesia the perioperative nurse should track and monitor the amount of anesthetic agent given. The maximum recommended dose of 1% lidocaine without epinephrine for adults is 300 mg (4.5 mg/kg). The maximum recommended dose of lidocaine with epinephrine is 500 mg (7 mg/kg). The amount that is administered should be reported to the surgeon.
265. Nursing intervention for all patients who receive regional anesthesia should include preparation for toxic systemic reactions of the central nervous system and cardiovascular collapse. In addition to having resuscitation equipment immediately available, current cardiopulmonary resuscitation (CPR) certification is an essential requirement for the perioperative nurse.

Section Questions

Q52. During IV conscious sedation the patient should be sedated enough not to respond to verbal stimuli. (Ref. 195)

True False

Q53. Morphine is the most common drug used in IV conscious sedation. (Ref. 199)

True False

Q54. List four undesirable effects of IV conscious sedation. (Ref. 202)

____

____

____

____

Q55. Patients who have had IV conscious sedation should be given written postoperative instructions because the medications they received may diminish their recall ability. (Ref. 210)

True False

Q56. Respiratory and cardiac systems remain relatively stable under regional anesthesia. (Ref. 212)

True False

Q57. Regarding spinal anesthesia (Ref.213, 217, 218, 219, 222):

a. the level of anesthesia is influenced by the patient's position immediately following administration
b. injection is at or above L2–L3
c. the primary nursing responsibility is assistance in positioning and support
d. is always administered with the patient in a sitting position
e. a sudden rise in blood pressure is a complication of spinal anesthesia

Q58. Total spinal anesthesia is an emergency. Explain why. (Ref. 224)

____

____

Q59. A headache 24 to 48 hours after spinal anesthesia is usually the result of an increase in cerebrospinal pressure. (Ref. 225)

True False

Q60. Epidural anesthesia is useful for labor and delivery. (Ref. 229)

True False

Q61. Intravenous block (Ref. 235, 237, 238):

a. is useful for procedures on the shoulder
b. includes the injection of lidocaine into a vein

c. includes the application of a tourniquet to an extremity
d. is useful for procedures of the hand

Q62. Nerve blocks (Ref. 239, 240):
a. are useful in patients with chronic pain
b. are useful for abdominal procedures
c. involve application of a tourniquet

Q63. The perioperative nurse who assists the anesthesia care provider during a nerve block may be asked to inject the local anesthetic. This is an appropriate responsibility. (Ref. 244)

True False

Q64. When lidocaine with epinephrine is administered as a local anesthetic, absorption of the drug is _____ and as a result, a _____ dose may be given than can be given when lidocaine without epinephrine is used. (Ref. 247, 266)
a. accelerated/lower
b. slowed/higher

Q65. During a procedure under local anesthetic the perioperative nurse should monitor the patient's cardiac rate and rhythm and mental status. (Ref. 250)

True False

Q66. Topical anesthetics are absorbed slowly by mucous membranes and are therefore safe. (Ref. 255)

True False

NOTES

Association of Operating Room Nurses (AORN). (1995). *Standards and recommended practices*. Denver: AORN.

Atkinson, L.J., & Kohn, L. (Eds.). (1986). *Berry and Kohn's introduction to operating room technique* (6th ed.). New York: McGraw-Hill.

Beck, C. (1994). Malignant hyperthermia: Are you prepared? *AORN Journal*, *59*(2), 367–390.

Bennett, S.N., et al. (1995, July). *New England Journal of Medicine*, 333, 147–154.

Brooks-Braun, J.A. (1995, Sept.). Postoperative atelectasis and pneumonia. *American Journal of Critical Care*, *4*(5), 340–347.

Donnelly, A. (1994). Malignant hyperthermia: Epidemiology, pathophysiology, treatment. *AORN Journal*, *59*(2), 393–405.

Gruendemann, B., & Fernsebner, B. (Eds.). (1995). *Comprehensive perioperative nursing*. Boston: Jones and Bartlett.

Litwack, K. (1995). *Post anesthesia nursing care*. St. Louis: Mosby Year Book.

Mathias, J. (1995, Oct.). FDA clears sevoflurane for use. *OR Manager*, *11*(10), 36.

McCormack, J. (1995, Sept.). Warming devices pay off for surgical patients—and the budget. *Materials Management*, *4*(9), 44–46.

McKinney, M. (1993). Anesthetized patients may hear, understand conversations. *AORN Journal*, *57*(6), 1467–1470.

Meeker, M., & Rothrock, J. (Eds.). (1995). *Alexander's care of the patient in surgery*. St. Louis: Mosby Year Book.

Messina, B.A. (1994). Pulse oximetry: Assuring accuracy. *Journal of Post Anesthesia Nursing*, *9*(4), 228–231.

Roth, R.A. (Ed.). (1995). *Perioperative nursing care curriculum*. Philadelphia: W.B. Saunders.

Somerson, S., et al. (1995, June). Insights into conscious sedation. *American Journal of Nursing*, 22–26.

Stein, R. (1995). The perioperative nurse's role in anesthesia management. *Journal of the Association of Operating Room Nurses*, *62*(5), 794–804.

Appendix 11-A

Chapter 11 Post Test

1. Possible patient injury related to anesthesia includes a compromised airway, an untoward drug reaction, an alteration in cardiac output, and an ineffective breathing pattern. List two additional possible injuries related to anesthesia. (Ref. 3)

   ____

   ____

2. An anesthesiologist, a certified nurse anesthetist, or an perioperative nurse may be responsible for monitoring the patient who is receiving IV conscious sedation. (Ref. 11)

   True False

3. Because patient assessment in preparation for anesthesia is performed by an anesthesiologist or a CRNA, it is not necessary for the perioperative nurse to also perform an assessment. (Ref. 12)

   True False

4. During the assessment it is important that the patient be asked about family history with anesthetics. Explain why this information is important. (Ref. 20)

   ____

   ____

5. Preoperative teaching should include encouraging a patient who smokes to refrain from smoking prior to surgery because to do so may reduce the risk of postoperative pulmonary complications. (Ref. 24)

   True False

6. List six factors that influence selection of anesthesia agents and technique. (Ref. 30)

   ____

   ____

   ____

   ____

   ____

   ____

7. The primary goal of preoperative medication is to put the patient to sleep. (Ref. 40, 51)

   True False

8. Agents that promote gastric emptying and lower stomach pH, such as sodium citrate (Bicitra) and metoclopramide (Reglan) should be given 90 minutes or more before surgery. (Ref. 41)

   True False

9. Match the items. (Ref. 43, 45, 48, 49, 50)

a. midazolam (Versed)	___ raises gastric pH
b. ranitidine (Zantac)	___ reduces anxiety, provides some amnesia
c. glycopyrrolate (Robinul)	___ decreases oral secretions
d. droperidol (Inapsine)	___ relief from pain
e. fentanyl (Sublimaze)	___ antiemetic

10. Monitoring for all patients who receive anesthesia should include (Ref. 54, 55):
    a. ECG
    b. blood pressure
    c. heart rate
    d. oxygen saturation

11. Some anesthetic agents, such as isoflurane and halothane, dilate blood vessels or interfere with the temperature-regulating mechanism in the hypothalamus and can cause the patient's temperature to drop. (Ref. 88, 89, 96)

    True False

12. An internal esophageal probe may be used to monitor patient temperature. (Ref. 75)

    True False

13. Nitrous oxide (Ref. 82, 83, 84, 107):
    a. is sufficient for most surgeries
    b. is a potential hazard to operating room staff
    c. is used in combination with other inhalation agents
    d. is a neuromuscular blocker

14. Match the items. (Ref. 114, 118, 119)

a. thiopental sodium (Sodium Pentothal)	___ nonbarbiturate induction agent
b. propofol (Diprivan)	___ barbiturate
	___ minimal aftereffects such as vomiting
	___ medium supports bacterial growth
	___ short-acting induction agent
	___ rapid loss of consciousness

15. Fentanyl is a powerful narcotic that provides relief from pain and is given during surgery as an adjunct to other drugs and to relieve pain in the postoperative period. (Ref. 125, 126)

    True False

16. Succinylcholine (Anectine and Quelicin), atracurium besylate (Tracrium), tubocurarine chloride (curare), mivacurium (Mivacron), pancuronium bromide (Pavulon), and vecuronium bromide (Norcuron) are neuromuscular blockers. Name the one that is a depolarizing agent and causes fasciculation. (Ref. 137)

    ____

17. Neuromuscular blockers (Ref. 111, 134, 135, 136, 138, 140):
    a. are useful to relax the jaw and larynx at intubation
    b. are delivered from the anesthesia machine
    c. cause paralysis
    d. are all short acting
    e. are given to facilitate tissue manipulation intraoperatively

18. The aspiration of stomach contents can be fatal. List three immediate interventions that the perioperative nurse should be prepared to take in the event of regurgitation. (Ref. 158, 159)

____

____

____

19. The Sellick maneuver is an appropriate intervention for the patient with a hiatal hernia. (Ref. 159, 160)

True False

20. It is a nursing responsibility to ensure that the anesthetized patient is properly positioned. (Ref. 163, 164, 165, 166)

True False

21. List four symptoms other than muscle rigidity that may be seen in malignant hyperthermia. (Ref. 174, 175)

____

____

____

____

22. _____ is usually one of the first signs of malignant hyperthermia crisis. (Ref. 175)
   a. rapid rise in temperature
   b. increased end tidal CO_2 volume
   c. profuse sweating

23. The treatment drug for malignant hyperthermia is ____________ and it is administered at ____________ mg/kg until the patient responds or a maximum of 20 doses is given. (Ref. 182, 186, 188)

24. Goals of IV conscious sedation are to allay patient fear and anxiety, to maintain consciousness, to elevate the pain threshold, and to maintain vital signs. (Ref. 197)

True False

25. Naloxone hydrochloride (Narcan) enhances the effect of narcotics. (Ref. 200)

True False

26. It is appropriate to have resuscitative equipment available when local infiltration, nerve block, and intravenous block are being administered because cardiovascular collapse is a possible adverse reaction to these forms of anesthesia. (Ref. 236, 248, 249, 250)

True False

27. List three reason why regional anesthesia might be more appropriate for a patient than general anesthesia. (Ref. 211)

____

____

____

28. Describe the benefit derived by encouraging the patient to arch the back and lower the chin in preparation for spinal anesthesia. (Ref. 218)

____

____

29. The perioperative nurse should remain in contact with the patient during spinal anesthesia administration in the lateral position because the patient may feel in danger of falling from the table. (Ref. 219)

    True False

30. Explain why patients under spinal anesthesia are at risk for neurologic or integumentary injury. (Ref. 227)

____

____

31. Epidural anesthesia can be delivered as a single dose, or a small catheter may be left in place for continuous infusion and pain management. (Ref. 232)

    True False

32. Appropriate anesthesia technique for a cataract surgery is (Ref. 242):
    a. nerve block
    b. intravenous block (Bier)

33. What reaction should the perioperative nurse suspect if a patient receiving local anesthesia states he or she feels lightheaded, hears voices, or is restless, and what interventions should the nurse be prepared to take? (Ref. 248)

    Reaction:

____

    Intervention:

____

____

34. The nurse who is monitoring the patient who is receiving local anesthesia must be able to recognize and interpret normal baseline data and changes that occur. These data include blood pressure. List five additional data. (Ref. 263)

____

____

____

____

____

Appendix 11–B

Competency Checklist: Anesthesia

Under observer's initials enter initials upon successful achievement of competency. Enter N/A if competency is not appropriate for institution.

NAME ____________________________________

	OBSERVER'S INITIALS	DATE
Preoperative assessment		
1. Assesses patient/chart for anesthetic considerations (as applicable):		
a. coexisting disease	________	________
b. NPO status	________	________
c. allergies to medications, contrast dyes, tape, latex	________	________
d. current medications	________	________
e. previous surgeries	________	________
f. patient/family history of anesthesia complications	________	________
g. current medications	________	________
h. substance abuse	________	________
i. pregnancy	________	________
j. diagnostic testing	________	________
k. response to preoperative medications	________	________
l. anxiety level	________	________
m. knowledge level	________	________
2. Verifies that patient is in compliance with preoperative instructions.	________	________
3. Communicates assessment data to surgical team as appropriate.	________	________
4. Provides emotional support (answers patient concerns, provides reassuring touch, etc.) to patient/family.	________	________
5. Provides information as needed to patient/family.	________	________
6. Reinforces preoperative teaching with patient/family.	________	________
General Anesthesia		
7. In preparation for induction:		
a. checks suction and places for easy access to patient's mouth	________	________
b. applies monitoring equipment (ECG leads, blood pressure cuff)	________	________
c. places IV line	________	________

NAME ________________________________

	OBSERVER'S INITIALS	DATE
d. applies safety strap	________	________
e. limits patient exposure	________	________
f. maintains quiet atmosphere	________	________
g. remains at patient side at head of table, provides reassurance	________	________
8. At induction assists in intubation as needed (provides endotracheal tube, applies cricoid pressure, suctions, inflates cuff, etc.)	________	________
9. Following induction:		
a. checks position and pressure points and provides protective devices as needed	________	________
b. applies warming devices as appropriate (lengthy procedure, large/deep incision, etc.)	________	________
10. Monitors fluid output and replacement and irrigating fluid.	________	________
11. During emergence and extubation:		
a. checks suction and places for easy access to patient's mouth	________	________
b. remains at head of OR table by patient	________	________
c. assists anesthesia care provider as needed (suction, ambu, O_2, etc.)	________	________
12. Provides report to postanesthesia care unit (e.g., patient name and age, surgical procedure, surgeon and anesthesiologist, anesthesia technique, estimated blood loss, fluid and blood administration, urine output, response to surgery/anesthesia, lab results, chronic and acute health history, drug allergies, expected problems/ suggested interventions, discharge plan).	________	________
Regional Anesthesia		
13. Implements procedures to alert others that patient is awake.	________	________
14. Assists in positioning patient for administration of regional anesthetic (e.g., provides stool for feet, instructs patient).	________	________
15. Provides safe environment for patient during positioning for administration of regional anesthetic (e.g., remains with patient).	________	________
16. Patient exposure limited during prep.	________	________
17. Monitors and reports amount of local anesthetic agent administered.	________	________
Monitoring		
18. Demonstrates ability to apply and use monitoring device and interpret data for:		
a. blood pressure	________	________
b. cardiac rate and rhythm	________	________

NAME ____

	OBSERVER'S INITIALS	DATE
c. respiratory rate	________	________
d. oxygen saturation	________	________
e. mental status/level of consciousness	________	________
19. Demonstrates airway management, including use of oxygen delivery devices and equipment.	________	________
20. Demonstrates ability to use resuscitative equipment.	________	________
Emergency Preparations		
21. Retrieves malignant hyperthermia supplies without hesitation.	________	________
22. Explains protocol for malignant hyperthermia crisis.	________	________
23. Ensures immediate availability of resuscitative equipment (IV conscious sedation and local procedures).	________	________
24. Reports changes in patient condition and implements appropriate interventions.	________	________
Documentation		
25. Documents data as required by institutional policy.	________	________

OBSERVER'S SIGNATURE INITIALS

____ ____________

ORIENTEE'S SIGNATURE

____

Appendix A

Glossary

Active electrode: An accessory used in electrosurgery to deliver current from an electrosurgical generator to a patient for the purpose of hemostasis and/or cutting during surgery.

Aeration: A process utilizing warm air circulating in an enclosed cabinet to remove residual ethylene oxide from sterilized items. The length of the process is determined by the composition of the sterilized items and the amount of residual ethylene oxide. The process generally takes from 8 to 12 hours.

Aldrete postanesthesia scoring system: A scoring system used to evaluate the recovery of patients who have received general anesthesia. It evaluates patient activity, respiration, circulation, and oxygen saturation.

Antiseptic: A germicidal agent used on skin and tissue to destroy and prevent growth of microorganisms.

Asepsis: Absence of pathogenic microorganisms.

Aseptic technique: The practices by which contamination from microorganisms is prevented.

Atraumatic suture: Suture that is attached to the needle during manufacture. The needle and suture are a continuous unit in which needle diameter and suture diameter are matched as closely as possible, thereby creating minimal trauma as the needle and strand are pulled through tissue.

Autoclave: A steam sterilizer.

Back table: Also referred to as an instrument table. A stainless-steel table covered with a sterile drape on which sterile surgical instruments are arranged for use during surgery.

Barrier (sterile): Material, such as a sterile drape or wrapper, that is used to protect sterility of items by preventing the entry or migration of microorganisms from an unsterile surface or area. Sterile barriers are gowns, drapes, and package wrappers.

Biological monitor: A sterilization monitor consisting of a known population of resistant spores that is used to test the sterilizer's ability to kill microorganisms.

Bonewax: Bonewax is made from beeswax and is used to stop bleeding from bone. It is used most often in neurosurgery and orthopedic surgery.

Bovie: Dr. Bovie was instrumental in developing the first spark-gap vacuum tube generator that produced cutting with hemostasis. Modern electrosurgical units are still often referred to as "Bovies." The more accurate term is *electrosurgical unit.*

Bowie-Dick Test: A test designed to test the steam sterilizer's ability to remove air from the chamber.

Capacitive coupling: The transfer of electrical current from the active electrode through the coupling of stray current into other conductive surgical equipment. Capacitive coupling can cause a burn injury, such as bowel perforation, during laparoscopic surgery that may go unnoticed and lead to peritonitis.

Capnography: The measurement of the percentage of carbon dioxide exhaled during mechanical ventilation.

Chemical (process) indicator: A device used to monitor one or more process parameters in the sterilization cycle. The device responds with a chemical or physical change (usually a color change) to conditions within the sterilization chamber. It is usually supplied as a paper strip, tape, or label that changes color or as a pellet that melts when the parameter has been met.

Circulating nurse: A perioperative nurse who is present during a surgical procedure, is not scrubbed, and is responsible for managing the nursing care of the patient and for coordinating and monitoring other activities during the procedure.

Clean wound: A wound in which the gastrointestinal (GI), genitourinary, or respiratory tract is not entered. No inflammation is encountered and there is no break in aseptic technique. Examples of clean surgical procedures include hernia repair, carpal tunnel repair, and total joint replacement.

Clean contaminated wound: A wound in which the GI, genitourinary, or respiratory tract is entered under planned, controlled means. No spillage occurs and no infection is present. Examples of clean contaminated procedures include cholecystectomy, cystoscopy, and colon resection.

Closed gloving: A method of donning sterile gloves in which the arms are inserted into the gown only until the hands reach the proximal edge of the gown cuff. Gloving is accomplished without the fingers or hands extending beyond the proximal edge of the gown. Only after the glove is donned are the fingers extended beyond the gown edge and inserted into the finger slots.

Contaminated: Soiled or potentially soiled with microorganisms. All items opened for surgery, whether or not they were used, are considered to be contaminated.

Contaminated wound: A wound in which nonpurulent inflammation, gross spillage from the GI tract, a traumatic wound, or a major break in aseptic technique is encountered. Examples of contaminated procedures include gunshot wound, rectal procedures, and colon resection with GI spillage, and inflamed but not ruptured appendix.

Cottonoid pattie: A small sponge made of compressed cotton. Often used in neurosurgery. There are a variety of sizes ranging from ¼ × ¼ inch to 1 × 6 inch.

Critical item: An item that is introduced beneath a mucous membrane or into a vascular space. Critical items *must* be sterile.

Decontamination: A process of cleaning, disinfecting, or sterilizing that renders items safe for handling where they are no longer capable of transmitting infectious particles. Decontaminated items are NOT considered sterile.

Desiccation: An electrosurgical method of coagulation whereby an active electrode is in direct contact with tissue.

Dirty wound: A wound in which an old traumatic wound with dead tissue exists or an infectious process is present. Examples of dirty or infected procedures include colon resection for ruptured diverticulitis and amputation of a gangrenous appendage.

Disinfectant: An antimicrobial agent used on inanimate surfaces to destroy microorganisms.

Disinfection: Process that kills many or all living microorganisms with the exception of spores. High-level disinfection kills all bacteria, viruses, and fungi. Intermediate-level disinfection kills most bacteria, viruses, and fungi. Certain bacteria and viruses, such as tubercle bacilli and HBV, are resistant. Low-level disinfectant kills vegetative bacteria and the least resistant viruses and fungi.

Dispersive electrode: An accessory used in electrosurgery, that is in contact with the patient, and returns electrosurgical current from the patient to the generator.

Electrosurgery: A method of hemostasis that is provided when radio frequency electrical current is passed through the patient's body. The energy is supplied from an electrosurgical generator. It is delivered to the patient from an active electrode and returned to the generator via a dispersive electrode. Electrosurgery is used for purposes of cutting tissue or coagulating bleeding points.

Endogenous source of infection: A source of infection that arises from within the body.

Ethylene oxide sterilization: A method of sterilization that utilizes ethylene oxide gas as the sterilant. It is used primarily for items that cannot tolerate the heat and moisture of steam sterilization.

Exogenous source of infection: A source of infection from outside the body.

Fasciculation: Skeletal muscle contractions that occur when groups of muscles that are innervated by the same neuron contract simultaneously. The contractions appear as twitching. Fasciculation following administration of depolarizing muscle relaxants progresses in a cephalocaudal sequence.

Flash sterilization: A steam sterilization process for sterilizing items that are needed immediately. Flash sterilization is utilized when there is insufficient time to process an item in the prepackaged method. Items that are flash sterilized are unwrapped.

Fluid proof: Prevents the penetration of fluids through an intact barrier.

Fluid resistant: Resistant to the penetration of fluids. Over time, fluids will penetrate.

Fulguration: An electrosurgical method of coagulation whereby sparking is used to coagulate large bleeders. The active electrode does not contact tissue. Sparks contact the tissue, causing superficial coagulation followed by deep necrosis. The purpose is to destroy tissue.

Gelatin sponge (Gelfoam): A sponge, resembling Styrofoam, made from purified gelatin solution and used for hemostasis.

Hemoclip: *See* ligating clip.

Indicator: *See* chemical (process) indicator.

Induction: The period from the beginning of anesthesia through loss of consciousness.

Integrator: A device used to monitor more than one process parameter of the sterilization process. Usually supplied as a wicking paper that melts and progresses along the paper over time when the desired parameters have been achieved. The results are displayed in a window along the strip that indicates that the process is acceptable if the wicking reaches the target area on the strip.

Intraoperative: The period begins when the patient is transferred to the operating room bed and ends with transfer to the recovery area.

Iodophor: A complex of free iodine combined with detergent that is used to kill microorganisms.

IV conscious sedation: *See* monitored anesthesia care.

Kitner: A small roll of heavy cotton tape that is usually clamped to a forcep and used for dissection or absorption.

Laminar air flow: A high-powered unidirectional air flow. The intended purpose is to reduce airborne contamination.

Lap pad (tape): A square or rectangular gauze pad used for absorption where moderate or large amounts of blood or fluid are encountered.

Ligating clip: A stainless steel, titanium, or tantalum clip used to permanently clamp a vessel.

Local standby: *See* monitored anesthesia care.

Malignant hyperthermia: An emergency complication of general anesthesia that is characterized by a rapid rise in temperature (temperatures as high as 109.4°F [43°C] have been reported), extraordinary oxygen consumption, rapid uncontrolled muscle metabolism, and production of heat and carbon dioxide. Malignant hyperthermia is a crisis and the patient will most likely die if not treated.

Mayo stand: A stand on top of which fits a removable stainless-steel tray. The legs of the stand slide under the operating room table and the tray extends over the patient. Instruments that are frequently used are placed on the Mayo stand. The scrub person hands instruments from the Mayo stand to the surgeon during the procedure.

Memory: A characteristic that causes a material to return to the state in which it was originally folded or placed.

Microfibrillar collagen (Avitene): A fluffy, white, absorbable material made from purified bovine dermis used to provide hemostasis. Its application is topical. It is used for oozing or friable tissue.

Monitored anesthesia care: Medications are administered intravenously to provide sedation, systemic analgesia, and depression of the autonomic nervous system. This anesthesia technique may not require the presence of an anesthesia care provider. In the absence of an anesthesia care provider the patient is monitored by the perioperative nurse.

Open gloving: Technique for donning sterile gloves. In this procedure, the fingers of the scrubbed person extend beyond the cuff on the gown sleeve. Scrubbed hands touch only the inside of the gloves.

Oxidized cellulose: Oxidized cellulose (Oxycel, Surgicel, and Surgicel Nu-Knit) is a specially treated gauze or cotton that is applied directly to an oozing surface to control bleeding.

Passivation: A process used in making surgical instruments. In passivation the instrument is immersed in a nitric-acid bath solution that removes carbon steel particles and promotes the formation of a chromium oxide coating on the surface.

Peanut: A very small sponge approximately the size of a peanut that is commonly used for blotting blood. It is also used for dissection.

Peel pack: A see-through pouch made of plastic and paper or plastic and Tyvek that is used to contain items during sterilization and to maintain them in a sterile state during storage.

Perfusionist: A member of the surgical team who is a highly skilled technician and who is responsible for operating the cardiac bypass equipment during open heart-surgery.

Perioperative: Encompasses the three phases of the surgical experience: preoperative, intraoperative, and postoperative. Perioperative nursing activities are activities that occur in any or all of the three phases.

Plasma (sterilization): Plasma is a fourth state of matter that is a cloudlike mixture of charged ions and molecular species and is capable of killing microorganisms. Plasma, created by the application of radio frequency energy upon a hydrogen peroxide gas within a vacuum, is used for sterilization purposes.

Pledget: Small piece of felt used as a support under friable tissues.

Postoperative: The period begins when the patient is transferred to the recovery room until resolution of surgical sequelae.

Preoperative: The period begins when the decision to have surgery is made until the patient is transferred to the operating room bed.

Prep: *See* surgical prep.

Raytex: Gauze sponge of which common sizes are 4 × 4 or 4 × 8. It is used where a small amount of blood or fluid is encountered.

Restricted area: An area within the operating room department where surgical procedures are performed and where sterile supplies are unwrapped. Surgical attire and hats are required in this area. The Association of Operating Room Nurses (AORN) also recommends masks in this area.

Scrub: *See* surgical scrub.

Scrub person: A person who performs a surgical scrub on arms and hands, dons sterile attire, stands within the sterile field, and provides sterile instruments and other items to the surgical team during surgery. The scrub person is a member of the sterile team and is either a nurse or surgical technician/technologist.

Sellick maneuver: Manual compression of the esophagus between the cricoid cartilage and the vertebral column for the purpose of visualization of the tracheal lumen and the prevention of regurgitation and aspiration during intubation.

Semicritical item: An item that makes contact with an intact mucous membrane but is not introduced below the membrane. Semicritical items may be sterilized but *must* be disinfected when used on patients.

Semirestricted area: An area within the operating room department where surgical attire and hats are required. It includes peripheral support areas where clean and sterile supplies are stored. Traffic is limited to authorized personnel in surgical attire and to patients.

Shelf life: The amount of time an item may be assumed to be sterile. Shelf life is related to events and not to actual time. The longer an item remains on a shelf the greater will be the possibility that an event will occur that will cause contamination.

Skin prep: *See* surgical prep.

Spore: An inactive or dormant, but viable, state of a microorganism that is difficult to kill. Sterilization methods are monitored by their ability to kill known populations of highly resistant spores.

Steam sterilization: Process of sterilization that uses steam to kill all forms of microbial life.

Sterile field: The area immediately surrounding the patient into which only sterile items may be entered. A sterile field is created by placing sterile barriers over nonsterile items. The sterile field includes the area around the site of the incision and may include furniture covered with sterile drapes and personnel attired in sterile gowns and gloves.

Sterilization: A process that kills all living microorganisms including spores.

Sterilizer (steam):
Gravity displacement: A type of steam sterilizer in which steam displaces air through an outlet port by means of gravity.
Prevacuum: A type of steam sterilizer in which a vacuum is created to remove air at the beginning of the cycle.
Pulse pressure: A type of steam sterilizer in which a series of steam flushes and pressure pulses at above-atmospheric pressure removes air from the chamber.

Strike-through: An event that occurs when liquids soak through a barrier from a sterile to an unsterile area or from an unsterile area to a sterile area. Strike-through renders items contained within the barrier unsterile.

Styptic: An agent used to cause blood vessel constriction. An example is epinephrine.

Superheating: Occurs when fabrics that are dehydrated are subject to steam sterilization. The temperature of the fabric exceeds the temperature of the steam. Superheating destroys cloth fibers.

Surgical conscience: An inner commitment to strictly adhere to aseptic practice, to report any break in aseptic technique, and to correct any violation whether or not anyone else is present or observes the violation. A surgical conscience mandates a commitment to aseptic practice *at all times*.

Surgical counts: The counting of sponges, sharps such as blades and needles, and instruments that are opened and delivered to the field for use during surgery. Counting is a safety mechanism to decrease the risk of items that are used during the surgery from being retained in the patient.

Surgical prep: Preparation of the patient's skin at the incision site. The patient's skin is cleansed with an antimicrobial agent to reduce the number of microorganisms at the incision site to as low a level as possible and to prevent rebound growth for as long as possible. The prep may or may not include hair removal at the incision site.

Surgical scrub: A process of cleansing the hands and arms for the purpose of removing as many microorganisms as possible from the hands and arms prior to donning a sterile gown and gloves.

Suture ligature: A tie with an attached needle that is used to anchor the tie through the vessel for purposes of hemostasis.

Tape: *See* lap pad (tape).

Tensile strength: The amount of tension or pull that a suture will withstand when knotted before it breaks. The tension or pull is expressed in pounds. Tensile strength determines the amount of wound support that the suture provides during the healing process.

Terminal disinfection sterilization: Processes used to destroy microorganisms. Processes are conducted at the end of a surgical procedure and may be accomplished in a washer-sterilizer, washer-decontaminator, or by manual cleaning, and are followed with disinfection or sterilization.

Thrombin: An enzyme made from dried beef blood that is used to control capillary bleeding. It is supplied as a white powder and may be mixed with water or saline to form a thrombin solution.

Tie: A strand of material that is tied around a vessel to occlude the lumen for purposes of hemostasis.

Tonsil sponge: Cotton-filled gauze in the shape of a ball with a long attached tape. It is used in the mouth for absorption of blood. The tape extends outside the mouth.

Universal precautions: A method of infection control that requires that the blood and body fluid of all humans (patients and personnel) be considered infectious and that the same safety precautions be taken whether or not the patient is known to have a bloodborne infectious disease. The practice of universal precautions is a method of infection control that protects patients and operating room personnel.

Unrestricted area: An area within the operating room department where street clothes are permitted. Includes a control point where communication between the semirestricted and restricted areas is coordinated.

Washer-decontaminator: A machine that is used to wash instruments for the purpose of decontamination.

Washer-sterilizer: A machine that is used to wash instruments for the purpose of decontamination. The final cycle is a sterilization cycle. Following processing in a washer-sterilizer, items are dried and stored, or dried, packaged, and sterilized.

Wound dehiscence: A partial or complete separation of the wound edges after wound closure as a result of failure of the wound to heal or failure of the suture material to secure the wound during healing.

Wound evisceration: The protrusion of the abdominal viscera through the incision as a result of failure of the wound to heal or failure of suture to secure the wound during healing.

Wound healing:

Primary intention: Wound healing by primary union. It occurs when all layers of the wound are approximated, aseptic technique is maintained, and tissue is handled gently.

Secondary intention: Wound healing that occurs by wound contraction. Wound edges are not approximated. The wound is left open and healing occurs from the bottom upward. Granulation tissue forms in the wound and gradually fills in the defect.

Third (tertiary) intention: Wound healing that occurs when the wound is sutured several days after surgery. Wound suturing is delayed for several days to permit an area, where gross infection or extensive tissue was removed, to wall off or seal.

Appendix B

Answers to Section Questions

CHAPTER 3

Q1. Delayed recovery, increased suffering, death, extended hospital stay

Q2. Provides a portal of entry for pathogenic microorganisms

Q3. Surgery interrupts skin integrity, which is the body's first line of defense.

Q4. a, b

Q5. Sterilization, disinfection

Q6. A process that kills all living microorganisms including spores

Q7. A process that kills many or all living microorganisms except spores

Q8. An inactive or dormant but viable state of a microorganism

Q9. Sterilization

Q10. False

Q11. a

Q12. False

Q13. Steam

Q14. False

Q15. b

Q16. Compatibility of item with sterilization process, configuration of item, required equipment, cost, availability, safety, packaging, length of sterilization cycle

Q17. Autoclave

Q18. a, d, f, g

Q19. False

Q20. 250°F (121°C)

Q21. True

Q22. Improper placement within the autoclave or improper preparation can prevent steam contact with all surfaces.

Q23. Readily available, economical, compatible with most in-house packaging materials, no toxic residuals (safe for patient and employee), environmentally safe, suitable for wide range of materials, rapid

Q24. False

Q25. False

Q26. True

Q27. a

Q28. When steam enters the chamber there is instant contact with items to be sterilized because air has been removed and a vacuum created.

Q29. To test whether air is effectively being eliminated from the chamber

Q30. False

Q31. To sterilize an item that is needed immediately and for which there is no replacement immediately available

Q32. Transfer is difficult because of a lack of protective packaging.

Q33. c, d, e

Q34. a, c

Q35. a, b, d, e

Q36. When items cannot tolerate the temperature and moisture of steam sterilization

Q37. a, b, c

Q38. Effective against all types of microorganisms, does not require high heat, is noncorrosive, effectively penetrates large bundles

Q39. Cycle time is longer than with steam; highly flammable; diluents being phased out; more expensive than steam; requires lengthy aeration times; can cause eye irritation, nausea, vomiting, nasal and throat irritation, shortness of breath, tissue burns; hemolysis; personnel must be provided personal protective equipment and instruction in the hazards associated with EO; requires monitoring devices that produce alarm in the event of EO exposure; concentration of EO must be identified in the areas where EO sterilization occurs; some states have abatement requirements.

Q40. A spore used to biologically monitor ethylene oxide sterilizers

Q41. a

Q42. a, b, d

Q43. True

Q44. b, c, d

Q45. *Bacillus subtilis niger*

Q46. True

Q47. b

Q48. b

Q49. False

Q50. True

CHAPTER 4

Q1. a, c

Q2. True

Q3. b, c

Q4. True

Q5. Heavy-duty rubber gloves, a waterproof coverup, cap, mask, protective eyewear

Q6. Powered surgical instruments, delicate instruments, heat-sensitive instruments

Q7. c, d

Q8. False

Q9. False

Q10. The porous material permits entry of the sterilant, contact of the sterilant with all surfaces, and exit of the sterilant.

Q11. a

Q12. b

Q13. To prevent superheating, which destroys linen

Q14. 12

Q15. Ethylene glycol

Q16. c

Q17. False

Q18. a, b, d

Q19. a, b, d, e

Q20. Placement of a towel in the bottom and underneath the instrument tray during packaging

Q21. Inexpensive, permits visualization of item, lint free, provides an effective barrier, suitable for small items

Q22. b, c, d

Q23. False

Q24. Contents, initials of person who packaged items, lot control number (sterilization date)

Q25. b, c, d

CHAPTER 5

Q1. a, b, e

Q2. Old age, poor nutritional status, obesity, compromised immune system, preexisting disease, presence of infection, burns, history of smoking, presence of catheters or drains

Q3. True

Q4. False (*Staphylococcus*)

Q5. True

Q6. False

Q7. a, b, c, d, e, f

Q8. Masks, gloves, protective eyewear, gowns

Q9. An inner commitment to strictly adhere to aseptic practice, to report any break in technique, and to correct any violation whether or not anyone else is present or observes the violation; a commitment to aseptic practice at all times

Q10. Front—chest to level of the sterile field

Arms—from 2 inches above the elbow down to the top edge of the cuff

Q11. True

Q12. c

Q13. When liquids soak through a barrier from a sterile to an unsterile surface or vice versa. Strike-through allows the passage of microorganisms through the barrier and the contents must be considered contaminated.

Q14. False

Q15. b, c

Q16. To prevent growth of microorganisms in nicks and scratches that can be left by a razor. Incidence of postoperative wound infection increases in relation to the length of time before surgery that the shave is performed.

Q17. Effectively cleanses, rapidly reduces microbial count, broad-spectrum activity, easy to apply, nonirritating, nontoxic, provides residual protection

Q18. b

Q19. a, b

Q20. Crossing the ties will cause a gap to form that will permit unfiltered exhaled air to escape out the sides.

Q21. b

Q22. b, c, d, e

Q23. a

Q24. True

Q25. True

Q26. To remove glove powders, which can incite an inflammatory response and delay healing if introduced into the patient

Q27. a, c, d

Q28. Drapes are used to prevent passage of microorganisms between sterile and unsterile areas.

Q29. To reduce airborne contamination. Dust and microorganisms settle on lint, which, if airborne, may be introduced into the operative site.

Q30. False

Q31. The points of the towel clip will have been contaminated and moving the clip would contaminate the field.

Q32. a, b, c, d

Q33. True

Q34. Shipping cartons may harbor insects and dirt.

Q35. False

Q36. False

Q37. Disposal of infectious waste is significantly more expensive than disposal of noninfectious waste.

Q38. True

Q39. False

CHAPTER 6

Q1. Integumentary, respiratory, circulatory, musculoskeletal, nervous (neuromuscular)

Q2. No postoperative evidence of cramping or pain in joints or muscles, no evidence of inability to resume preoperative range of motion without pain, no evidence of weakness in extremities, no evidence of tingling or numbness, no evidence of uncompensated sensory deficit

Q3. The lung can become engorged with blood and decrease space for alveoli expansion; amount of oxygenated blood is reduced; lung compliance and expansion is decreased and amount of air taken in is reduced, which can lead to hypoventilation, hypoxia, hypercarbia; diaphragm is less able to work against pressure from abdominal contents.

Q4. a

Q5. True

Q6. Joint dislocation

Q7. b

Q8. Because of its superficial position and close proximity to bony structures

Q9. True

Q10. c

Q11. If the elbow slips off the mattress onto the metal edge of the table and is compressed between the table and the medial epicondyle, if the arm is allowed to rest on a fixed elbow with the forearm pronated across the ventral trunk, a malfunctioning blood-pressure cuff that does not allow sufficient time between compressions

Q12. True

Q13. a, b, d

Q14. True

Q15. False

Q16. False

Q17. True

Q18. b, c, d, e, f, g, h

Q19. b

Q20. Donut

Q21. False

Q22. False

Q23. True

Q24. False

Q25. A small pillow may be placed under the lumbar curvature.

Q26. Occiput, spinous processes, scapulae, styloid process of the radius and ulnar, olecranon process, sacrum, calcaneus

Q27. To allow the body enough time to adjust to the change in blood volume, respiratory exchange, and displacement of abdominal contents

Q28. True

Q29. False

Q30. Five hundred to 800 mL of blood is rapidly diverted from the visceral area to the extremities, which can result in sudden hypotension.

Q31. Pressure from the thighs on the abdomen and pressure from the diaphragm on the abdominal viscera restrict thoracic expansion. Lung tissue becomes engorged with blood; vital capacity and tidal volume are decreased.

Q32. The sitting position causes negative venous pressure in the head and neck and the patient is at risk for air embolism. The central venous pressure line with a Doppler ultrasound flowmeter will detect an air embolism.

Q33. b

Q34. True

Q35. c

Q36. A pillow is placed under the ankles

Q37. b (b and c are also correct)

Q38. True

Q39. False

Q40. False

Q41. Alignment, extremities not hyperextended, bony prominences padded, pressure relieved from nerves, respiratory and circulatory efforts restricted as little as possible, positioning devices appropriately positioned and padded as needed, no excessive restriction

Q42. a, b, c

Q43. Assessment considerations for positioning; preoperative and postoperative skin condition; position, placement of extremities; placement of positioning devices, rolls, and padding; restraints; precautions to protect eyes; changes in positioning; presence of safety strap

CHAPTER 7

Q1. Sponges, sharps, instruments

Q2. True

Q3. True

Q4. a

Q5. a, b, d, e

Q6. A radiopaque strip or thread

Q7. Lap pads, gauze sponges (Raytex and swabs), peanuts, Kitners, tonsil sponges, patties, pledgets

Q8. b, c

Q9. False

Q10. False

Q11. a, b

Q12. False

Q13. b, c

Q14. True

CHAPTER 8

Q1. a, c, e, f

Q2. a, b, d, e

Q3. d
e
c
b
a

Q4. Bonewax

Q5. To force blood from an extremity by compressing superficial blood vessels

Q6. Chemical burn from prep solutions, bruise, blister, nerve damage

Q7. a, b, c

Q8. To occlude blood flow at a lower pressure

Q9. a, b, d

Q10. False

Q11. a, b, c, d, e

Q12. Cut, coagulate

Q13. Safer

Q14. Deliver current from the generator to the operative site

Q15. a, b, d, e

Q16. True

Q17. Foreign body reaction, tissue sloughing, healing by first intention does not occur

Q18. True

Q19. Fulguration uses sparking to coagulate large bleeders. The active electrode does not contact the tissue. The intent is to cause tissue necrosis. Desiccation results in hemostasis without necrosis. In desiccation the electrode is in contact with tissue.

Q20. a, b

Q21. True

Q22. False

Q23. b, c

Q24. No evidence of burn at dispersive electrode site or alternate current path site, no evidence of burn at unintended site, no evidence of burn at entrance site of laparoscopic instrumentation, no evidence of fever or abdominal pain associated with peritonitis

Q25. a, b, c, d, f, g

Q26. Preoperative skin assessment, identification of electrosurgery equipment, site of dispersive electrode placement, person who applied electrode, postoperative skin assessment

CHAPTER 9

Q1. b

Q2. Tearing of tissue, retention of an instrument part, infection

Q3. False

Q4. False

Q5. a, d

Q6. a, b, c

Q7. c
a
b
d

Q8. True

Q9. Frazier, Yankauer, Poole

Q10. Laser

Q11. a, c, e

Q12. Alignment

Q13. Four

Q14. Held to the light and observed for clarity

Q15. Infection

Q16. Protective gloves, waterproof aprons, face shields

Q17. a, c

Q18. a, c

Q19. Oil-based lubricants prevent steam contact, which will inhibit sterilization.

CHAPTER 10

Q1. Dehiscence or evisceration

Q2. False

Q3. a

Q4. b

Q5. a

Q6. True

Q7. True

Q8. b

Q9. a, b, c, d

Q10. Absorbable

Q11. Nonabsorbable

Q12. True

Q13. Capillarity allows tissue fluid to be soaked into the suture and carried along the strand. Microorganisms may be carried along the strand and cause infection to occur.

Q14. False

Q15. a, b

Q16. Anemic, malnourished, protein deficient, debilitated, existing infection

Q17. b, c

Q18. Less tissue reaction, minimally affected by presence of infection, minimally affected by type of tissue, minimally affected by patient's state of health, absorption time is predictable, loss of tensile strength is predictable

Q19. a, c, d

Q20. True

Q21. Coated with lubricant

Q22. False

Q23. Taper, cutting, blunt

Q24. Blunt

Q25. Atraumatic, swaged

Q26. The bulk of two strands causes tissue trauma

Q27. To obliterate dead space, remove harmful materials including fluids

Q28. Hemovac or Jackson Pratt drains are self-contained and do not provide a pathway for microorganisms to enter the wound.

Q29. Ensuring that the correct needle is delivered to the field or to the surgeon so as to minimize tissue trauma

CHAPTER 11

Q1. a, b, c, e

Q2. False

Q3. a, c, d, e

Q4. Normal temperature, unimpeded air exchange, adequate ventilation, maintenance of cardiac output and fluid volume, electrolyte fluid balance, absence of allergic reaction, unimpaired thought process

Q5. Aldrete

Q6. True

Q7. a, b, c, d, f

Q8. Procedure, surgeon and anesthesiologist, anesthetic technique, intraoperative medications, estimated blood loss, fluid and blood administration, urine output, response to surgery/anesthesia, lab results, chronic and acute health history, drug allergies, expected problems/suggested interventions, discharge plan

Q9. False

Q10. False

Q11. a, b, c, d, e, f

Q12. a, b, c, d, e, f

Q13. True

Q14. True

Q15. b, c

Q16. False

Q17. True

Q18. a

Q19. Reduce anxiety; provide sedation, analgesia, and amnesia; prevent nausea and vomiting; reduce gastric acidity and volume; facilitate induction; reduce potential for allergic reaction; decrease secretions

Q20. True

Q21. True

Q22. Prevent nausea and vomiting

Q23. True

Q24. Monitor cardiac rate and rhythm and breath sounds

Q25. a, c, d, f

Q26. Anesthetic agents, patient exposure, open surgery, irrigating solutions that have cooled

Q27. True

Q28. True

Q29. a, e

Q30. Green

Blue

Q31. Anesthetic waste gases pose a serious health hazard to operating room staff.

Q32. True

Q33. True

Q34. b, d, e, f

Q35. Hallucination

Q36. True

Q37. Patient may appear to be awake and alert but may suddenly hypoventilate. Narcotics are respiratory depressants.

Q38. b

Q39. a, c, d

Q40. a, b, d

Q41. Limit patient exposure, shut doors, keep unnecessary personnel out

Q42. a, b, c

Q43. True

Q44. False

Q45. a, b

Q46. a, b, c

Q47. False

Q48. Succinylcholine

Q49. Dantrolene sodium (Dantrium); 2.5

Q50. Cold wound irrigation, cold IV solutions, surface cooling with ice, cold gastric lavage, cold rectal lavage

Q51. Bring cooling blanket into room, bring malignant hyperthermia cart (supplies) into the room

Q52. False

Q53. False

Q54. Nystagmus, slurred speech, unarousable sleep, hypertension, agitation, combativeness, respiratory depression, airway obstruction, apnea

Q55. True

Q56. True

Q57. a, c

Q58. Paralysis of the respiratory muscles, respiratory distress

Q59. False

Q60. True

Q61. b, c, d

Q62. a

Q63. True

Q64. b

Q65. True

Q66. False

APPENDIX C

Answers to Chapter Post Tests

CHAPTER 1

1. Responsibilities of the perioperative nurse include providing care in the pre- and postoperative period as well as the intraoperative period.

2. True

3. True

4. Patient confirms consent, patient describes sequence of events in the perioperative period, patient expresses feelings about surgical experience

5. Absence of infection—absence of elevated temperature, absence of redness, absence of heat, absence of unusual pain, absence of purulent drainage, absence of swelling

6. The patient's skin integrity is maintained.

   The patient is free from injury related to positioning, extraneous objects, or chemical, physical, and electrical hazards.

   The patient's fluid and electrolyte balance is maintained.

   The patient participates in the rehabilitation process.

   The patient's pain is managed.

   The patient's dignity and privacy are maintained.

   The patient's normal body temperature is maintained.

7. False

8. False

9. a, c

10. a, b, c, e

CHAPTER 2

1. Patient assessment, patient/family teaching, emotional support, planning care, communicating information

2. True

3. True

4. a, b, d, e

5. False

6. Knowledge deficit, anxiety

7. True

8. True

9. Patient confirms consent, patient describes sequence of events, patient expresses feelings about the surgery, patient indicates knowledge of expected surgical outcomes, patient confirms procedures to be followed upon discharge

10. Additional time may be needed, additional reinforcement may be needed, hearing deficit may be present requiring the nurse to speak more loudly, special instructional materials

11. True

12. True

13. True

CHAPTER 3

1. True

2. Freedom from infection

3. c

4. b

5. Semicritical items contact unbroken mucous membranes and do not penetrate body surfaces.

6. b, d

7. a, b

8. False

9. Steam will be prevented from contacting the item to be sterilized.

10. True

11. Steam, ethylene oxide, peracetic acid, gas plasma

12. Condensate can form and make the package wet and microorganisms can penetrate wet items.

13. In a gravity-displacement autoclave steam displaces air by gravity; in a prevacuum autoclave a pump removes air from the chamber prior to steam injection.

14. False

15. Flash

16. 10

17. Times and temperatures achieved during conditioning, exposure, and exhaust

18. a, b, c

19. c

    a

    b

20. b, d, e

21. c

22. a, b, e

23. c

24. 1 million

25. a, b, c

26. a, b, e, f

27. a

28. True

29. False

30. a, c, d

31. 0.2

32. a, b, d

CHAPTER 4

1. True

2. a, b, c

3. True

4. To prevent splashing, aerosolation, and the spread of airborne contaminants

5. True

6. c

7. True

8. b, c, d

9. Allows steam contact with the entire surface of the material

10. Laundered between use (laundered prior to sterilization)

11. Cloth has a limited life and after repeated use will lose its barrier qualities.

12. True

13. Cover items completely, permit penetration of sterilant, allow for air removal, resist tears and punctures, impervious to penetration of microorganisms, visually tamper proof, allow for aseptic delivery of contents to the sterile field, permit labeling, permit display of evidence of sterilization.

14. False

15. Blown dry

    Ethylene oxide in contact with water forms ethylene glycol, which is toxic.

16. True

17. b

18. False

19. b, c

CHAPTER 5

1. True

2. b, c, d, e

3. False

4. True

5. Skin, which is the first line of defense against infection, is not intact

6. True

7. Ordinary glasses do not have side guards

8. True

9. False

10. a, c, d

11. a, c

12. c

13. Rapid reduction in microbial count, broad spectrum, easy to apply, provides residual protection

14. Alcohol is flammable and electrosurgery could supply a spark capable of igniting the alcohol.

15. a, b, c

16. True

17. False

18. True

19. a

20. False

21. b

22. False

23. True

24. b

25. b

26. True

27. a, b, c

28. Personnel are a major source of microorganisms.

29. True

30. True

31. c

32. False (should only be deposited in color-coded bag if the waste is infectious)

CHAPTER 6

1. a, b, c, d

2. True

3. Principles of anatomy and physiology, anatomical changes and physiologic changes related to anesthesia and surgical positions, surgical procedure to be performed, proper positioning techniques, appropriate positioning equipment and its use

4. True

5. a, b, d, e, f

6. True

7. False

8. Check that equipment is not resting or exerting pressure on the patient.

9. b, c, d

10. a, b, c

11. c

12. True

13. c

14. b

15. b

16. Side rails, bumper pads, canopy

17. One team member to receive the patient, another to assist in transfer and prevent stretcher from moving away from operating table during transfer

18. True

19. a, c, d, e

20. a

    b

    c

21. d

22. Supine

23. True

24. To prevent fingers and hands from being crushed in table mechanism

25. b

26. Supine position, table tilted with head higher than feet

27. Application of antiembolectomy stockings, elastic bandage, or sequential-compression device

28. Padded armboards, donut, body rolls or laminectomy frame, pillows, padding

29. To prevent stretching of anterior tibial nerve and prevent pressure on the toes that can cause plantar flexion and footdrop

30. Prone

31. True

32. True

33. b, c, d, e

34. a

35. True

36. a, d
37. Assessment considerations for positioning; pre- and postoperative skin condition; position, placement of extremities; placement of positioning devices, rolls, padding; restraints; precautions to protect the eyes; changes made in positioning during the procedure; presence and position of safety strap

CHAPTER 7

1. False
2. Pain, possible readmission or extended hospital stay, additional surgery, delayed healing
3. False
4. Results of counts and persons who performed counts
5. True
6. b (or a and b)
7. Suture needles, hypodermic needles, cautery blades and needles, safety pins
8. a, c
9. False
10. a, b, c, d, e

CHAPTER 8

1. Fibrin
2. Oxidized cellulose (Oxycel, Surgicel, Surgicel Nu-Knit), microfibrillar collagen (Avitene), styptic, pressure, instrument, suture ligature, ligating clip, bonewax, tourniquet, electrosurgery
3. b
4. c
5. a
6. Chemical burn from prep solutions, bruise, blister, nerve damage
7. Accurate pressure, connections, gas in tank, fasteners
8. c
9. Webril or stockinette material
10. a
11. Chemical burn
12. False
13. Intravascular thrombosis
14. True
15. Skin assessment prior to and following tourniquet use, location of cuff, cuff pressure, time of inflation and deflation, identification number of equipment used, identification of person who applied cuff
16. Cut, coagulate
17. Dr. Bovie was instrumental in the development of the first spark-gap vacuum generator that produced cutting with hemostasis. This was the precursor for today's electrosurgery units.
18. Delivers current from the generator to the operative site
19. a
20. b, c
21. Grounding pad, inactive electrode, patient plate, "Bovie pad," return electrode
22. a, c
23. Current that enters the patient is measured and compared with current returning to the dispersive electrode. If they are not sufficiently balanced, the unit will alarm and deactivate. This allows less chance for burn injury.
24. a, c
25. a, b, c

26. True

27. No evidence of burn at dispersive electrode site or alternate current path site, no burn at unintended site, no burn at entrance of laparoscopic instruments, no fever or abdominal pain associated with peritonitis

28. In the case of accidental activation the active electrode will not cause an incidental burn or fire.

29. Bony prominence, scar tissue, area of excessive hair, fatty undervascularized areas

30. Verify patient contact with dispersive electrode

31. True

32. Use a smoke evacuator or suction

CHAPTER 9

1. Patient injury (retained instrument part or tissue trauma), infection

2. False

3. In an emesis basin

4. Metzenbaum, Mayo

5. Elevate or remove tissue from bone or other tissue

6. Hemostats

7. Kocher

8. a

9. Retraction

10. True

11. Titanium

12. Secure the needle in the jaws, lock the holder in the second ratchet, and test whether the needle can be easily moved. If it can, it is not functioning correctly.

13. Insulation flaw or crack

14. False

15. False

16. b
a
d
c
f
e

CHAPTER 10

1. Dehiscence, evisceration

2. True

3. d
a
a
c
b

4. b

5. Tensile

6. Absorbable

7. Coated

8. a, b

9. a, b, c, d

10. b

11. b, c

12. c

13. b

14. Suture material, trade name, generic name, product number, size, length, color, number of sutures in the package, description of needle, whether monofilament or braided, coating material, manufacturer, date of manufacture and expiration

15. c, d

16. A suture (strand of material) attached to the needle during manufacture so as to create a continuous unit between needle and suture

17. True

18. True

19. a, b, c

CHAPTER 11

1. Electrolyte and fluid imbalance, alteration in thought process, ineffective thermoregulation

2. True

3. False

4. If family history indicates a problem with anesthesia there is a possibility that the patient is susceptible to malignant hyperthermia.

5. True

6. Age, medical history, current physical status, intended procedure, patient preference, expected length of recovery from anesthesia, surgeon preference and requirements, anesthesia care provider expertise and preference, patient's previous anesthesia history, whether elective or emergent, considerations for postoperative pain management

7. False

8. False

9. b
   a
   c
   e
   d

10. a, b, c, d

11. True

12. True

13. b, c

14. b
    a
    b
    b
    a, b
    a, b

15. True

16. Succinylcholine

17. a, c, e

18. Provide suction, turn the patient's head to the side, adjust the table into Trendelenburg, assist anesthesia provider

19. True

20. True

21. Inappropriate tachycardia with tachypnea, unstable blood pressure, metabolic and respiratory acidosis, increased end-tidal CO_2, fever, profuse sweating, cyanotic mottling of the skin, dark unoxygenated blood in the field

22. b

23. Dantrolene sodium (Dantrium); 2.5

24. True

25. False

26. True

27. Full stomach, metabolic disease, renal disease, hepatic disease

28. Facilitates correct needle insertion by exposing the desired interspaces

29. True

30. Sensory pathways are blocked and the patient cannot feel improper positioning or pressure.

31. True

32. a

33. Toxic. Establish and maintain airway, assist or control ventilation, administer sedation

34. Cardiac rate and rhythm, oxygen saturation, respirations, skin condition, mental status, drug actions/reactions

Index

J

K

L

M

N

O

P

R

S

T

U

V

W